ACUPUNCTURE

IN

OBSTETRICS AND GYNECOLOGY

by

VALENTIN TUREANU, M.D.   **LUMINITA TUREANU, M.D.**
Obstetrician-Gynecologist   Obstetrician-Gynecologist

WARREN H. GREEN, INC.
St. Louis, Missouri, U.S.A.

Published by

WARREN H. GREEN
8356 Olive Boulevard
St. Louis, Missouri 63132, U.S.A.

ISBN No. 0-87527-525-7

Printed in the United States of America

ACUPUNCTURE

IN

OBSTETRICS AND GYNECOLOGY

VALENTIN TUREANU, M.D.
Obstetrician-Gynecologist

LUMINITA TUREANU, M.D.
Obstetrician-Gynecologist

TABLE OF CONTENTS

III Gynecology

FOREWORD

Valentin and Luminita Tureanu, husband and wife, are practicing obstetricians and gynecologists. Both have been superbly trained in the contemporary principles of European medical practice. Over the years, however, they developed a strong interest and enthusiasm for acupuncture and for the use of this singular therapeutic tool in obstetrics and gynecology. In the course of exploring this technique, they have authored many articles on acupuncture in national and international journals and have published a book (originally in Romanian) entitled "Acupuncture in Obstetrics and Gynecology." Consequently, they now are recognized as acclaimed theoreticians in the field of alternative medicine.

The English edition of "Acupuncture in Obstetrics and Gynecology" offers a very informative clinical update on the role that acupuncture can play in the management of many aspects of the female reproductive physiology and pathology. This exceptional new resource concentrates not only upon the therapeutic aspects of acupuncture, but also upon the pathophysiology of pregnancy and gynecological disorders from the perspective of Chinese traditional medicine.

The authors trace the applications of acupuncture from basic concepts through clinical evaluation and effective management. In each chapter, the reader is taken step-by-step through all the practical applications of acupuncture that are relevant to current obstetrical and gynecological practice: pregnancy, birth, postpartum, analgesia, gynecological conditions, sexual disturbances, and urological problems.

This comprehensive guide presents the reader with a well-balanced combination of western and eastern medical concepts. The wealth of quality information that is contained in this new book will provide the experts in acupuncture with new insights into the field. The same attributes will make the book very interesting reading for any obstetrician and gynecologist.

In these times of increasing preoccupation with cost containment in medicine and a more responsible utilization of resources and technology, the application of acupuncture to well selected and suitable clinical cases might represent a more economic and very reasonable alternative.

Alex C. Vidaeff, M.D., FACOG
Clinical Instructor in Obstetrics, Gynecology
and Reproductive Biology
Harvard Medical School

ABOUT THE AUTHORS

Valentin and Luminita Tureanu are both graduates of the Institute of Medicine and Pharmacy, Faculty of Medicine, Cluj-Napoca, Romania. They received their residency training in Obstetrics and Gynecology at "Prof. Dr. Panait Sirbu" University Hospital of Obstetrics and Gynecology, Bucharest and have over 12 years, and respectively, 9 years, experience in the field. They have received postgraduate training and achieved competence in acupuncture, ultrasound, and laparoscopic surgery. They have both served as lecturers of the Institute of Postgraduate Training and Continuous Education of Physicians and Pharmacists, Bucharest, coordinating diploma papers in obtaining the competence in acupuncture.

The Drs. Tureanu have professional memberships in: New York Academy of Sciences, American Academy of Medical Acupuncture, International Society for Ultrasound in Obstetrics and Gynecology, and International Society for Gynecologic Endoscopy.

They have written many articles on acupuncture in national and international journals, several published in American journals (American Journal of Acupuncture, Alternative Health Practitioner and Clinical Bulletin of Myofascial Therapy) and have published 2 books in Romanian entitled "Acupuncture in Obstetrics and Gynecology" and "Microsystems, Optimum Time and Extraordinary Vessel Points in Acupuncture."

Over the years staying current in their field has been a major preoccupation for Drs. Tureanu. By attending courses, seminars and workshops, congresses and conferences in several European countries and the United States, they have acquired knowledge that they have successfully used in their daily activities.

INTRODUCTION

Terms such as alternative, complementary, unconventional and nontraditional are often used to designate types of treatment outside the realm of western or allopathic medicine. Although these designations suggest a divergence from the norm, it is important to note that 80% of the world's population is using one of the so-called alternative therapies.

Increasingly physicians all over the world are reconsidering alternative therapies as a different approach to health and disease states. Consequently, Chinese traditional medicine and acupuncture are enjoying more widespread acceptance as methods of diagnosis and treatment, which can complement western medicine or serve as an alternative to it when allopathic procedures are contraindicated.

Diagnostic techniques and therapeutic options in obstetrics and gynecology are technologically complex. From hormonal dosing to imaging modalities and scanning procedures through in-vitro fertilization, the complex methods of drug treatment and diverse surgical procedures can explain why a practitioner of obstetrics and gynecology with western medicine training attaches less interest to acupuncture.

Why consider acupuncture? Because it has great therapeutic potential undiminished up to the present. Because it is economic, with little or no side effects and limited contraindications. In careful selected cases, mainly with functional diseases, valuable results can be obtained.

The present book can thus be helpful to specialists in obstetrics and gynecology who are interested in understanding and use of acupuncture as an alternative approach, to enhance clinical skills and increase their practice and also to all enthusiasts of Chinese traditional medicine who have found not only a way of healing but an entire "new" medicine in approaching disease and its healing.

We have considered it useful to present general notions concerning energetic structures involved, physiology, pathology and symptomatology, pulse and tongue diagnosis. The following chapters present medical illnesses during pregnancy, labor and postpartum period, gynecological illnesses, aspects of sexual dysfunction, diseases of the urinary tract, acupuncture analgesia, particularly in obstetrics and gynecology and in the end the acupoints location on Regular Channels and Extraordinary Vessels. For ease, pathology is presented: definition in western medicine, definition, etiopathology, symptoms and principles of treatment from the perspective of Chinese traditional medicine along with an explanation about each acupoint action and the stimulation methods used.

We wish to thank Professor Dr. Dumitru Constantin, vice-president of the Romanian Society of Acupuncture and Professor Dr. Jean Bossy, from the Medicine Faculty of Montpellier-Nimes, France, and all those who have supported and guided us in our acupuncture practice.

Also, we want to thank the entire staff lead by Professor Dr. Bogdan Marinescu, from "Prof. Dr. Panait Sirbu" University Clinic of Obstetrics and Gynecology in Bucharest where we trained in our specialty, Obstetrics and Gynecology.

And not last, we wish to thank Alex C. Vidaeff, M.D., Clinical Instructor in Obstetrics, Gynecology and Reproductive Biology at Harvard Medical School for his appreciation and support of our activity.

We hope this book will be an interesting experience for all those physicians or just readers who consider health as an energetic balance consequence and are interested in knowing more about acupuncture and thus a different approach to healthcare.

The Authors

ACUPUNCTURE

IN

OBSTETRICS AND GYNECOLOGY

VALENTIN TUREANU, M.D.
Obstetrician-Gynecologist

LUMINITA TUREANU, M.D.
Obstetrician-Gynecologist

CHAPTER 1

GENERAL NOTIONS

PHYSIOPATHOLOGY

All of the phenomena of the universe reflect the Yin-Yang duality. The Chinese theory of Yin and Yang, applied to the analysis of natural phenomena, establishes the essential laws that govern evolution as a whole: opposition, integration, mutual completion, transformation and infinite divisibility of Yin and Yang.

The individual, an ephemeral presence in the energetic universe, submits to this fundamental law of duality, which initially is reflected in the existence of the two sexes: the man, Yang, and the woman, Yin. That same Yin and Yang bipolarity is continually rediscovered in the process of understanding human physiology.

From the perspective of Chinese traditional medicine, the development and evolution of woman consists of a succession of stages defined by the number seven and its multiples. In seven-year-old girls, the Kidney Qi is becoming strong, dentition changes and hair grows. At fourteen years of age, the Extraordinary Vessels Ren Mai and Chong Mai become functional, menstruation and possible fertility appear. At twenty-one years old, the Kidney Qi reaches its complete manifestation. At twenty-eight years old, the musculoskeletal system is completely developed and the whole body achieves its functional potential. At thirty-five years old, the complexion begins to fade, hair falls out. At forty-two years old, the three Yang channels of the hand get weak, the face dries and hair becomes gray. At forty-nine years old, the Extraordinary Vessels Ren Mai and Chong Mai become weak, the body is exhausted, and menstruation and fertility cease.

The same progression is true for the evolution of man, which is marked by the number eight and its multiples. At eight years old, the Zheng (Normal) Qi nourishes the whole body, dentition changes and hair grows. At the age of sixteen, Zhen Qi becomes strong; sexual activity can begin in conjunction with an evolved procreative ability. At twenty-four years of age, Zhen Qi reaches its maximal functional level, the musculoskeletal system is developed and the process of dentition is concluded. At thirty-two years old, the male has attained his full developmental capacity. At forty-years old, the Kidney begins to get weak, the hair falls out and teeth decay. At forty-eight years old, Yang decreases in the upper part of the body, the complexion fades and hair becomes gray. At fifty-six years old, the Liver Qi weakens, sexual life reduces in intensity, the sperm rarify and the whole physique changes. At sixty-four years old the Kidney Qi weakens, physical size reduces, walking becomes difficult, the whole body is perceived as heavy and procreation ceases.

Female physiology and pathology are under the sign of Yin, which signifies a prevalence of blood. This contrasts with man, who is Yang, and in whom there is a prevalence of Qi. The complementary nature of the two sexes is obvious.

The woman's whole life, including both the normal physiological phenomena — menstruation, pregnancy, lactation, and menopause — and the pathological ones, is based upon the fundamental notion of a Qi/blood balance. This dialectical aspect particularly holds in obstetrics and gynecology. The following main elements are involved in female physiology and pathology:

- Qi and blood
- Uterus
- Zang-Fu organs
- Extraordinary Vessels

Qi and Blood

Qi, blood and body fluids, as fundamental elements, are the basis of activity in the human body.

Changes in, and movement of, Qi explain all of its physiological effects, as " Qi is the root of human body." Qi influences many bodily functions: growth and development, activity of the Zang-Fu organs, and distribution of bodily fluids.

Defensive Qi (Wei Qi) is involved in controlling temperature and defensive actions. Qi controls blood, perspiration, urination, excretion and seminal discharge. Nourishing Qi (Ying Qi) as a constitutive part of blood, circulates within the channels.

The Spleen and Stomach, in Middle Jiao, transform the Essence in blood. Other Zang-Fu organs, such as the Heart, Lung, Liver and Kidney, contribute to blood formation. The Qi of the Heart controls blood circulation in the channels. The Liver stores blood, controls its volume and ensures the proper circulation of Qi. Zang-Fu organ dysfunction reflects upon the circulation of blood.

Blood nourishes the tissues and organs of the entire body and sustains psychic activities. Between the Yang Qi and the Yin blood, there is a mutual relationship, with major consequences for physiology, pathological manifestation and the differentiation of syndromes.

"Qi is the commander of blood and blood is the mother of Qi." This statement also explains the manifestations of the different pathological conditions that affect the female reproductive system. The material component of menstruation is represented by blood, but the formation, circulation and control function are dependent upon Qi. In woman, the blood must arrive in the "Sea of blood" and concentrate premenstrually within the uterus. When Qi controls blood, the menstrual flow is regular, normal in aspect and quantity. When Qi is deficient, blood cannot be maintained in the channels, a state which may result in hemorrhage, uterine bleeding, or blood loss during pregnancy. The stagnation of Qi may cause tachymenorrhea, amenorrhea, dysmenorrhea, infertility, or insufficient lactation. The collapse of the Kidney Qi causes uterine prolapse.

The dysfunction of blood can manifest as deficiency, stagnation and Heat or Cold in the blood. Blood deficiency in women, whatever its cause, may lead to amenorrhea, dysmenorrhea, infertility, or insufficient lactation and is consequent to a deficiency of Qi (i.e., "Qi follows the blood in exhaustion"). Stagnation of blood leads to metrorrhagia, pelvic inflammatory disease, afterpains, and eclampsia. Heat in the blood is a possible pathogenic factor in spaniomenorrhea, metrorrhagia, vicarious menstruation, blood loss during pregnancy, and postpartum fever, whereas Cold in the blood can manifest as amenorrhea, dysmenorrhea, and a variety of other conditions.

Qi and blood are absolutely essential; they condition each other, which is why their pathological manifestations involving the female reproductive system influence each other.

Uterus

The uterus, also called Baozang or Zigong, is considered an extraordinary organ from the perspective of Chinese traditional medicine. Called the "Cover of Yin," the uterus, often compared to the lotus flower, contains the seeds of a new life. Its function is to control menstruation, and to supervise and nourish the fetus.

The functions of the uterus are governed by the Extraordinary Vessels—Ren Mai and Chong Mai—and the three Yin channels of the foot, (Spleen, Liver, Kidney) as well as the Heart.

The Kidney Qi dominates the reproductive function. Its relationship with the Extraordinary Vessels and the five Zang organs explains why uterine functions can be affected by any energetic dysfunction involving these structures.

When the Qi of the Kidney is strong, Qi and blood circulation within Ren Mai and Chong Mai Vessels is unobstructed and menstruation is normal, as are the functions of reproduction and gestation.

The effects of the Zang organs on uterine function relate to their respective roles in circulation: the Heart controls, the Liver stores, and the Spleen produces and contains the blood. Pathological changes of these organs have repercussions for the uterus. Thus, a deficiency of the Heart and Spleen will result in a deficiency of blood and of Qi, which may lead to cessation of menstruation. A weakened Spleen can no longer contain blood, causing uterine bleeding and other symptoms.

The stagnation of the Liver Qi causes irregular menstruation. An excess of Qi (creating a Qi/blood imbalance) or a deficiency of blood caused by weakness of the Spleen during pregnancy may lead to miscarriage.

Menstrual Cycle

From puberty to menopause, menstruation is evidence of a harmonious female body balance. The two phases of the menstrual cycle, follicular and luteal, are governed by lunar rhythms. The menstrual cycle can be considered a sequence of four periods, each of seven days. Menstruation, the most Yin part of the cycle, is dependent upon the Ren Mai Vessel. The other phases are ruled by the Yin Wei Mai Vessel with the three branches:

- The Spleen branch governs the maturation of the ovary until ovulation.
- The Liver branch governs the migration of the ovum.
- The Kidney branch prepares the uterine trophicity for a possible pregnancy.

Normal menstruation is a manifestation of blood of which "Qi is the commander." Yuan (Congenital) Qi, whose origin is the Kidney, circulates primarily within the Ren Mai and Chong Mai Vessels and, less so, within the Du Mai and Dai Mai Vessels.

Any dysfunction of the circulation of Qi within these channels, will impede the regular onset of menstruation and give rise to disorders of the menstrual cycle.

The Physiology of Pregnancy

The creation of the individual is the expression of the male Yang and female Yin union. The spermatozoon is considered a manifestation of Yang energy, because of its mobility and capacity to penetrate the ovum. The ovum—a receptor of sperm energy and less mobile than sperm—is considered a manifestation of Yin.

The developed embryo is the future individual in whom the same Yin and Yang polarity will be found. Maintaining the energetic balance will allow a harmonious development, though there is a displacement of this balance during pregnancy in favor of blood, because "the blood of the mother provides the growing of the fetus." Pregnancy will cause an accumulation of blood and body fluids in the pelvis (mainly in the uterus), with the direct involvement of the Chong Mai and Ren Mai Vessels. Nourishment and development of the uterus, the placenta and the fetus are also provided.

The source of blood formation is represented by maternal organs such as the Liver, the Spleen and the Kidney: The Liver stores the blood, the Spleen produces and controls the blood, and the Kidney is the source of congenital and acquired Essence. The maternal Kidney comes into contact with the fetus through the Chong Mai Vessel. In this manner the ancestral program contained in the inherited Yuan and Jing energies is transmitted to the future individual. Normal development of the pregnancy is possible when the structures most involved in that process are in harmony:

- Maternal blood and Qi
- Fetal blood and Qi
- Free circulation of Qi among the Chong Mai and Ren Mai Vessels
- Maternal Zang organs: the Kidney, the Liver and the Spleen

A lack of energetic balance affecting one of these components will generate various pathological manifestations of pregnancy. In addition to receiving nourishment through the maternal energetic line, the fetus creates its own circulation. The point of origin of this circulatory flow is RM 8 (Shenque), which is also the end point after the energy has circulated through the Ren Mai and Du Mai Vessels. The organs of the fetus are thought to develop from the fetal Kidney in a sequence conforming to that of the Five elements. Each organ is associated with a lunar month of pregnancy (Liver, Gall Bladder, Heart, Small Intestine, Spleen, Stomach, Lung, Large Intestine, Urinary Bladder). The Urinary Bladder (organ and channel) are the last structures to develop.

At the end of the gestational period, the energetic system of the fetus is almost entirely developed. At birth, the Ren Mai and Du Mai Vessels join at the level of the mouth and RM 8 effaces and forms the navel.

Lactation

Toward the end of pregnancy, a reorganization of the Qi and blood balance occurs. Throughout labor, birth, and the postpartum period (through lochia) there is a great loss of Qi and blood. Simultaneously, the Chong Mai and Ren Mai Vessels relinquish control and nourishment of the fetus. The circulation of Qi is free within the channels and the energetic balance prior to pregnancy is reestablished.

It is in this context that lactation begins, with an upward push of fluids. Corresponding to ancient texts, milk forms from Qi and blood, obtained from the nutritive substance of food or acquired Essence.

Milk is the blood returned to the Lung, which turns to white when it reaches the breast. When nursing is finished, milk returns to the Lung, then reaching the uterus, turns red and is removed at menstruation.

Lactation that is normal, in both amount of milk production and time of onset (approximately 48-72 hours after birth) allows eutrophic development of the newborn and assumes the following conditions:

- Adequate feeding and hydration during pregnancy and the postpartum period.
- A physiological amount of blood loss during labor and the postpartum period.
- The energetic balance of the most involved structures: the Stomach, the Liver and the Spleen.
- The free circulation of Qi, uninterrupted by surgical scars (Pfannenstiel incision for Cesarean section, episiotomy) or by

Liver Qi stagnation caused by depressive factors.

Any disturbance of these conditions has repercussions for the nursing process and may result in insufficient lactation.

Menopause

Menopause marks the decline of woman's reproductive functions: definitive ceasing of menstruation and loss of childbearing capability. The fundamental element of the onset of menopause is the depletion of ovarian follicles. The decrease of the circulating estrogens is evidenced by a variety of clinical manifestations, among the most frequent being: vulvar and vaginal atrophy, hot flushes, osteoporosis, and psychical disturbances.

From the perspective of Chinese traditional medicine, the energetic context of the onset of menopause is dominated by the exhaustion of Kidney Qi and the weakness of the Chong Mai and Ren Mai Vessels. The classical references on this subject point out that the deficiency of Kidney Yin is more important than the deficiency of Kidney Yang.

Observing the law of the Five elements, the deficiency of the Kidney Yin will cause a Yang excess of the Liver and the Heart, with specific symptomatology in the upper part of the body: face redness, hot flushes, vertigo, tinnitus, hypertension, nervousness, and insomnia associated with menstrual cycle disorders. A red tongue with a thin coating and a fine, rapid pulse may also be noted.

If the Qi of the Kidney Yang is deficient, the Spleen will be damaged and the symptomatology of Yin type appears: apathy, edema, and polyuria. The woman may also present with a pale, white-coated tongue and a deep, weak pulse.

The weakness of the Kidney Qi that interferes in the fluids metabolism and governs the bones explains the development of osteoporosis during menopause.

ZANG — FU ORGANS

Zang-Fu organs are the source of Qi and blood. The Liver, Spleen, Kidney, Heart, Stomach and Lung are the organs involved in female physiology and pathology.

The Liver

The Liver is located in the right hypochondriac region. Its main function is to store blood and regulate the volume of the circulating blood according to the needs of the human body. The Liver is so closely related to all other organ activity that, observing the law of the Five elements, pathological influences are easily exchanged.

The activity of the Liver to store blood interferes with menstrual cycle physiology. Oligomenorrhea and amenorrhea may be caused by an impairment of the Liver's ability to store blood.

Another Liver function is to ensure the unobstructed flow of Qi within the channels, preventing Qi and blood stagnation. Conditions favorable to the proper progression of pregnancy, birth and lactation are thus created.

Liver Qi stagnation caused by depression or anxiety may lead to symptoms indicative of: premenstrual syndrome, irregular menstrual cycle, metrorrhagia, amenorrhea, vicarious menstruation, dysmenorrhea, leukorrhea, pelvic tumoral masses, or insufficient lactation.

Excessive Liver Qi attacks the Stomach and injures its ability to digest nutrient substances, thus vomiting during the first trimester of pregnancy appears. Ascendance of the Liver Fire with accompanying dizziness, headache, and muscular contractions generates psychical disorders during pregnancy, the postpartum period and menopause.

The deficiency of the Liver Qi, together with Qi/blood imbalance, causes sexual disorders (decrease of libido, frigidity) and menstrual cycle disorders. Associated symptoms can be: visual disturbances, dizziness, numbness, insomnia, bitter taste, dry mouth.

The Kidney

The main function of the Kidney is to store the Jing Essence. The Essence of the Kidney is congenital and inherited, the result of the transformation of food by the Spleen and Stomach.

Reproduction, growing and development capability are related to the Kidney's level of energy. The Kidney is closely related to the uterus and the Chong Mai and Ren Mai Vessels. The Kidney Essence grows at puberty, concurrent with the onset of menstruation and fertility. It decreases with age, generating the weakness of the entire body, with lack of reproductive capability and restriction of the sexual life.

The Kidney controls the metabolism of water. An impairment of this function generates edema and urinary disorders (polyuria or oliguria).

The Kidney also dominates "the anterior and posterior orifices." The term "anterior orifice" refers to the urethra and the external genitalia. A dysfunction of the Kidney Qi causes frequent urination, enuresis, oliguria and infertility. The "posterior orifice" is the anus. A Qi deficiency of the posterior orifice can cause: loose stools, constipation, or rectal prolapse.

The Kidney is the "House of the Water and Fire," site of the Yin Essence called Kidney Yin, and of Yang Qi called Kidney Yang. A dynamic physiological balance exists among these components.

A deficiency of the Kidney can cause: menstrual cycle disorders, uterine bleeding, amenorrhea, dysmenorrhea, leukorrhea, miscarriage or infertility. The deficiency may be caused by excessive sexual activity, early onset of sexual activity, or multiparity, or it may be congenital. The deficiency of the Kidney Yin due to exhaustion generates an inability to control Yang, which becomes excessive. The symptomatology is characteristic of excess: heat in the chest, palms and foot; afternoon fever; nocturnal sweating; sexual dreams in women; reddish, malodorous leukorrhea; vertigo; insomnia; palpitations; dry mouth; red tongue with a thin coating; and a thready, rapid pulse.

If the Kidney Yang is deficient, symptoms may include lumbar pain or weakness in the lumbar region; aversion to cold; cold extremities; sexual disorders (frigidity, decrease of libido); leukorrhea; pale complexion; pale tongue with a white coating and a deep, weak, slow pulse.

The Spleen

The Spleen is located in the Middle Jiao and has an internal-external relationship to the Stomach. The function of the Stomach is to receive; the Spleen transports and transforms the food and water. Both organs are sources of Qi and blood. The Spleen controls blood, keeping it within the vessels and preventing extravasation. The Spleen also is involved in water metabolism, providing adequate hydration to the tissues, transporting the excessive fluid from the channels and transforming Damp.

A deficiency of the Spleen Qi results in symptoms such as: lack of appetite, abdominal distension, asthenia, pelvic pain that spreads toward the lumbar region, menstrual cycle disorders (e.g. uterine bleeding), and prolapse of the internal organs (uterine, rectal).

The storage in the Lower Jiao and transformation into Damp cause white, abundant, odorless leukorrhea; the tongue is pale with a white coating, and a weak, slow pulse may be detected.

Normally the Stomach influences the Qi/blood balance and the physiological relationship with the Chong Mai and Ren Mai Vessels, producing a regular menstrual cycle, physiologic pregnancy and lactation.

When the Spleen and Stomach are deficient, they are unable to nourish the Chong Mai and Ren Mai Vessels, a condition which may result in infertility or may cause vomiting during pregnancy. An excess of the Spleen may lead to hypomenorrhea or amenorrhea.

The Heart

The Heart is a Zang organ, located in the thorax, having an internal - external relationship with the Small Intestine. The main function of the Heart is to control the blood and vessels and to promote the circulation of blood.

When the Qi of the Heart is strong, the entire body is adequately nourished. The complexion and the pulses reflect the Heart's energy level.

The Heart dominates mental activity ("Heart is the house of the spirit"), memory, and sleep. Consciousness and thinking are also related to the Heart.

The dysfunction of the Qi of the Heart generates psychical disorders. Thus, the deficiency of the Kidney Yin existing during pregnancy, the postpartum period or menopause will cause an excess of the Yang of the Heart. Under these circumstances the following symptoms may appear: insomnia, lack of memory, palpitations, and tinnitus.

A deficiency of the Heart and Spleen may cause a deficiency of Qi and blood manifested by late menstruation, scanty menstrual flow or even amenorrhea.

A close structural relationship exists between the Heart and the tongue with ramifications for both physiology and pathology. The Heart dominates taste and speech, as well as the appearance of the tongue, which reflects the normal function of the Heart (i.e., the "Heart opens in the tongue" and the "tongue is the mirror of the Heart").

The Lung

The Lung is located in the thorax, in an upper position among the Zang organs, and has an internal - external relationship with the Large Intestine.

The main functions of the Lung are to dominate the Qi and control respiration, to support the distribution of the Qi, to dominate the skin and hair, and to regulate the passage of the water. The Lung opens into the nose.

The Lung cooperates in its functions with those of all the other organs of the body, because "all types of Qi belong to the Lung." The deficiency of Qi of the Lung may cause hypermenorrhea (as Qi is "the commander of the blood").

From the perspective of Chinese traditional medicine, the uterus establishes connections with the Lung and the breast. It is believed that the menstrual blood, the fetal blood and the milk are distributed by the same vessel. The milk is the blood that has nourished the fetus, returns to the Lung and becomes white when it reaches the breast. In this way the Lung is involved in the onset of lactation.

EXTRAORDINARY VESSELS

The Extraordinary Vessels are part of the channels and collaterals system, large vessels which connect and harmonize the circulation of Qi in the twelve Regular Channels. In contrast to the Regular Channels, the Extraordinary Vessels do not have an exact course and are regarded as "functions." They are not directly related to the Zang-Fu organs and are not part of any system. Except for the Du Mai and Ren Mai, these vessels do not have their own points. Arising from the Kidney-Urinary Bladder system, they transport and issue the Zong Qi (Ancestral Qi) to the entire body.

By serving to connect the other channels, the Extraordinary Vessels control, store and regulate the Qi and blood in each channel. In this way they are indirectly connected, through their source point and Confluent point, with the Regular channels. The direction of the Qi circulation is considered to be centripetal, though it seems to be more a continuous wave-like movement through the channels that makes possible the transference of energy to the human body needs.

The Extraordinary Vessels are also involved in the development of the fetus. Through a continuous approach of the "ancestral project" they participate in the process of cellular multiplication and regulate the function of reproduction.

In the case of pathological conditions of excess or deficiency in the Regular channels, the Extraordinary Vessels can take or concede energy, maintaining the physiological energetic balance.

The following Extraordinary Vessels are involved in female physiology: Chong Mai, Ren Mai, Dai Mai, Du Mai, Yin Wei Mai and Yin Qiao Mai.

Chong Mai - SEA OF XUE

An Extraordinary Vessel of major importance, Chong Mai is also called "pathway," "crossroad," and "Strategist." Derived from a common trunk with the Kidney, together with the Ren Mai and Du Mai, the Chong Mai Vessel is bilateral and symmetrical.

The course of Chong Mai starts in the interior of the lower abdomen, descending towards the perineum. A posterior branch ascends in the interior along the spine. It exteriorizes at the point Qichong (ST 30) and communicates with the Kidney channel, borrowing its points, from Henggu (K 11) to Youmen (K 21). Ascending along the abdomen, it reaches the neck and surrounds the lips.

Also referred to as "the Sea of the twelve channels" or "the Sea of blood," the Chong Mai Vessel:
- Has a trophic function, as Chong Mai is considered to be "the Mother of the 5 Zang and 6 Fu organs," to which the vessel provides energy.
- Coordinates and communicates, influencing the anterior-posterior and up-down balance of the body through the distribution of its three branches: anterior, posterior, inferior.
- Controls the body temperature.
- Controls the body fluids.
- Controls fecundity and sexual development.

At puberty the Ren Mai Vessel becomes functional and the Chong Mai Vessel consolidates; in this way "Sea of blood" becomes available for the onset of menstruation and the woman is able to reproduce. When a woman reaches the age of 49, Qi and the functions of Chong Mai Vessel weaken, causing menstruation to cease and the reproductive phase of life to end. It is believed that, in women, the Chong Mai Vessel has more energy than blood, which is eliminated as menstrual flow.

The main connections of Chong Mai are established with the Ren Mai Vessel, the Stomach and the Kidney channels.

Chong Mai and Ren Mai govern the menstrual cycle and pregnancy, They are considered to be "Mother of the uterus Qi and blood." Although their influence on the female reproductive tract is shared, the Chong Mai Vessel serves more a trophic function, whereas the primary role of the Ren Mai Vessel is to supply energy.

The Stomach channel is responsible for the transformation of food and the distribution of Qi necessary to the production of menstrual blood. Qichong (ST 30) is the source point of Chong Mai and the crossing point of the Stomach channel with the Chong Mai Vessel. Providing the Qi to the Chong Mai and Ren Mai Vessels, the Kidney is also involved in reproduction and development through its other functions.

Injury of the Chong Mai Vessel can cause the following pathology: abdominal distension; lower abdominal and lumbosacral pain and spasms; infertility; uterine malpositions; uterine prolapse; vaginitis; leukorrhea; or urethritis. During pregnancy such injury may cause miscarriage; intrauterine demise of the fetus; intrauterine growth retardation; fetal malformations; retention of the placenta; or insufficient lactation. In cases where there is a disturbance of the course of the Chong Mai Vessel pilosity or hair loss may occur.

Ren Mai — SEA OF YIN
(Conception Vessel, Directing Vessel)

The Ren Mai Vessel has its origin in the common pelvic trunk. Along its course, it intersects with all of the Yin channels and, consequently, is called "the Sea of the Yin" channels.

The course of the vessel starts in the interior of the lower abdomen and exteriorizes at the perineum. It approaches the pubic region, then ascends midline along the abdomen to the neck, surrounds the lips, passes through the cheeks and enters the infraorbital region at the point Chengqi

(ST1). The direction of circulation within the vessel is upward.

Ren Mai becomes active at puberty and weakens at menopause. The main role of the Ren Mai Vessel is to control the Yin functions of the entire body. The ancestral Yin energy, the blood and body fluids depend upon Ren Mai. Ren Mai is considered to be "the commander vessel of women," controlling, together with the Chong Mai Vessel, the reproductive function. Ren Mai establishes close relations with the uterus and the three Yin channels of the foot (the Liver, the Kidney and the Spleen), fostering normal energetic circulation within the channels which makes possible menstrual regularity and physiologic pregnancy.

Ren Mai also interacts with some of the endocrine glands: the thyroid, adrenals, gonads, and pancreas. The functions of the parasympathetic nervous system and the memory are considered to be coordinated by this vessel.

The pathology of Ren Mai manifests as failure to conceive (without apparent cause), miscarriage, or intrauterine demise of the fetus. If the disturbance is one of deficiency, the following symptoms may be observed: disorders of the menstrual cycle, leukorrhea, pelvic tumoral masses, menopause disorders, and insufficient lactation.

An excess of Qi within the vessel causes dysmenorrhea. Other manifestations may be associated, including lumbar weakness sensation; epigastric, pelvic and periumbilical pains spreading towards the pubis; pains of the external genitalia; and trophic disturbances along the course of the Ren Mai Vessel.

Dai Mai
(Girdle Vessel)

The course of the Dai Mai Vessel begins near the L4 vertebra, then surrounds the body between the waist and abdomen, passing on the right and left hypochondriac areas. Dai Mai receives and distributes the Qi of the Kidney through the Divergent channels and is directly related to the Gall Bladder channel, from which it borrows some of its acupoints.

The Regular channels, passing on this level, "are forced to arrange their course." By its location, the Dai Mai Vessel surrounds and maintains the channels that cross it (the Gall Bladder, Urinary Bladder, Spleen, Liver, Kidney, Ren Mai and Du Mai) influencing the up-down, right-left and front-back energetic balance, with major repercussions for reproductive physiology and pathology.

Damage to the Dai Mai Vessel manifests as a sensation of fullness and abdominal distension, the feeling of "sitting in the water," a sensation of cold in the buttocks area, spasms caused by dysfunction of the circulation of Yin, or lumbar pains with girdle spreading.

Through their course, the Chong Mai, Ren Mai and Du Mai Vessels depend upon Dai Mai, which is why it is said that this channel "cures the bads from the woman's abdomen and lactation disorders." The reference to reproductive system symptomatology includes menstrual cycle disorders such as late menstruation, metrorrhagia, and dysmenorrhea as well as pelvic congestion, or leukorrhea.

Du Mai
(Governor Vessel)

This Extraordinary Vessel originates from the pelvic common trunk and has its own acupoints. It starts at the perineum and extends along the spine, enters the brain in the point Fengfu (DM 16), ascends towards the vertex and descends on the forehead towards the tip of the nose.

The Du Mai Vessel controls all of the Yang functions of the body; consequently, it is called "the Sea of the Yang channels." The ancestral Yang energy is distributed through the back Shu points towards the Zang-Fu organs. Together with the Ren Mai Vessel, Du Mai ensures the Yang/Yin balance and the free circulation of Qi and blood, thus it affects reproduction and lactation physiology and the regular onset of menstruation.

Du Mai interacts with the sympathetic nervous system and the anterior hypothalamus. By its course, the vessel makes possible the contact between Zong Qi and Shen Qi.

The female reproductive symptomatology associated with the Du Mai Vessel manifests as menstrual cycle disorders, infertility, urinary disorders, constipation, and pelvic pain that spreads towards the cardiac region.

Yin Wei Mai

The Yin Wei Mai vessel, also called "the Yin Vessel of Connection," ensures the distribution of Qi in the Yin area, dominating the internal body.

Because the vessel does not have its own points, it borrows points from the Kidney, the Spleen, and the Liver channels and from the Ren Mai vessel. The point of origin for Yin Wei Mai is Zhubin (K 9). The vessel then ascends along the internal aspect of the thigh to the abdomen, thorax and neck towards the tongue and reaches the point Lianquan (RM 23).

Yin Wei Mai acts in conjunction with the parathyroid, adrenals and ovaries. The vessel primarily influences the point Fushe (SP 13), where it crosses the Spleen and Kidney channels.

During pregnancy, the Yin Wei Mai Vessel acts to balance the Chong Mai Vessel and its three branches (the Spleen, the Kidney and the Liver). It also governs the first, second and third trimesters of pregnancy. This explains the necessity of treating Yin Wei Mai when it is damaged, selecting points located on the branch that correspond to a chronological sequence (i.e., of the three, thirteen-week periods of gestation). For example, when treating morning sickness, points along the Spleen branch are selected.

The disorders of Qi and blood distribution within the Yin spaces— particularly in the pelvis—have the following principal manifestations: metrorrhagia, dysmenorrhea, lower abdominal pain and distension, pain and a sensation of heaviness in the external genitalia, with the classical association of precardiac pain.

Different authors postulate that the point Zhubin (K 9)— the origin of the Yin Wei Mai Vessel in the energetic balance of pregnancy— has an important role in the prevention of miscarriage, in the treatment of premature labor, and in prophylactic therapy with cases in which there is a history of hypertension during pregnancy.

Yin Qiao Mai
(Vessel of Force and Movement)

The Yin Qiao Mai Vessel is considered, on the whole, to be an annex of the Kidney channel, from which it borrows many of its points. Its course starts on the posterior aspect of the navicular bone, at the point Zhaohai (K 6), then ascends towards the internal malleolus and along the internal aspect of the thigh towards the external genitalia.

The vessel progresses upward on the thorax to the supraclavicular fossa. It then proceeds along the neck, past the point Renying (ST 9) and the zygomatic area. It advances towards the internal angle of the eye, at the point Jingming (BL 1), and communicates with the Yang Qiao Mai Vessel.

The function of Yin Qiao Mai is to control the circulation of Yin Qi on the lateral aspect of the body and to stimulate Zong Qi towards the Yin areas. Also of note is the point Jiaoxin (K 8), the "Crossing point of the menstruation," which influences the female reproductive system and the pelvic area.

The following symptomatology is associated with the Yin Qiao Mai vessel: spontaneous pelvic pains that worsen or improve during the night (the Yin time of the day) according to the excess or deficiency of Qi within the channels; menstrual cycle disorders, dysmenorrhea, leukorrhea, infertility, frigidity, miscarriage, and postpartum hemorrhage.

The Extraordinary Vessels, Yang Wei Mai (the Connection Yang vessel) and Yang Qiao Mai (the Yang vessel of force and movement) are not described in the classical literature as having particular influence on female reproductive pathology.

PULSE DIAGNOSIS

From the perspective of Chinese traditional medicine, palpation of the pulse is a valuable method of diagnosis. The quality of the pulse can show the energetic imbalances of the body and, therefore, the condition of Qi and blood and of the Zang-Fu organs can be evaluated.

The location of pulse palpation is the radial artery of the wrist. Considering the styloid process of the radius, three areas of palpation, corresponding to San Jiao, are described:

AREA	superficial	deep	superficial	deep
	left		right	
Cun	SI	H	LI	L
Guan	GB	LV	ST	SP
Chi	BL	K	SJ	PC

- Cun   - point L 9   - Upper Jiao: Heart, Lung
- Guan   - point L 8   - Middle Jiao: Spleen, Stomach, Liver
- Chi   - point L 7   - Lower Jiao: Urinary Bladder, Kidney

Superficial palpation assesses the energetic condition of the Fu Yang organs, whereas deep palpation evaluates the Zang organs. Left pulses are Yang and right pulses are Yin.

The relationship of the pulses to the Zang Fu organs is depicted on the above chart.

The Technique of Radial Pulse Palpation

The palpation of the pulse is performed with the patient relaxed, in a sitting position, with the arms at the same level as the heart. Examination upon awakening is preferred, when Yin is not yet disturbed and Yang has not dispersed. It is also important to avoid sudden variations of light or sound that can modify the pulse.

Palpation of the pulse is achieved by placing the middle finger at the level of the styloid process of the radius at L8 (Guan), then the index finger at L 9 (Cun) and, finally, the ring finger at L7 (Chi). Based on the amount of pressure applied, the pulse may be felt at either a superficial or deep level.

The character of the pulse varies with patients' morphology (e.g., tall or small, fat or thin) and temper (asthenic or dynamic). The following characteristics of the pulse need to be evaluated:

- depth: superficial or deep
- speed: rapid or slow
- force: strong or weak
- type: full or thready, soft or hard
- rhythm: regular or irregular

Peripheral Pulse Palpation

For a more thorough assessment of the energetic condition of the body, palpation of the pulse at locations other than the radial artery should be considered.

Corresponding to the three levels of the human body—Sky, Man, and Earth— there are three levels for palpation of pulses:

- Level Sky - at the head; the pulse is palpated at the following points:
  GB 5 (Xuanlu) - at the temporal artery

SJ 23 (Sizhukong) - at the facial artery

BL 2 (Zanzhu) - at the superior orbital artery

SI 18 (Quanliao) - at the facial artery

ST 9 (Renying) - at the external carotid artery

Palpation of the pulse at point ST 9 allows us to appreciate the superficial Yang energy, the condition of the Fu organs and that of the upper part of the body.

- Level Man - at the upper limb; the pulse is palpated at the following points:

L 9 (Taiyuan) - at the radial artery

H 7 (Shenmen) - at the cubital artery

PC 7 (Daling) - at the interosseous artery

LI 4 (Hegu) - at the perforating artery

Palpation of the pulse at point L 9 allows us to appreciate the deep energy and the condition of the Zang organs.

- Level Earth - at the lower limb; the pulse is palpated at the following points:

K 3 (Taixi) - at the posterior tibial artery

SP 12 (Chongmen) - at the femoral artery

LV 11 (Yinlian) - at the femoral artery

LV 3 (Taichong)

ST 42 (Chongyang) - at the dorsal artery of foot

Palpation of the pulse at point ST 9 evaluates the circulation of blood. Palpation of the pulse at point L 9 on the right wrist assesses the condition of Qi. Palpation of the pulse at point K 3 provides information about the body's general level of energy; as long as the pulse is strong and easily palpated, the prognosis for recovery from a certain disease is good. If, on pulse palpation at points ST 42 and LV 3, an agitation is felt within the arteries, it is indicative of the onset of menstruation.

Physiological Pulse

Normally, the pulse is regular, smooth, even and forceful, with a frequency of four beats during an inspiration-expiration cycle. It is slightly stronger on the left than the right wrist. It decreases in strength from Guan to Cun and then Chi.

The physiological variations of the pulse are determined by the following factors: age, sex, constitution, emotional condition, and climatic disturbances.

Seasonal Variations of the Pulse

Depending upon the season, the energy of one of the five Zang organs is prevalent. If the pulse corresponds properly to the season, it will reflect the energy of the dominant organ. During the spring, for example, a strained pulse is normal and not pathologic.

An early or late onset of the season has repercussions for the quality of the pulse. For this reason it is said that "when the season is antedated, the pulse keeps the nature of his mother. When the season is postdated, the pulse takes the nature of the son."

Pulse of Spring

This pulse corresponds to the Chinese astronomic spring that lasts for 73 days, beginning February 6. Spring may be early or late in its arrival.

The pulse associated with this season is strained (as a "violin string" that vibrates under the fingers), long and forceful, and signifies the excess of Liver Qi that occurs during spring.

But spring is also associated with Wind, an exogenous pathogenic factor that causes allergies, infections and parasitosis. If the Wind enters the body through the point GB 44 (Zuqiaoyin), it can damage the Liver. As a consequence, the pulse develops exaggerated characteristics and becomes very superficial and stretched. Without treatment, the pulse becomes large, indicative of the prolonged damage to the Liver.

Pulse of Summer

Heart energy is, as a normal condition, in excess during the summer. The summer pulse is broad and forceful on the upstroke—a wave that comes and goes without filling the reflux. On palpation, the movement of a wave can be felt. If excessive Heart energy enters the body through the point LI 1 (Shangyang), the pulse becomes forceful, hard and large, symptomatic of the damage to the Heart when no treatment is given.

Pulse of the Ending Summer

The fifth season is dominated by the Spleen Qi. The pulse is sliding and slightly slow, with less than four beats per breath. This pulse expresses the Yin/Yang balance. The entry of excessive Damp through the point ST 45 (Lidui) can change the pulse, which then becomes weaker, soft and fine. The long pulse is associated with untreated injury to the Spleen.

Pulse of Autumn

During autumn, lung energy is, physiologically, in excess. The pulse is as light as a "feather" and very shallow. It is felt immediately upon superficial palpation and easily disappears with deep palpation. It is the pulse of Yangming, characterized by Dryness. The excessive dryness that enters the body through the point L 11 (Shaoshang) is pathogenic and may change the pulse, causing it to become irregular, slow and lacking in uniformity. As the disease progresses untreated, the pulse will accelerate to six beats per breath.

Pulse of Winter

The excess of the Kidney energy during winter is a normal physiological finding. The pulse becomes deep and hard and is felt only upon deep palpation. The invasion of pathogenic Cold through the point K 1 (Yongquan) can damage the Kidney, causing the pulse to become rapid, then soft and weak.

Pathological Pulses

With the exception of normal physiological variations, a change in any of the characteristics of a normal pulse indicates a lack of energetic balance. Twenty-eight types of pathological pulses are described in the classical literature (by Wang Shu He, 3rd century B.C.).

1) Superficial Pulse (Fu) is:
- Very superficial, seems to float; disappears with application of pressure
- A Yang pulse
- The normal pulse during autumn
- A sign of exterior syndromes caused by invasion of exogenous pathogenic factors
- A sign of the deficiency of antipathogenic Qi (Wei Qi)
- A sign of disease progression, when the pulse remains weak during prolonged diseases of endogenous origin

2) Deep Pulse (Chen) is:
- Felt only upon deep palpation
- A Yin pulse
- The normal pulse during winter
- Related to the Kidney, the diseases of the organs and Yin channels
- A sign of interior syndromes
- Symptomatic, when strong, of a syndrome of excess type; when weak, suggests a syndrome of deficiency type

3) Slow Pulse (Chi) is:
- Very slow, less than 3 beats per breath, and small
- A sign of Cold syndromes with Qi and blood stagnation
- A sign of Yin excess, when strong
- A sign of Yang deficiency, when weak
- The pulse of diseases that often are incurable

4) Rapid Pulse (Shu) is:
- An accelerated pulse with more than 6 beats per breath and with a regular rhythm
- A Yang pulse
- The normal pulse of little children
- A sign of Heat syndromes
- Symptomatic of an internal excess of Yang, when strong

5) Hollow Pulse (Xu) is:
- A slow, soft pulse; hardly perceptible; disappears with application of pressure
- A sign of Qi and blood deficiency
- A sign of approaching death, in the presence of a chronic disease

6) Excess Type Pulse (Shi) is:
- Ample, forceful; a large pulse
- A Yang pulse
- An index of Zong Qi
- A sign of syndromes of excess type: an accumulation of Heat in San Jiao, an excess of Fire in Shaoyang

7) Surging Pulse (Hong) is:
- Superficial, extremely broad on palpation
- Wave-like; strong as it approaches the apex, weak as it subsides

- Characteristic of summer; the pulse "in iron of lance"
- A Yang pulse
- A sign of Heat excess
- Indicative, when strong, of the invasion of exogenous pathogenic Fire
- Indicative of the deficiency of Heart blood and an unfavorable prognosis, when soft

8) Thread Pulse (Xi) is:
- Soft, thin "as hair," a clear, perceptible pulse
- The pulse of overstrain
- A sign of deficiency of Qi and blood; also symptomatic of a deficiency of Qi caused by aggression of Damp

9) Weak Pulse (Ruo) is:
- A deep, weak, soft and slow pulse, felt during light palpation
- A Yin pulse
- Associated with a continuous condition of restlessness
- A sign of syndromes of Qi and blood deficiency and exhaustion of Yang
- A pulse of gravity

10) Retarded Pulse (Roan) is:
- A regular, soft pulse (4 beats per breath)
- Felt when very light pressure is applied
- Related to the Spleen and associated with the fifth season
- A Yin pulse
- A sign of diseases caused by the deficiency of Spleen and pathogenic Damp

11) Tense Pulse (Jin) is:
- A rapid pulse, like the "twisted string of a violin"
- A Yin pulse
- A sign of aggression of pathogenic Cold; present in pain syndromes that result from Cold
- Associated with the retention of food

12) String-taut Pulse (Xuan) is:
- A long, straight, string-like pulse (e.g., like a "violin string")
- Associated with the spring and the Liver
- A sign of excess of the element, Wood
- Indicative of Yang in Yin

- Symptomatic of diseases of the Liver and Gall Bladder
- Associated with pain syndromes
- Accompanies throat pains
- Indicative, when hard, of the gravity of disease; when soft, it
  suggests a disease with a smooth progression

13) Sliding Pulse (Hua) is:
- A superficial, light pulse, which roll under the fingers as "pearls
  roll on a plate"
- A normal pulse in pregnant women
- Indicative of Yin in Yang
- Associated with the retention of food and phlegm
- A sign of an excess of Heat in the Stomach and of blood accu-
  mulation in the lower part of the body

14) Dicrotic Pulse (Ku) is:
- A superficial, large and soft pulse
- Perceived as hollow in the middle and full along the borders,
  gives the impression, on palpation, of "onion leaves"
- Indicative of Yin in Yang
- A sign of blood deficiency (e.g. hemorrhagic syndrome)
- Associated with the invasion of pathogenic Fire in the Yang
  channels and with an excess of Heat in Taiyang

15) Hard Pulse (Lao) is:
- A full, big, large, straight pulse; is felt in response to deep palpa-
  tion
- Indicative of Yang in Yin
- A sign of interior syndromes of excess and stagnation of Qi
- Felt in chronic diseases caused by cold and characterized by pain
- Associated with diseases that are hard to cure

16) Broad Pulse (Chang) is:
- A long and broad pulse; capable of being palpated in a larger
  than expected area
- Considered a normal pulse, if regular
- A Yang pulse
- A sign of Heat in Yangming
- Indicative, when stretched, of a Yang disease

17) Short Pulse (Duan) is:
- Hardly perceptible; felt on palpation at "Cun" and "Chi" only

- Very short; its area of palpation is smaller
- A Yin pulse
- A sign of Yang Qi deficiency of the Stomach, stagnation of food and obstruction of San Jiao

18) Spread Pulse (San) is:
- A superficial, stretched pulse that disappears on pressure
- A Yin pulse
- A sign of exhaustion of Yin, of Yang and of Kidney Qi
- Indicative of a need to reserve prognosis
- Felt on palpation during miscarriage

19) Hidden Pulse (Fu) is:
- A very deep pulse, located close to the bony plane
- A Yin pulse
- A sign of inward invasion of exogenous pathogenic factors
- Associated with damage to the Qi circulation
- Found in cases with severe pains, diarrhea

20) Separated Pulse (Ge) is:
- Perceived, on palpation, as a vibrating "drum leather"
- Felt on the surface; feels hollow with deep palpation
- A Yang pulse
- A sign of Yin exhaustion
- A sign of metrorrhagia, premature labor

21) Vast Pulse (Da) is:
- A large and forceful pulse (vast as "the wave of ocean on calm weather" that covers everything without any damage)
- A sign of health, when it occurs with a normal pulse
- A sign of Yang excess
- A sign of unfavorable prognosis, when it accompanies pathological manifestations

22) Agitated Pulse (Dong) is:
- Palpated at "Guan" only; represents the fight between Yin and Yang
- Perceived, during palpation, as "a ball that rolls"
- A Yang pulse
- The pulse of pain and fear
- A sign in women, when felt at Shaoyin, of conception

- A sign of Qi deficiency or obstruction

23) Hurried Pulse (Cu) is:

- A rapid pulse with intermittent interruptions, frequently felt at "Cun"
- A Yang pulse
- A sign of excess of Heat, Qi and blood stagnation, also related to retention of Damp or food
- Associated with an excess of Yang that destroys Yin
- Indicative, when weak, of exhaustion

24) Rough Pulse (Se) is:

- A slow, weak pulse; perceived, during palpation, as "passing the fingers over knots of bam bao"
- A Yin pulse
- A sign of Qi and blood stagnation, a weakness of Essence and blood deficiency
- Indicative, in pregnant woman, of threatened abortion
- A pulse of gravity

25) Intermittent Pulse (Dai) is:

- A slow and weak pulse, with regular pauses
- A Yin pulse
- An indicator that 100 days of pregnancy have elapsed; at 70 years old this pulse is considered a sign of long life
- A sign of exhaustion of Qi of the Zang organs
- Associated with syndromes of Wind, painful syndromes and disease caused by emotional factors (e.g., fear) and traumatic factors (e.g., strains, luxations)
- A sign of obstruction of Qi circulation in the channels

26) Knotted Pulse (Jie) is:

- A slow pulse with irregular pauses
- A sign of Yin excess, accumulation of Qi and retention of Cold-Damp
- A Yin pulse
- Related to the stagnation of blood
- A sign that a disease has dire prognosis

27) Small Pulse (Wei) is:

- A very small and soft pulse; hardly perceptible; seems to float and disappears with the application of pressure

- A Yin pulse
- Associated with all syndromes of deficiency
- Symptomatic of Qi and blood deficiency
- Associated, in women, with reproductive system diseases caused
  by deficiency

28) Soft Pulse (Ru) is:
- A superficial and fine pulse, which disappears during deep palpation; it gives the impression of a "silk dress floating on water"
- A Yang pulse
- A sign of exhaustion of "Sea of Marrow", signals a collapse of Yin
- Indicative of the need to reserve prognosis

Pulses and Pregnancy

Certain pulses are believed to be related to pregnancy. Some of them are normal, indicating a physiologic progression of the pregnancy, others are abnormal indicating a pathological development of pregnancy such as threatened abortion, premature labor or fetal distress.

If the pulse, during palpation of point L 7 (Lieque) at "Chi," is very strong and different from the pulse palpated on L 8 (Jingqu) and L 9 (Taiyuan), pregnancy is diagnosed. Pregnancy is also indicated when the pulse of Heart, palpated at "Cun" on the left wrist, is very fluent and when the pulse at point ST 42 (Chongyang) is much stronger than the pulse palpated on the carotid artery at point ST 9 (Renying).

In the third month of pregnancy, pulses felt at "Cun" are rapid, sliding and tense, regardless of the depth of palpation. In the fifth month of pregnancy, pulses felt at "Cun" and "Chi" are no longer sliding but remain rapid, irrespective of the depth of palpation.

It is possible to determine the gender of the fetus during pulse palpation. If pulses felt at "Cun" and "Chi" on the left wrist are more rapid than those on the right wrist, the child is male; if the pulses are more rapid on the right wrist, the child is female.

The following pulses are characteristic of pregnancy:

Sliding Pulse (Hua)

This is a rapid, fluid pulse, which "slides under fingers as balls of abacus." It gives an impression of gentleness, which rolls as "pearls on a platen." This pulse is a sign of Qi/blood balance and abundance and suggests a favorable prognosis when felt in pregnant women.

Certain qualities of this pulse can also help to establish the gender of the fetus. When the "rolling ball" is perceived as sharp, it indicates that the child is male; if the impression is of a round ball, the child is female.

Separated Pulse (Ge)

Again, this pulse is said to give the impression of "drum leather," because it is felt on the surface but feels hollow upon deep palpation. This pulse is associated with an exhaustion of Yin and, thus, a blood imbalance. The deficient blood is not able to assure proper development of the fetus. The separated pulse is indicative of a pregnancy in which the woman may experience miscarriage or premature labor.

Spreaded Pulse (San)

This is a superficial, vast pulse that disappears with the application of pressure "as flowers of poplar, leaves no traces." It is a sign of Qi and blood deficiency and of Kidney Qi deficiency. This pulse in also an indicator of miscarriage during pregnancy.

Rough Pulse (Se)

This is a Yin pulse , which is slow, rough on palpation, and which gives the impression of "passing the fingers on knots of bamboo." It is a sign of Qi and blood stagnation. The presence of this pulse during pregnancy is a sign of fetal distress.

TONGUE DIAGNOSIS

From the perspective of Chinese traditional medicine, tongue diagnosis is a method of diagnosis by inspection.

Physiology of the Tongue

As is the case with all of the sense organs, the tongue is directly or indirectly related to Zang-Fu organs through the channels. Each organ is associated with a specific area of the tongue: the Kidney localizes at tongue root, the Spleen and Stomach in the middle, the Heart at the tip of the tongue, the Liver and Gall Bladder on the left border and the Lung on the right border toward the tip. Normal functions and pathological changes of the different organs will manifest on the tongue.

The examination of the tongue will establish the size, motility and color of the tongue proper (muscular tissue) as well as the nature and color of its coating, which is produced by the Qi of the Stomach. Tongue inspection must be performed in daylight. The patient is asked to stick out his tongue so that characteristics of the tongue proper and the coating can be noted. The tongue should appear normal in size, should move freely, and should be moist. It is light red in color and has a thin white coating.

Pathologic Changes

Tongue Proper

a) Color

- Pale tongue: occurs in deficiency syndromes and syndromes of Cold caused by a deficiency of Qi and blood or a deficiency of Yang Qi; a bright pink tongue indicates a collapse of Yin, or an excess of Yang; a dry, bright pink tongue suggests a deficiency of bodily fluids; if the tongue also has purplish spots, Heat has injured the Pericardium.

- Red tongue: occurs in Heat syndromes related to excess or in syndromes caused by Yin deficiency; a dry, red tongue indicates an excess of Heat with deficiency of the body fluids; a faded, but moist tongue suggest an obstruction of the Upper jiao.

- Deep red tongue: occurs in instances of extreme Heat. In exogenous febrile diseases, this symptom represents the pathogenic Heat invasion of Qi and blood. In endogenous diseases it is a sign of excessive Fire caused by a deficiency of Yin.

- Purplish tongue: indicates the stagnation of blood. The tongue's dry and dull appearance is related to Heat, the pale and moist aspect is related to Cold. Dark purplish spots, apparent on the tongue's surface, suggest the existence of a toxic condition. Purplish spots are also a sign of blood stagnation.

b) Shape of Tongue Proper

A thick, pale tongue with teeth prints on the border indicates a Yang deficiency of the Spleen and Kidney and an excess of Damp caused by impaired fluid circulation. If the tongue is thick, red and occupies the buccal cavity, an excess of Heat of the Heart and Spleen is indicated.

A thin and pale tongue is a sign of the deficiency of Qi and blood. When the tongue is thin, dark red and dry, excessive Fire caused by a deficiency of Yin and a depletion of bodily fluids is suggested.

A dark red, cracked tongue, indicates excessive Heat and a depletion of body fluids. A pale, cracked tongue is associated with a deficiency of blood. Congenital cracked tongue should be ruled out, as it can be normal in some individuals. In these cases, however, the cracks are not deep and their aspect does not change over time.

Thorny tongue, characterized by hypertrophic papilla and a red color is a sign of the internal hyperactivity of pathogenic Heat. The degree of hypertrophic papilla and roughness is related to the severity of the syndrome. A deviated tongue indicates the attack of the Wind relative to an injured Liver and may be considered an early diagnostic sign.

A rigid tongue with restricted motility (as in febrile diseases) is a sign of Heat invasion of the Pericardium or of a depletion of bodily fluids caused by excessive pathogenic Heat. In endogenous diseases, the rigid tongue may be a precocious sign of Wind attack.

A flabby tongue indicates a deficiency of Qi and blood and a lack of nourishment. A pale appearance is a sign of Qi and blood deficiency; whereas a dark, red tongue is a sign of Yin collapse.

Tongue Coating

The tongue's coating is considered thick when the tongue proper can't be seen through it and thin when it can be seen. Characteristics of the tongue's coating can indicate the severity of the action of pathogenic factors and the progress of disease.

In acute, superficial diseases and in illnesses caused by a deficiency of antipathogenic Qi, the tongue coating is thin.

If the tongue coating is thick, it is a sign of disease that has entered a chronic stage and has evolved inward. The thickening of the tongue coating is a sign of disease aggravation, whereas thinning is a sign of the progressive removal of pathogenic factors.

The balance of bodily fluids can be assessed by observing whether the tongue's coating is moist or dry. Normally the coating of the tongue appears moist and bright. A dry, rough coating signals depletion of bodily fluids as a result of excessive Heat or a deficiency of the Yin fluids. When the coating appears too moist and the tongue becomes slippery, excessive water and Damp are indicated. A thick, sticky tongue coating is frequently observed in syndromes of Damp and Phlegm or food retention. When the coating is clammy, either an excess of Yang Heat has caused impure Qi of the Stomach to ascend or there retention of Phlegm or food.

The occurrence of "geographic tongue," with exfoliated parts of the tongue coating, is a sign of the consumption of Qi and of Stomach Yin. If the exfoliation is complete, the tongue becomes bright, indicating an exhaustion of the Yin of the Stomach and severe injury to the Stomach Qi. A coating that is white and thin in appearance is associated with syndromes of external Cold. A thick white coating suggests syndromes of internal Cold. A yellowish coating indicates Heat and interior syndromes. The deeper the yellow color of the coating, the greater is the severity of pathogenic Heat.

A greyish coating is to be found in interior syndromes; it has a yellow cast and is dry when excessive Heat consumes the bodily fluids. It appears moist and whitish when an internal accumulation of Cold Damp or Phlegm retention has occurred. A blackish coating is to be found in interior syndromes of extreme Heat or Cold. Many times the black color of the coating represents a transformation from grey or yellow and is a sign of gradual aggravation of the disease. A pale, bright, darkish coating, is indicative of excessive Cold caused by a deficiency of Yang. A yellowish, dry, darkish coating, indicates a depletion of bodily fluids as a result of excessive Heat.

Correlating findings from the examination of the tongue proper and its coating usually indicates a diagnosis. For example, in syndromes of deficiency, the tongue is pale with a white, moist, thin coating. In cases when the data obtained from the inspection of the tongue proper do not correspond to those from inspection of the tongue's coating, an attentive analysis may lead to a correct diagnosis. It is important to recall, however, that evaluation the color, thickness and moistness of the tongue's coating, must take into account the patient's food intake and the time of the examination.

SYNDROMES

In traditional Chinese medicine the differentiation of the syndromes is a method of diagnosing and establishing an adequate therapy.

The method is based upon the symptoms and signs observed in the course of applying the four diagnostic techniques. From these the etiology and pathogenesis are established, as are the possible interrelationships and evolution of the disease.

The differentiation of the syndromes according to the theory of Qi and blood and the theory of Zang-Fu organs is presented in succession.

THE DIFFERENTIATION OF THE SYNDROMES ACCORDING TO THE THEORY OF QI AND BLOOD

SYNDROMES OF QI

The pathogenic manifestations determined by the disturbances of Qi are described in four syndromes:
- The deficiency of Qi
- The sinking of Qi
- The stagnation of Qi
- The perversion of Qi

The Syndrome of Qi Deficiency

The pathogenic manifestations are determined by the hypofunction of Zang-Fu organs.

Etiopathogenesis

Deficiency of Qi is caused by chronic diseases, overstrain (e.g. exhausting labor), inadequate food intake, and weakness associated with old age.

A dysfunction in the circulation of Qi influences blood circulation, as "Qi is the commander of blood." The blood is not able to sustain and properly nourish the upper extremity and dizziness and vision disturbances appear. The deficiency of Wei Qi (the antipathogenic Qi) will affect the contraction and expansion of pores, the hydration of the skin and hair, regulation of the body temperature and warming of the Zang-Fu organs. The consumption of Qi, upon exertion, aggravates the symptoms.

The insufficiency of Qi affects the functions of Chong Mai and Ren Mai Vessels. The weakened Qi can no longer command blood and, consequently, disorders of the menstrual cycle appear.

Clinical Manifestations

The primary symptoms of Qi deficiency include dizziness, visual disturbances, asthenia, lack of desire to speak, spontaneous sweating, palpitations, and pale complexion. A pale tongue with a thin coating is typical, as is a weak, forceless pulse.

Pathology

Menstrual cycle disorders (short menstrual cycle with excessive flow), uterine bleeding, blood loss during pregnancy, threatened abortion, prolonged and exhausting labor, and an abnormal presentation of the fetus represent the types of pathology associated with this syndrome.

The Syndrome of Sinking of Qi

This syndrome is caused by a worsening of the deficiency of Qi. It is called "the sinking of the Middle jiao Qi" because the Middle jiao is more frequently involved.

Etiopathogenesis

The circumstances are the same with those associated with a deficiency of Qi. The pathological manifestations caused by a loss of the sustaining ability of Qi exacerbate the symptoms of Qi deficiency.

Clinical Manifestations

The primary symptoms associated with the syndrome of sinking Qi include dizziness, visual disturbances, asthenia, abdominal distension and a "bearing down" sensation (comparable to the sensation of bearing a child). After some time, ptosis and prolapse of different organs are possible. The syndrome is accompanied by a pale tongue and a weak pulse.

Pathology

Pathological findings include uterine prolapse, prolapse of the urinary bladder, urinary incontinence, rectal prolapse, and renal or gastroptosis.

The Syndrome of Qi Stagnation

The syndrome results from disorders of Qi circulation, with retardation or obstruction of Qi in certain areas of the body or at the level of the Zang-Fu organs.

Etiopathogenesis

The stagnation of Qi can be caused by emotional factors (most frequently, depression and anxiety), inadequate food intake, the attack of exogenous pathogenic factors (Cold, Wind), and traumatic factors (strains, sprains). The retardation in the circulation of Qi generates obstruction, with distension and pain. Persistent stagnation may cause the appearance of tumoral masses at different locations.

Clinical Manifestations

The primary symptoms include distension and pain. The distension is more severe than pain, but neither has a fixed position. Belching, flatulence, or frequent hiccup can alleviate the symptoms, which are accompanied by a dark red tongue and a string-taut, sliding pulse.

Other signs and symptoms of the affected Zang-Fu organs may by observed. The most frequently involved organ is the Liver.

Pathology

Pathological findings associated with this syndrome include menstrual cycle disorders (i.e., irregular menstrual cycle, excessive menstrual flow with clots, dysmenorrhea, and amenorrhea); infertility; threatened abortion; uterine dystocia; psychological disorders during the postpartum period; postpartum hemorrhage; constipation; mastitis; insufficient lactation; and ovarian cyst.

The Syndrome of Perversion of Qi

This is a disturbance in the upward and downward movement of Qi caused by pathological changes in the organs. The disturbance typically involves the Lung, the Stomach and the Liver.

Etiopathogenesis

The retention of food, fluids or Phlegm in the Stomach or the invasion of the Stomach by exogenous pathogenic factors (Heat-Damp, Cold) will damage the Qi of the Stomach. Obstruction of Qi circulation occurs and the Stomach's ability to facilitate descent of the Qi is affected.

Persistent disturbance of emotional factors (or an anger attack of the Liver) can cause an ascent of Liver Qi and its transformation into Fire, with resulting symptoms of excess in the upper extremity.

Clinical Manifestations

The primary manifestations are:
- Symptoms related to a disturbance of the Stomach Qi: nausea, vomiting, hiccup, belching.
- Symptoms related to a disturbance of the Liver Qi: headache, dizziness, vertigo and coma, hemoptysis and hematemesis in severe cases. The tongue is white with a thick coating. A sliding pulse can usually be palpated.

Pathology

Pathological findings include morning sickness and eclamptic attacks.

SYNDROMES OF BLOOD

The pathogenic manifestations determined by the disturbances of blood are described in three syndromes:

- The deficiency of blood
- The stagnation of blood
- Heat in the blood

The Syndrome of Blood Deficiency

This syndrome is caused by insufficient blood that can not properly nourish the Zang-Fu organs and the channels.

Etiopathogenesis

The source of blood is considered to be the Spleen/Stomach couple. A deficiency of the Spleen and Stomach will result in insufficient blood. Excessive blood loss, chronic hemorrhage or severe emotional changes that consume the Yin of the body may cause insufficient blood. Consequently, the Zang-Fu organs, the channels and their related regions are not properly nourished. Because blood supports the mental activities, a blood deficiency may cause mental disorders.

Clinical Manifestations

The primary symptoms are a pale or dark-colored complexion, pale lips, dizziness, visual disturbances, palpitations, insomnia, numbness of the limbs. A pale tongue and thready pulse usually accompany these symptoms.

Pathology

Pathological findings include menstrual cycle disorders (e.g., a long menstrual cycle with scanty menstrual flow); dysmenorrhea; infertility; insomnia; abdominal pain during pregnancy; threatened abortion; insufficient lactation; and constipation.

The Syndrome of Blood Stagnation

Retardation in the circulation of blood, with blood storage in different regions of the body, or lack of dispersion of the extravasated blood, defines the syndrome of blood stagnation.

Etiopathogenesis

The causes of blood stagnation vary and may include traumatic factors (strains, contusions), hemorrhage, and invasion by exogenous pathogenic factors (Cold, Heat).

As "Qi is the commander of blood," a retardation of the Qi circulation will generate a retardation of blood circulation. The stagnant blood leads to obstruction with consequent pain.

The accumulation of the stagnant blood in certain areas causes tumoral masses to appear. Obstruction of the blood vessels affects normal blood circulation and causes hemorrhage.

Clinical Manifestations

The primary symptoms are pain with a fixed location and lancing quality; fixed tumoral masses, which feel firm and consistent on palpation; and repeated hemorrhage with dark blood and clots. A dark red tongue with purplish spots is frequently observed as is a deep, wiry pulse.

Pathology

Pathological findings include menstrual cycle disorders (long menstrual cycle with a dark-colored flow and clots), amenorrhea, dysmenorrhea, metrorrhagia, salpingitis, abnormal presentation of the fetus, dystocic labor, and eclampsia.

The Syndrome of Heat in the Blood

This syndrome refers to symptoms caused by pathogenic Heat or Heat in the blood.

Etiopathogenesis

Heat in the blood can be exogenous in nature (e.g. consequent to an exposure to high temperature, activity in insufficiently ventilated spaces, or excessive exposure to sun) or of endogenous origin (e.g., caused by the transformation of Liver Qi obstruction into Fire). Heat is a Yang pathogenic factor characterized by ascending movement which results in a disturbance of mental faculties. Heat consumes the Yin body fluids and accelerates the circulation of blood, creating a potential for injury to the blood vessels.

Clinical Manifestations

The primary symptoms are mental restlessness, mania (in severe cases), dry mouth, lack of desire to drink, nasal bleeding, hematuria, hematemesis, hemoptysis, and metrorrhagia. A dark, red tongue and a wiry, rapid pulse are also observed.

Pathology

Pathological findings include menstrual cycle disorders (short menstrual cycle with excessive menstrual flow), metrorrhagia, vicarious menstruation, and blood loss during pregnancy.

THE DIFFERENTIATION OF THE SYNDROMES ACCORDING TO THE THEORY OF ZANG-FU ORGANS

The differentiation of the syndromes according to this theory is based upon clinical manifestations associated with the dysfunction of Zang-Fu organs, Qi, blood and body fluids. Used in conjunction with the eight principles of diagnosis and the theory of Qi and blood, this type of differentiation of the syndromes is of real help in establishing a precise diagnosis and adequate therapy.

The main syndromes involved in gynecological and obstetrical pathology are presented below.

The Deficiency of the Kidney Qi

The Kidney has several functions: it stores the Essence, controls reproduction and development, dominates the metabolism of water, dominates the bones and produces the marrow. The Kidney opens in the ears, in the anterior orifices (urethra and genitalia) and in the posterior orifice (anus). Thus, deficiency of the Kidney Qi will have major pathological consequences.

Etiopathogenesis

The deficiency of the Kidney Qi may be congenital or may be a consequence of old age. Other precipitating factors may be overstrain, stress, or chronic disease. The deficient Kidney causes lumbar symptoms. The weakness of the Kidney Qi leads to the inability of the urinary bladder to control urination and urinary disorders appear. The functions of the genital apparatus are also affected.

Clinical Manifestations

The primary symptoms are pain, weakness in the lumbar region and knee joints, pollakiuria with clear urine, urinary incontinence or enuresis, and clear leukorrhea. A pale tongue with a white coating and a weak, thready pulse are also commonly observed.

Pathology

Pathological findings include leukorrhea, menopause syndrome, urinary incontinence, urinary tract infections, blood loss during pregnancy, threatened abortion, and edema.

The Deficiency of the Kidney Yang

The Kidney Yang is the basis of Yang for the whole body, It warms and sustains Zang-Fu organs and tissue functions.

Etiopathogenesis

The deficiency of the Kidney Yang may be constitutional or a function of old age, chronic diseases, or excessive sexual activity (associated with early marriage and multiparity). As a result of this deficiency, the function of warming is damaged and the brain, marrow, bones and ears have no nutritive support. The Yang deficiency affects reproductive ability and the function of the Dai Mai and Ren Mai Vessels.

Clinical Manifestations

The primary symptoms are a pale complexion, cold limbs, an aversion to cold, lumbar pain and a sensation of weakness in the knees, dizziness, tinnitus, asthenia, palpitations, and infertility. A pale tongue with a white coating and a deep and weak pulse will also be noted.

Pathology

Pathological findings include leukorrhea, infertility, frigidity, urinary retention, constipation, edema of the lower limbs, and abdominal pain during pregnancy.

The Deficiency of the Kidney Yin

The Kidney Yin is the basis of the Yin body fluids that moisten and nourish Zang-Fu organs and tissues.

Etiopathogenesis

This syndrome may be caused by chronic diseases, excessive sexual activity, or by consumption of the Yin during fevered diseases. The deficiency of Yin leads to a weakening in the Kidney's ability to produce marrow, to nourish the brain and to dominate the bones. When the Kidney Yin is deficient, Yang becomes hyperactive and symptoms of excess appear.

Clinical Manifestations

The primary symptoms of this syndrome are dizziness, tinnitus, insomnia, memory disturbances, lumbar pain and weakness in the knee joint, nocturnal emission, dry mouth, afternoon fever, flushed face, night sweating, oliguria, and constipation. A red tongue with a thin coating and a rapid, thready pulse also accompany the symptoms.

Pathology

Pathological findings include metrorrhagia, dysmenorrhea, leukorrhea, and menopausal disorders.

Damp-Heat in the Urinary Bladder

The Urinary Bladder functions of storing and excreting the urine are supported by the Kidney Qi.

Etiopathogenesis

Damp-Heat can be exogenous in nature (i.e., caused by exogenous pathogenic Damp-Heat invasion) or endogenous (e.g., resulting from the excessive intake of hot, greasy and sweet food). As a pathogenic factor, Damp-Heat is characterized by heaviness and descending movement. The accumulation of Damp-Heat in the urinary bladder will damage the urinary bladder function, causing urinary disturbances, calculi formation, and urinary tract infections. Damp-Heat can injure the vessels and hematuria may appear. When the Kidney—the related organ—is also damaged, there will be lumbar symptoms.

Clinical Manifestations

The primary symptoms of this syndrome are frequent urination, dysuria, turbid urine or hematuria, urinary calculi, lumbar pain, a sensation of abdominal fullness and distension. The tongue coating is sticky and yellow. A rapid pulse can be palpated.

Pathology

Pathological findings include urinary disorders, urinary tract infections, and urinary retention.

The Stagnation of the Liver Qi

The Liver has many functions: it maintains the free circulation of Qi, dominates the tendons and opens in the eyes. Injury to the Liver affects the circulation of Qi and leads to a variety of symptoms.

Etiopathogenesis

Liver Qi stagnation is most frequently caused by a disturbance of the emotional factors. The retardation of Qi circulation generates characteristic symptoms. Because the Liver and Spleen are closely related in the overacting cycle, the excess of the Liver causes a deficiency of the Spleen/Stomach couple. Consequently, there is obstruction of the Qi circulation and digestive symptoms appear. Interference with the Qi circulation results in an accumulation of Damp and its transformation into Phlegm. Qi dysfunction leads to impaired blood circulation with injury to the Chong Mai and Ren Mai Vessels. The prolonged stagnation of Liver Qi may cause the formation of tumoral masses.

Clinical Manifestations

The primary symptoms associated with this syndrome are depression, irritability, a sensation of painful distension in the hypochondriac and thoracic regions, painful distension of the breasts, fullness in the chest and frequent hiccup, loss of appetite, belching and, possibly, the sensation of a foreign body in the throat, dysmenorrhea, and tumoral masses. The tongue will appear dark red or dark red with purplish spots and a string-taut, wiry pulse can be palpated.

Pathology

Pathological findings include menstrual cycle disorders (irregular menstrual cycle), dysmenorrhea, premenstrual syndrome, infertility, insomnia, morning sickness, abdominal pain and blood loss during pregnancy, threatened abortion, eclampsia, insufficient lactation, and mental disorders during the postpartum period.

Flare Up of the Liver Fire

Etiopathogenesis

This syndrome may be caused when obstructed Liver Qi ascends and is transformed into Fire or may result from the accumulation of Heat from excessive smoking, indulgence in alcoholic drinking or greasy food.

Fire is a Yang pathogenic factor characterized by ascending movement which causes symptoms of excess in the upper part of the body. Fire can accumulate in the Liver channel or can attack the ear through the Gall Bladder channel, given the close relationship of the Liver and Gall Bladder. Fire can injure the blood vessels, causing hemorrhagic symptoms.

Clinical Manifestations

The primary symptoms of this syndrome are dizziness; vertigo; headache with a sensation of painful distension; conjunctival congestion; flushed face; bitter taste; dry mouth; irritability; pain with a burning sensation in the hypochondriac and costal regions; tinnitus with sudden onset (and a wavelike pattern), which is not alleviated with the application of pressure; hematemesis, nasal bleeding; hemoptysis; constipation; and yellow urine. A red tongue with a yellow coating and a rapid, string-taut pulse may be observed.

Pathology

Pathological findings include vicarious menstruation, morning sickness, eclampsia, insomnia, and mental disorders during the postpartum period.

The Deficiency of the Liver Blood

Etiopathogenesis

The Liver blood can become insufficient because of insufficient production of blood, excessive blood loss or consumption of blood as a function of chronic disease. The deficiency of the Liver blood damages the nutritive support of the Heart and eyes, the tendons and the extremities. The insufficient blood empties the "Sea of blood" and menstrual cycle disorders appear.

Clinical Manifestations

The primary symptoms are a pale complexion, dizziness, vertigo, visual disturbances, numbness of the extremities, muscular spasms, scanty menstrual flow, a pale tongue, and a thready pulse.

Pathology

Pathological findings include hypomenorrhea and amenorrhea.

Damp-Heat in the Liver and Gall Bladder

Etiopathogenesis

Damp-Heat may be caused by the invasion of exogenous pathogenic Damp-Heat or by excessive indulgence of greasy food, with endogenous production of Damp-Heat. Stagnation characterizes Damp-Heat, leading to an accumulation in the Liver and Gall Bladder which interferes with the Liver's ability to facilitate free circulation of Qi. The ascending Qi of the Gall Bladder generates a bitter taste. Damp accumulation damages the Yang Spleen creating dysfunction of the Stomach-Spleen couple and digestive symptoms. The effect upon the Urinary Bladder causes urinary disorders. Because the Liver channel course is in the area of the external genitalia, the accumulation of Damp-Heat in the channel leads to vulvar pruritus and leukorrhea.

Clinical Manifestations

The primary symptoms of this syndrome include painful distension in the hypochondriac region, bitter taste, inappetence, nausea, vomiting, abdominal distension, and oliguria with yellow urine. Jaundice and fever, vulvar pruritus and yellowish, malodorous leukorrhea may also occur. A red tongue with a sticky, yellow coating and a rapid, string-taut pulse are typical.

Pathology

Pathological findings include vulvar pruritus, leukorrhea, and urinary disorders.

The Deficiency of the Spleen Qi

Etiopathogenesis

The Qi of the Spleen can be damaged by chronic disease, overstrain, stress, and inadequate nutrition (e.g., excessive intake of greasy and sweet food). The weakness of the Spleen will damage its functions of transporting and transforming water, food and Damp.

The Spleen-Stomach couple is the source of blood. Thus, a Spleen deficiency will cause an insufficiency of blood and Qi and an inability to adequately nourish the organs. The deficiency of Spleen in controlling the blood generates an excess of Yin and causes edema. The insufficient Spleen results in an excess of the Liver. Body weakness caused by chronic disease impedes the upward movement of Qi. As Qi sinks, organ prolapse and visceral ptosis are possible.

Clinical Manifestations

The primary symptoms of this syndrome are a pale complexion, emaciation, asthenia, lack of desire to speak, inappetence, abdominal distension, edema, loose stools, pelvic pain with lumbar spreading, and menstrual cycle disorders (long menstrual cycle with a scanty menstrual flow and light red, fluid blood). A sensation of "bearing down" (comparable to the sensation of bearing a child); vertigo; visual disturbances; uterine, urinary bladder and anal prolapse; renal and gastroptosis may occur in association with the primary symptoms. A pale tongue with a thin, white coating and a weak and slow or soft, thready pulse may also be noted.

Pathology

Pathological findings include hypomenorrhea, morning sickness, threatened abortion, edema and hypertension.

The Spleen Dysfunction in Controlling Blood

Etiopathogenesis

The Spleen function in controlling blood may become weak as a result of overstrain, stress, or chronic disease. The weakened Spleen is an insufficient source Qi and blood. Without the control of the Spleen, the blood extravasates and hemorrhagic symptoms appear.

Clinical Manifestations

The primary symptoms include a pale complexion, asthenia, lack of desire to speak, purplish spots, bloody stools, hematemesis, excessive menstrual flow a pale tongue and a weak, thready pulse.

Pathology

Pathological findings include hypermenorrhea and abnormal uterine bleeding.

Consumption of the Large Intestine Fluid

Etiopathogenesis

This syndrome describes the consumption of bodily fluids that may occur during labor and the postpartum period, in fevered diseases or in old age. Insufficient fluid in the Large Intestine causes dryness, with constipation as a result.

Clinical Manifestations

The primary symptoms are constipation and a dry mouth and throat, A red tongue, barely moist tongue or one with a dry, yellow coating may be observed. A thready pulse can be palpated.

Pathology

Constipation is a pathological finding associated with this syndrome.

COMPLICATED SYNDROMES OF ZANG-FU ORGANS

The notion of complicated syndromes refers to the clinical manifestations caused by the simultaneous or consecutive dysfunction of two or more organs.

In the obstetrical and gynecological pathology presented in the book, the following syndromes are involved.

Disharmony Between the Heart and Kidney

Etiopathogenesis

Chronic, overstrain and stress, or excessive sexual activity can damage the Yin of the Heart and Kidney. The emotional factors that cause the obstruction of Qi, and its transformation into Fire, can also cause disharmony between the Heart and Kidney. The Heart Fire becomes excessive in the upper part of the body and insufficient in the lower part, with imbalance between the Heart and Kidney. The insufficient Yin of the Kidney is not able to ascend and balance the Heart Fire that becomes hyperactive and disturbs mental functioning.

At the same time, consuming the Kidney Essence empties the "Sea of marrow" causing the lumbar region to have no nutritive support.

Clinical Manifestations

The primary symptoms are insomnia with frequent dreams, anxiety, memory disturbances, dizziness, tinnitus, dry throat, and night sweating. Associated symptoms may include a sensation of lumbar weakness and long, irregular menstrual cycles with scanty menstrual flow. A red tongue with a thin coating and a rapid, thready pulse may also occur.

Pathology

Pathological findings include insomnia and psychological disorders during menopause.

Yin Deficiency of the Liver and Kidney

Etiopathogenesis

This syndrome may result from injury to the Yin blood caused by severe emotional changes, overstrain, and stress or may relate to consumption of the Liver and Kidney Yin as a function of chronic disease or old age. The deficiency of Yin gives no nutrient support to the upper extremity. The insufficient Yin creates endogenous Heat and clinical manifestations of false excess appear. The Chong Mai and Ren Mai Vessels are also injured, causing menstrual cycle disorders.

Clinical Manifestations

The primary symptoms are headache; vertigo; visual disturbance; tinnitus; flushed face hot flushes with a sensation of heat in the chest, palms and feet; night sweating; and dry mouth. Associated symptoms include a sensation of lumbar weakness, constipation, scanty menstrual flow, a red tongue with a thin coating and a thready, rapid pulse.

Pathology

Pathological findings include menopausal disorders, insomnia, psychological disorders during the postpartum period.

Yang Deficiency of the Spleen and Kidney

Etiopathogenesis

Chronic diseases can consume the Qi and injure Yang and, as a result, damage the Spleen and the Kidney. This syndrome may also be caused by a deficiency of the Kidney Yang that accompanies old age. The Kidney Yang deficiency generates an excess of Yin ,with injury to the Spleen.

The insufficient Yang of the Spleen can no longer warm the organs and tissues. The deficient Spleen is unable to transport and transform food and body fluids, leading to an accumulation of Damp and the onset of edema.

Clinical Manifestations

The primary symptoms of this syndrome are a pale complexion, apathy, cold extremities, aversion to cold, inappetence, and edema of the face and/or limbs. Associated symptoms include excessive menstrual flow, a sensation of lumbar weakness, frequent urination, loose stools, a pale tongue with a thin coating and a deep, weak pulse.

Pathology

Pathological findings include edema, and abnormal uterine bleeding during the perimenopause.

The Deficiency of the Spleen and Heart

Etiopathogenesis

The blood of the Heart can be consumed and the Spleen Qi can be weakened as a result of chronic disease, chronic hemorrhage, overstrain, or stress. The blood of the Heart also can be insufficient because of a Spleen deficiency, leading to an inability to produce enough blood. The deficiency of Spleen affects the function of transporting and transforming food. The Qi and blood deficiency injures the Chong Mai Vessel and causes disorders of the menstrual cycle. The Spleen's inability to control blood results in metrorrhagia.

Clinical Manifestations

The primary symptoms are a pale complexion, asthenia, insomnia and dream-disturbed sleep, memory disorders, inappetence, palpitations, abdominal distension, and belching. Associated symptoms may include disorders of the menstrual cycle with amenorrhea or metrorrhagia, loose stools, a pale tongue with a thin, white coating, and a weak, thready pulse.

Pathology

Pathological findings include abnormal uterine bleeding during perimenopause and psychological disorders during postpartum.

CHAPTER 2

OBSTETRICS

PREGNANCY PATHOLOGY

MORNING SICKNESS

During the first four months of pregnancy symptoms such as nausea, vomiting, and anorexia are frequently observed. The etiology of these symptoms is not completely known, and factors other than the hormonal changes and physical condition of pregnancy should be considered. In western medicine, treatment seeks to alleviate symptoms and in most cases some symptom reduction is obtained.

From the perspective of Chinese traditional medicine, these symptoms are explained within the context of Qi/blood balance changes of pregnancy: the Qi of the uterus is obstructed, forcing the Liver Qi to ascend. The Qi of the Stomach gets weak and blood stagnates in order to nourish the fetus.

Etiopathogenesis

a) The Stagnation of the Liver Qi

As the Liver blood circulates to nourish the fetus, the Liver blood deficiency results in an excess of the Liver Qi. Transforming into Fire injures the Stomach, which can no longer perform the function of descending the Qi. This inability leads to Qi obstruction in the epigastrium and symptoms of nausea, vomiting and distension in consequence.

b) Heat in the Stomach

This condition is considered a reaction to the development of the fetus: the Qi of the fetus is influenced to ascend by the obstructed Qi of the uterus. Heat in the Stomach may also be caused by constitutional internal Heat. The Heat will accumulate above, preventing the Qi of the Stomach from descending. Symptoms of the excess type appear.

c) Phlegm-Damp Affecting the Stomach

If the Stomach and Spleen are constitutionally deficient or there are Phlegm and Damp during pregnancy, the Qi of the Stomach ascends counter to the Qi of the Chong Mai Vessel, leading to a deficiency of Yang in the Middle Jiao and producing the symptoms of morning sickness.

Clinical Manifestations

The symptoms differ according to the etiopathogenesis:

a) The Stagnation of the Liver Qi

Main symptoms include belching, bitter or acid vomiting, epigastric distension and hypochondriac pain, depression, and dizziness. A thin white or white-yellowish tongue coating may be noted, as may a tense and slippery pulse.

b) Heat in the Stomach

Main symptoms include bitter or acid vomiting, dry mouth and lips, thirst, constipation, anxiety, and insomnia. The patient may present with a red tongue with a yellow coating and may have a slippery and rapid pulse.

c) Phlegm-Damp Affecting the Stomach

Main symptoms include watery vomiting, ptyalism, a sensation of thoracic distension, lack of taste, dizziness, palpitations, and dyspnea. A thick and white tongue coating may be observed, as may a slippery pulse.

Treatment

Acupuncture is given with the even movement method. The acupoints that are not to be stimulated during pregnancy must be avoided, as the fetus may be injured.

Adequate nourishment is maintained by eating repeated, small amounts and avoiding raw, cold and greasy food.

The main points are used: RM 12, SP 4, P 6.

RM 12 (Zhongwan) is the Influential point of the Fu organs, the Front-Mu point of the Stomach, regulates the Qi of the Stomach

SP 4 (Gongsun) is the Luo point of the Spleen channel and the Confluent point of Chong Mai Vessel, regulates the meridians and is indicated for nausea and vomiting

PC 6 (Neiguan) together with the points RM 12 and SP 4 improves thoracic distension and descends the counter-way Qi, arrests vomiting

Depending upon the different symptoms and etiopathogenesis, other points can be added.

a) The Stagnation of the Liver Qi

Therapeutic principle: clear the Liver, regulate Qi.

Prescription:

LV 3 (Taichong)   is the Shu-Source point of the Liver channel and regulates Liver functions, descending the Qi of the Stomach

ST 36 (Zusanli)   is the He point of the Stomach channel, harmonizes the Stomach by pacifying the ascending Qi

RM 17 (Shanzhong) is the Influential point of Qi, regulates the circulation of Qi

b) Heat in the Stomach

Therapeutic principle: cool and spread the Stomach Heat.

Prescription:

ST 44 (Neiting)   is the Ying point of the Stomach channel which, with the reducing methods, removes the Heat, improving Qi circulation

GB 34 (Yanglingquan) is the He point of the Gall Bladder channel, spreads the Fire of Gall Bladder and Liver, so Qi is no longer ascending in a counter-way

c) Phlegm-Damp Affecting the Stomach

Therapeutic principle: harmonize the Stomach, remove Damp and Phlegm.

Prescription:

ST 40 (Fenglong)   is the Luo point of the Stomach channel, transforms the Phlegm

Other points can be associated in individual cases: **SP 9** (Yinlingquan) in Damp-Heat, **BL 17** (Geshu) and **BL 18** (Ganshu) in Liver Qi stagnation, **BL 55** (Jianshi) in cases with vomiting caused by Heat in the Stomach, **BL 20** (Pishu) and **RM 4** (Guanyuan) in cases caused by the deficiency of the Spleen and Stomach.

Auricular Therapy: the points used are the Liver, Stomach, Shenmen, Subcortex, Sympathetic Nerve.

CONSTIPATION

There is a physiological predisposition for constipation during pregnancy. From the perspective of Chinese traditional medicine, the constipation is caused by the changes of the energetic balance during pregnancy, influenced by preexisting deficiencies of the organs or the onset of other symptoms that may occur in relation to morning sickness.

Etiopathogenesis

In general, constipation occurs when the transporting function of the Large Intestine has been affected. The Spleen, Stomach and Kidney are also involved. Different types of constipation found during pregnancy may be a result of the following circumstances:

a) The stagnation of Qi

b) Blood deficiency with dryness of the intestines

c) The deficiency of Kidney Yang and storing of the Cold

d) Heat in the Intestine because of Yin deficiency of the Stomach caused by vomiting in early pregnancy.

Clinical Manifestations

a) The Stagnation of Qi

Main symptoms include constipation, difficult and painful defecating, loss of appetite, bitter mouth, abdominal pain, and irritability. The patient may have a thin and white tongue coating and a string-taut pulse.

b) Blood Deficiency

Main symptoms include constipation, a pale and dry complexion with pale lips, palpitations, vision disturbances, and asthenia. The patient may have a pale tongue with a thin coating and a thready pulse.

c) The Deficiency of Kidney Yang

Main symptoms include constipation, aversion to cold, oliguria, coldness of the body, and a pale complexion. The patient may have a pale tongue with a moist coating and a slow, deep pulse.

d) Heat in the Intestine

Main symptoms include constipation with dry stools, belching, vomiting, dry mouth, thirst, oliguria, and anxiety. The patient may have a red tongue with a yellow coating and a slippery, rapid pulse.

Treatment

a) The Stagnation of Qi

Therapeutic principle: remove stagnation and resume the free circulation of Qi

Prescription:

RM 12 (Zhongwan) is the Influential point of the Fu organs, harmonizes Middle Jiao

ST 36 (Zusanli) strengthens the Spleen and Stomach and removes stagnation

LV 2 (Xingjian) is the Yang point of the Liver channel, removes stagnation and the Liver Fire, drains Middle Jiao

SJ 6 (Zigou) is the Jing point of the San Jiao channel, promotes the circulation of Qi in San Jiao and Fu organs

ST 44 (Neiting) removes stagnation

b) Blood Deficiency

Therapeutic principle: nourishes the blood for moistening the Intestine

Prescription:

BL 17 (Geshu) is the Influential point of blood, regulates and nourishes the blood

BL 20 (Pishu) is the Back-Shu point of the Spleen, nourishes the blood and fortifies the Spleen

SP 6 (Sanyinjiao) is the Crossing point of the three Yin channels of the foot (Spleen, Liver and Kidney), regulates Qi and blood

ST 36 (Zusanli) is the He point of the Stomach channel, strengthens the Spleen, has a generally fortifying effect

Acupuncture is given with the reinforcing method to promote the formation and nourishing of the blood.

c) The Deficiency of the Kidney Yang

Therapeutic principle: warm the Kidney Yang

Prescription:

BL 23 (Shenshu)	is the Back-Shu point of the Kidney, strengthens and promotes the functions of the Kidney
DM 4 (Mingmen)	tones the Kidney Yang, regulates the Qi
K 6 (Zhaohai)	is the Crossing point of the Kidney channel with Yin Qiao Mai Vessel and the main point in the treatment of constipation
ST 36 (Zusanli)	and
RM 12 (Zhongwan)	regulates the circulation of Qi
SP 15 (Daheng)	regulates the functions of the Large Intestine and the circulation of Qi in the Fu organs

Moxibustion can be used to stimulate the following points: BL 23, DM 4, RM 12 and ST 36.

d) Heat in the Intestine

Therapeutic principle: remove the Heat, moisten Intestine

Prescription:

LI 11 (Quchi)	is the Reinforcing point of the Large Intestine channel, removes the Heat
PC 3 (Quze)	cools and stimulates blood.

Acupuncture is given with the reducing method.

SP 6 (Sanyinjiao)	fortifies the Spleen and Stomach, restores the Qi/blood balance
K 6 (Zhaohai)	promotes the function of the Lower Jiao

Acupuncture is given with the reinforcing method.

PC 8 (Laogong)	is the Ying point of the Pericardium channel, regulates Qi and blood and nourishes the Yin of the Stomach

URINARY TRACT INFECTIONS IN PREGNANCY

Urinary tract infections, from asymptomatic bacteriuria to cystitis and acute pyelonephritis, are quite often seen during pregnancy. Cystitis is more commonly observed, with frequent and urgent urination, dysuria, and a sensation of fullness in the urinary bladder. In severe cases, chills, fever, and lumbar pain may be reported.

From the perspective of Chinese traditional medicine, the urinary tract infections are part of the Lin syndrome. Main symptoms are: dysuria, frequency and urgency of urination, dripping of urine, pain during urination, and frequent urination with a small volume each time.

Etiopathogenesis

a) The Deficiency of Qi

The syndrome is also called "Urinary Bladder deficiency-Cold" and is an inherited or acquired Kidney deficiency of Qi. The weakness of the Kidney impairs the Urinary Bladder's function of storing and discharging the urine.

b) The Deficiency of Yin

The deficiency of Yin causes an excess of Yang and results in a Heat syndrome of the Shi type.

c) Heat in the Blood

Heat in the blood is a syndrome of excess of the pathogenic Qi (Xie Qi), manifesting as urinary tract infections. The condition may develop the complications of stagnation of the Heat in the Liver and Heart channels and injury of the Small Intestine by the Fire of the Heart.

Clinical Manifestations

a) The Deficiency of Qi

Main symptoms include clear urine, lumbar pain and strain, and urinary incontinence. The patient may have a pale tongue with a normal coating and a slow, weak pulse.

b) The Deficiency of Yin

Symptoms besides those of the Lin syndrome include yellow urine, weakness, red cheeks, feverishness, dry mouth, thirst, restlessness, anxiety, insomnia, and dizziness. The patient may have a red tongue with no coating or a yellow coating and a rapid, hollow pulse.

c) Heat in the Blood

Main symptoms include yellow urine, maybe blood in the urine or clots, painful urination, flushed face, bitter and dry mouth, thirst, restlessness, insomnia, constipation, and yellow leukorrhea. The patient may have a red tongue with a sticky, thick coating and a sliding, rapid strong pulse.

If there is stagnant Heat in the Liver channel, the following symptoms may be found: vision disturbances, tinnitus, vertigo, dry and bitter mouth, irritability, and nervousness.

If the Heart channel and the Small Intestine channel are injured, the following symptoms may be associated: burning urethral sensation before urination, a flushed face, restlessness, anxiety, and insomnia. The patient may have a red tongue with a yellow coating and a rapid, strong pulse.

Treatment

a) The Deficiency of Qi

Therapeutic principle: Reinforcing and ascending the Qi.

Prescription:

BL 23 (Shenshu)	is the Back-Shu point of the Kidney, nourishes the Yin and strengthens the Yang of the Kidney
BL 25 (Dachangshu)	regulates the Qi of the Fu organs, and thus of the Urinary Bladder
BL 25 (Zishi)	strengthens the Kidney, increases the Jing Essence, regulates urination.
DM 4 (Mingmen)	tones the Yang of the Kidney, regulates the Qi
K 3 (Taixi)	is the Yuan-Source point of the Kidney channel, tones the Lower Jiao, regulates the Chong Mai and Ren Mai Vessels
K 4 (Dazhong)	is the Luo point of the Kidney channel, tones the Kidney channel, regulates Qi

For the effective treatment of Lin diseases, other points located on the Ren Mai Vessel can be used: **RM 1** (Huiyin), **RM 2** (Qugu), **RM 3** (Zhongji), **RM 4** (Guanyuan), **RM 6** (Qihai). During pregnancy, stimulation of certain points must be avoided.

Other points located on the Kidney channel can also be used: **K 11** (Henggu), **K 12** (Dahe), **K 13** (Qixue), **K 14** (Siman), **K 15** (Zhongzhu) and also **K 8** (Jiaoxin), **DM 2** (Yaoshu), **DM 3** (Yaoyanggguan).

b) The Deficiency of Yin

Therapeutic principle: nourish the Yin and cool the Heat.

Prescription:

DM 13 (Taodao)	is the Crossing point of the three Yang channels with the Du Mai Vessel, stimulates Qi circulation, sedates the mind
DM 14 (Dazhui)	is the Crossing point of Du Mai Vessel with the Urinary Bladder channel
H 6 (Yinxi)	is the Xi point of the Heart channel, regulates the Heart and mind, removes pathogenic Heat, cools the blood

These three points can be used together in intractable cases. Acupuncture is given with the reducing method.

K 2 (Rangu)	nourishes the Yin of the Kidney, cools the Heat
K 5 (Shuiquan)	regulates the Qi and blood of the Chong Mai and Ren Mai Vessels
SP 6 (Sanyinjiao)	regulates Qi and blood.

Acupuncture is given with the reinforcing method.

BL 17 (Geshu)	is the Influential point of the blood, strengthens the Spleen and regulates the blood
BL 13 (Feishu)	is the Back-Shu point of the Lung, nourishes the Yin, removes pathogenic Heat

c) Heat in the Blood

Therapeutic principle: eliminate the Heat

Prescription:

BL 28 (Pangguangshu)	is the Back-Shu point of the Urinary Bladder channel, tones the primary Qi, regulates Lower Jiao and removes Heat
BL 54 (Zhibian)	removes pathogenic Heat
BL 40 (Weizhong)	is the He point of the Urinary Bladder channel, removes Heat and detoxifies the blood
K 6 (Zhaohai)	is one of the eight Confluential points of the

Extraordinary Vessels, cools and regulates the functions of Lower Jiao.

SP 9 (Yinlingquan) is the He point of the Spleen channel, restores Qi functions, promotes urination and spontaneous discharge of urine

LV 8 (Ququan) is the He point of the Liver channel, removes pathogenic Heat, regulates Qi and blood, releases urinary bladder

Except for SP 6 and BL 40, acupuncture is given with the reducing method for the other points.

Other points can also be used: **SP 10** (Xuehai), **LV 2** (Xingjian), **K 2** (Rangu), **L 5** (Chize), **LI 11** (Quchi).

When there is Heat in the Liver channel, the following points can be used:

LV 2 (Xingjian) is the Ying point of the Liver channel, removes pathogenic Heat from the Liver and cools the blood

LV 4 (Zhongfeng) is the Jing-River point of the Liver channel, removes Heat from the Liver channel

SP 12 (Chongmen) is the Crossing point of the Spleen and Liver channels with Yin Wei Mai Vessel, regulates Qi circulation, removes the pathogenic Heat

LV 1 (Dadun) is the Jing point of the Liver Channel, decreases the Qi of the Liver and Gall Bladder channels

When there is Heat in the Heart channel the following points can be used:

DM 14 (Dazhui) stimulates the circulation of Qi, sedates the mind

BL 27 (Xiaochangshu) is the Back-Shu point of the Small Intestine, removes the Heat from Lower Jiao, regulates the excretory system

K 6 (Zhaohai) cools the Heart, clears the Lower Jiao, sedates the mind

PC 8 (Laogong) is the Ying point of the Pericardium channel, removes pathogenic Heat, cools the blood and

	sedates the mind
SI 2 (Qiangu)	is the Ying point of the Small Intestine channel, removes the Heat
SI 3 (Houxi)	is the Reinforcing point of the channel, together with
BL 40 (Weizhong)	removes the Heat from the blood

Other points can be added: **LV 3** (Taichong) and **SP 3** (Taibai) in cases with painful abdominal distension and lumbar spreading of the pain.

When there is blood in the urine, the following points can be used:

SI 5 (Yanggu)	is the Jing-River point of the Small Intestine channel, removes pathogenic Heat and calms the mind
H 8 (Shaofu)	is the Ying point of the Heart channel, regulates Qi circulation and has a sedative effect
SP 9 (Yinlingquan)	restores Qi functions and stimulates urination
SP 10 (Xuehai)	removes the Heat from the Lower Jiao and stops bleeding

INSOMNIA DURING PREGNANCY

Insomnia can become an annoying symptom during pregnancy, especially during the third trimester. Where it persists, insomnia can cause or aggravate different diseases.

From the perspective of Chinese traditional medicine, there are three mechanisms that explain the wakeful and sleep state alternation:

- defensive energy of Wei Qi, that circulates within the six Yin channels during the night, the Yang giving up the place to Yin
- passing from the wakeful state into sleep (Yang against Yin) depends upon the Yang Qiao Mai Vessel
- passing from sleep to wakeful state (Yin against Yang) depends upon Yin Qiao Mai Vessel

There are several patterns in which insomnia can manifest: difficulty falling asleep, early awakening, periods of wakefulness during sleeping, inability to sleep throughout the night.

The history should detail the specific problems with sleep.

a) Falling Asleep

If it is difficult to fall asleep, it means that the Yang does not easily cede its place to Yin. An anxiety condition, characterized by troublesome thoughts when falling asleep, is a sign of Shen disturbance.

b) Sleep Duration

It is necessary to specify if the duration of sleep is short, if there is a period time between falling asleep and awakening or if it is a compensatory insomnia, with short sleeping periods during daytime.

c) Awakening

Frequent awakenings with superficial sleep suggests a deficiency of Yin. Awakening at irregular hours correlates with Zang-Fu organs injury. Waking at 1 to 2 o'clock in the night indicates injury of the Lung, at 3 to 4 o'clock suggests Liver or Gall Bladder injury, and at 4 to 5 o'clock is a sign of a Spleen disturbance.

d) The Quality of the Sleep

An unrestful sleep reflects an inadequate depth of the Qi circulation. Thus, morning asthenia means injury of the Liver.

e) Dreams and Nightmares

If the sleep is restless because of nightmares, Heat is affecting the Stomach.

Frequent dreams are a sign of Spleen and Heart deficiency.

Dreams about water are caused by an excess of Yin.

Crossing large areas of water by foot with an accompanying sense of fear and anxiety suggests a Kidney deficiency.

Dreams about Fire are a sign of Yang excess.

Dreamscapes that include mountains, fire and smoke are a sign of Heart deficiency.

Dreams in which the subject is flying indicate an excess of the Lung.

Dreams with mountain abysses or oranges are a sign of Spleen deficiency.

Dreams in which the subject stands at the edge of an abyss suggest Kidney deficiency.

Dreams accompanied by a sense of fury indicate Liver excess.

Associated neuropsychological symptoms such as headache, dizziness, palpitations, and memory loss should be considered when establishing the diagnosis.

Etiopathogenesis

The causal factors of insomnia are correlated with the injury of Zang-Fu organs: Heart, Spleen, Liver, Kidney and Stomach.

Chinese traditional medicine describes four etiopathogenic types:

a) The Qi Deficiency of the Heart and Spleen

The Qi deficiency of these two organs is caused by anxiety and overstrain. Blood becomes deficient and unable to nourish the Heart. As the Heart is the "house of Shen," mentality is weakened and insomnia appears.

b) Disharmony Between the Heart and Kidney

This condition may be caused by chronic diseases, stress, overstrain, or excessive sexual activity which damages the Kidney Yin. The deficient Kidney can not control the Fire Heart and thus the excessive Yang of the Heart disturbs the mind.

c) Upward Disturbance of the Liver Fire

Mental depression is a possible cause of Liver Qi stagnation. Prolonged stagnation of Liver Qi may result in Fire which injures the mind and leads to insomnia.

d) Dysfunction of the Stomach

There is a retention of Phlegm and Damp during pregnancy, favored by inadequate food intake. The stagnation of Phlegm and Damp in the Middle Jiao, with Stomach dysfunction, may lead to insomnia.

Clinical Manifestations

a) The Qi Deficiency of the Heart and Spleen

Main symptoms include difficulty falling asleep, with easy awakening; dream-disturbed sleep; palpitations; asthenia; apathy; anorexia; a pale complexion; abdominal distension; and loose stools. The patient may have a pale tongue with a white, thin coating and a weak, thready pulse.

b) Disharmony Between the Heart and Kidney

Main symptoms include insomnia; restlessness; dizziness; palpitations; tinnitus; night sweating; dry mouth; a sensation of heat in the chest, palms and soles; and lumbar weakness. A red tongue and a rapid, thready pulse may be noted.

c) Upward Disturbance of the Liver Fire

Main symptoms include dream-disturbed sleep, irritability, dizziness, vertigo, headache, dry mouth with a bitter taste, tinnitus, redness of the eyes, distending pain in the costal and hypochondriac regions, and constipation. The patient may have a red tongue with a yellow coating and a rapid, string-taut pulse.

d) Dysfunction of the Stomach

Main symptoms include insomnia, a sensation of fullness and distension in the epigastrium, abdominal distension, belching, and constipation. A white, sticky, wet tongue coating and a slippery pulse may be noted.

Treatment

a) The Qi Deficiency of the Heart and Spleen

Therapeutic principle: tone the Heart and Spleen

Prescription:

BL 15 (Xinshu)	is the Back-Shu point of the Heart, nourishes the blood, calms and drains the Heart, sedates the mind
BL 20 (Pishu)	is the Back-Shu point of the Spleen, tones the Spleen Qi
SP 6 (Sanyinjiao)	is the Crossing point of the three Yin channels of the foot, strengthens the Spleen, soothes the mind
H 7 (Shenmen)	is the Yuan-Source point of the Heart channel, strengthens the Heart and sedates the mind
PC 6 (Neiguan)	is the Luo point of the Pericardium channel, nourishes the Heart and calms the mind

Acupuncture is given with the even movement method.

b) Disharmony Between the Heart and Kidney

Therapeutic principle: harmonize the Heart and Kidney.

Prescription:

SP 6 (Sanyinjiao) is the Crossing point of the Yin channels of the foot, tones the Kidney, regulates Qi and blood circulation, calms the mind

BL 15 (Xinshu) is the Back-Shu point of the Heart, nourishes the Heart, disperses the Fire of the Heart

BL 23 (Shenshu) is the Back-Shu point of the Kidney, nourishes the Yin and strengthens the Yang

H 7 (Shenmen) is the Yuan-Source point of the Heart channel, regulates the Heart, soothes the mind

K 3 (Taixi) is the Yuan-Source point of the Kidney channel, nourishes and fortifies the Kidney

Other points can be used in alternative prescriptions, and stimulation with the even movement is given.

K 1 (Yongquan) is the Jing-Well point of the Kidney channel, nourishes the Kidney and cools the Heat, calms the spirit

K 6 (Zhaohai) cools the Heart and calms the spirit.

c) Upward Disturbance of the Liver Fire

Therapeutic principle: calm the Liver, spread the Fire, soothe the mind.

Prescription:

BL 18 (Ganshu) is the Back-Shu point of the Liver, removes the Liver Qi stagnation, spreads the pathogenic Fire

BL 19 (Danshu) is the Back-Shu point of the Gall Bladder, removes pathogenic Heat from the Liver and Gall Bladder, strengthens the Spleen

LV 2 (Xingjian) is the reducing, Ying point of the Liver channel, removes pathogenic Heat and cools the blood, calms fear

LV 3 (Taichong)	is the Yuan-Source point of the Liver channel, removes pathogenic Fire from the Liver, stimulates Qi and blood circulation, cools the eyes
GB 23 (Zhejin)	is the Crossing point of the Gall Bladder and Urinary Bladder channels, removes Liver Qi stagnation
SP 6 (Sanyinjiao)	regulates Qi and blood, calms the mind
PC 6 (Neiguan)	calms the Heart and mind

Acupuncture is given with the reducing method and attention should be paid when stimulating SP 6 in order to avoid weakening the blood.

Other points can also be used to reduce Yang:

BL 17 (Geshu)	is the Influential point of blood, nourishes blood, increases Yin
K 5 (Shuquan)	regulates Qi and blood, restores Yin/Yang balance

The above acupoints are stimulated with the reinforcing method.

d) Dysfunction of the Stomach

Therapeutic principle: harmonize the Stomach and soothe the mind

Prescription:

ST 36 (Zusanli)	is the He point of the Stomach channel, regulates the Stomach functions and strengthens the Spleen
BL 21 (Weishu)	is the Back-Shu point of the Stomach, regulates the Stomach and strengthens the Spleen, removes pathogenic Damp
ST 40 (Fenglong)	is the Luo point of the Stomach channel, regulates the Stomach, reduces the Phlegm, sedates the mind
PC 6 (Neiguan)	calms the mind
C 7 (Shenmen)	sedates the spirit.

Acupuncture is given with the reducing method.

In cases of insomnia characterized by irregular awakening, other points can also be stimulated:

- awakening at 1 to 2 o'clock in the morning
Therapeutic principle: tone the Lung
Prescription:
L 7 (Lieque)   is the Luo point of the Lung channel, regulates Qi, regulates the circulation within the channels

BL 13 (Feishu)   is the Back-Shu point of the Lung, promotes Qi circulation, nourishes the Yin, removes pathogenic Heat

- awakening at 3 to 4 o'clock in the morning
Therapeutic principle: disperse the Liver
Prescription:
LV 3 (Taichong)   is the Yuan-Source point of the Liver channel, removes pathogenic Fire from the Liver

BL 18 (Ganshu)   is the Back-Shu point of the Liver, removes Liver Qi stagnation and the pathogenic Fire

- awakening at 4 to 5 o'clock in the morning
Therapeutic principle: promote the Spleen functions
Prescription:
SP 10 (Xuehai)   removes Heat from the blood

BL 17 (Geshu)   is the Influential point of blood, strengthens the Spleen and regulates the Stomach

In cases of insomnia with frequent nightmares, the following points can be useful:

ST 45 (Lidui)   is the Jing-Well point of the Stomach channel, promotes the mental functions

H 7 (Shenmen)   calms the spirit

SP 1 (Yinbai)   is the Jing-Well point of the Spleen channel, tones Qi and soothes the mind

ABDOMINAL PAIN DURING PREGNANCY

Abdominal discomfort and pain during pregnancy may have several causes: pressure, tension of the round ligament of the uterus, distension, flatulence and Braxton Hicks contractions. If contractions occur, the onset of premature labor should be ruled out. Usually these can be relieved with sedatives, such as Diazepam. Other disorders of the gastrointestinal, urinary or neurologic system should also be ruled out.

Etiopathogenesis

From the perspective of Chinese traditional medicine, four etio-pathogenic types are described:

a) The Deficiency of Yang Qi

Pregnancy may increase a congenital deficiency of Yang Qi. A deficiency also may be caused by an attack of exogenous pathogenic Cold.

Cold is characterized by constriction and stagnation, thus Qi and blood circulation are damaged. Abdominal pain and other signs of Yang deficiency appear.

b) The Deficiency of Blood

Because Qi and blood are inseparable and mutually related, a blood deficiency during pregnancy, frequently caused by the Spleen and Stomach weakness or emotional states that consume the Yin blood, will generate a stagnation of Qi that may cause pain.

c) The Stagnation of Damp

There is a physiological tendency to retain Phlegm Damp during pregnancy, especially during early pregnancy. Damp is sticky and stagnant. As a Yin pathogenic factor, it will injure the Yang and obstruct the circulation of Qi. The excess of Damp injures the Spleen function and a deficiency of blood will appear.

d) The Stagnation of Qi

When the Liver is injured, the disturbance in the circulation of Qi will cause an obstruction of the channels and give rise to abdominal pain and distension.

Clinical Manifestations

a) The Deficiency of Yang Qi

Main symptoms include a cold and painful abdomen with aversion to Cold, a pale complexion, cold skin, lack of appetite, loose stools, and frequent urination. The patient may have a pale tongue with a thin, white coating and a weak and slow pulse.

b) The Deficiency of Blood

Main symptoms include edema of the face, eyes and limbs; diarrhea; a sensation of heaviness in the body; a sensation of fullness in the thoracic and epigastric regions; and dizziness. The patient may have a sticky, white tongue coating and a soft, sliding pulse.

c) The Stagnation of Damp

Main symptoms include edema of the face, eyes and limbs; diarrhea; a sensation of heaviness in the body, a sensation of fullness in the thoracic and epigastric regions, and dizziness. The patient may have a sticky, white tongue coating and a soft, sliding pulse.

d) The Stagnation of Qi

Main symptoms include abdominal and thoracic distension, pain in the hypochondriac region, belching, acid regurgitation, and irritability. The patient may have a white, thin tongue coating and a wiry pulse.

Treatment

a) The Deficiency of Yang Qi

Therapeutic principle: Warm Yang, dispel the Cold

Prescription:

ST 36 (Zusanli)	is one of the four Dominant points and the He point of the Stomach channel, regulates the Qi of the Middle Jiao, regulates the Stomach
ST 25 (Tianshu)	is the Front-Mu point of the Large Intestine, regulates the Stomach and Spleen, promotes Qi circulation.
BL 29 (Zhonglushu)	warms Yang and dispels the Cold
RM 3 (Zhongji)	strengthens the Yang, regulates the Middle Jiao

b) The Deficiency of Blood

Therapeutic principle: support blood, promote Qi and blood circulation.

Prescription:

BL 17 (Geshu)	is the Influential point of blood, strengthens the Spleen, regulates blood and promotes Qi circulation

BL 20 (Pishu)	is the Back-Shu point of the Spleen, strengthens the Spleen, stimulates the formation of blood
ST 36 (Zusanli)	is the He point of the Stomach channel, tones the Stomach and strengthens the Spleen, supports blood
BL 43 (Gaohuangshu)	fortifies the functions of Qi, strengthens the Spleen
BL 53 (Baohuang)	reinforces the Qi of the Fu organs, tones the lumbar region and the spine. This point should be stimulated with care and caution.

c) The Stagnation of Damp

Therapeutic principle: dispel Damp, promote circulation of water.

Prescription:

ST 36 (Zusanli)	is the He point of the Stomach channel, regulates the Stomach, strengthens the Spleen, invigorates the Middle Jiao, has a fortifying effect
SP 9 (Yinlingquan)	is the He point of the Spleen channel, strengthens the Spleen and removes pathogenic Damp
SP 12 (Chongmen)	regulates the functions of Qi, is used in pregnancy edema
K 7 (Fuliu)	is the Reinforcing point of the Kidney channel, regulates the draining of the Lower Jiao, regulates body fluids and removes Damp
RM 9 (Shuifen)	strengthens the Spleen and removes pathogenic Damp

Acupuncture is given with the reinforcing method, except for SP 9, (which is stimulated with the reducing method) and SP 12 (with which the even movement method is used).

d) The Stagnation of Qi

Therapeutic principle: drain the Liver, remove the stagnation of Qi

LV 3 (Taichong)	is the Yuan-Source point of the Liver channel,

	promotes Qi and blood circulation, removes the stagnation of the Liver
LV 6 (Zhongdu)	is the Xi point of the Liver channel, removes Liver Qi stagnation, stimulates blood circulation
LV 13 (Zhangmen)	is the Front-Mu point of the Spleen and the Influential point of the Zang organs, removes Liver Qi stagnation, regulates the organs
RM 4 (Guanyuan)	tones and regulates Qi, regulates blood, regulates the circulation within the Chong Mai and Ren Mai vessels
PC 6 (Neiguan)	is the Luo point of the Pericardium channel, promotes Qi circulation and has a sedative effect

VAGINAL BLEEDING DURING PREGNANCY

Vaginal bleeding during pregnancy may have different causes. Major pregnancy complications, such as hemorrhage from placental separation or placenta previa, should be ruled out, as they can severely affect both mother and fetus, if diagnosis is not promptly established and therapy not immediately implemented.

Most often vaginal bleeding, accompanied by abdominal pain, is a sign of threatened abortion. Bedrest is mandatory; other therapies remain controversial.

In Chinese traditional medicine, vaginal bleeding during pregnancy is called Jijing, Tai Lou. Acupuncture should be used with precaution, preferably as an alternative therapy, and in conjunction with pharmacotherapy.

Etiopathogenesis

From the perspective of Chinese traditional medicine, four etiopathogenic types are recognized:

a) Heat in the Blood

This syndrome is caused by exogenous pathogenic Heat or endogenous Heat resulting from obstructed Liver Qi that has turned into Fire. The excessive activity of the Heat consumes the Yin from the blood, injures the blood vessels and thus, causes blood loss in the form of vaginal bleeding during pregnancy.

b) The Deficiency of Qi

The deficiency of Qi may be a result of inadequate food intake, overstrain, stress, or chronic diseases. The functions of the Zang-Fu organs will be damaged as will be the circulation of blood, which is closely related to Qi.

c) The Deficiency of Blood

The deficiency of blood is caused by a dysfunction of the Spleen-Stomach couple, with a consequent deficiency in the formation of blood. Other causes can be excessive blood loss or severe emotional changes that consume the Yin of the blood. The deficient blood cannot properly nourish the organs or channels and symptoms of deficiency appear.

d) The Injury of the Chong Mai and Ren Mai Vessels

Chong Mai and Ren Mai Vessels can be injured in cases of Qi and blood deficiency, deficiency of the Kidney or when there is Heat in the blood. The blood cannot be maintained to nourish the fetus and vaginal bleeding appears during pregnancy.

Clinical Manifestations

a) Heat in the Blood

Main symptoms include vaginal bleeding during pregnancy, a flushed face, red lips, dry throat and lips, nervousness, insomnia, a sensation of fullness in the thorax, a sensation of heat in the palms, feverishness, a preference for cold, oliguria, and constipation. The patient may have a red tongue with a yellow coating and a rapid, sliding pulse.

b) The Deficiency of Qi

Main symptoms include dark-colored vaginal bleeding after fecundation, apathy, asthenia, aversion to Cold, lack of appetite, pale complexion, frequent or urgent urination, and palpitations. The patient may have a pale tongue with a thin coating and a weak, hollow, sliding or slow pulse.

If there is an associated deficiency of blood the symptomatology is similar, except for the vaginal bleeding.

c) The Deficiency of Blood

Main symptoms include vaginal bleeding in small amounts, with light-colored blood; a pale-yellowish complexion; dizziness; insomnia; palpitations; a sensation of heat in the palms; dry mouth; night sweating; and constipation. A pale tongue with a thin coating or no coating and a rapid, thready or sliding pulse may be noted.

If there is an associated deficiency of the Kidney, it may lead to a sensation of lumbar weakness and pain.

d) The Injury of Chong Mai and Ren Mai Vessels

Main symptoms include vaginal bleeding during pregnancy, asthenia, exhaustion, lumbar weakness and pain, and a painful sensation in the lower abdomen. A pale tongue with a normal coating and a deep, forceless pulse may be observed.

Treatment

a) Heat in the Blood

Therapeutic principle: cool the Heat, nourish the blood.

Prescription:

SP 10 (Xuehai) removes Heat from the blood, regulates blood circulation

LI 11 (Quchi) is the He point of the Large Intestine channel, removes exogenous pathogenic Heat, regulates Qi and blood circulation, regulates the channels

BL 17 (Geshu) is the Influential point of blood, promotes blood functions

BL 43 (Gaohuangshu) strengthens the Spleen, fortifies the circulation of Qi

BL 20 (Pishu) is the Back-Shu point of the Spleen, strengthens the Spleen and supports blood

In cases with prolonged symptoms that aggravate, other points can, in time, be used in alternative prescriptions:

SP 1 (Yinbai) is the Jing-Well point of the Spleen channel, strengthens the Spleen, regulates blood, maintains the blood within the vessels, sedates the mind

RM 3 (Zhongji)	is the Crossing point of the Ren Mai Vessel with the Spleen, Kidney and Liver channels, removes internal Heat and regulates Lower Jiao
PC 6 (Neiguan)	is the Luo point of the Pericardium channel, nourishes the Heart and sedates the mind

In cases of internal Heat caused by Liver Qi stagnation, the following points can be used:

LV 1 (Dadun)	is the Jing-Well point of the Liver channel, promotes Liver Qi circulation, regulates Lower Jiao, calms the spirit
LV 6 (Zhongdu)	is the Xi point of the Liver channel, removes Liver Qi stagnation, stimulates the circulation of blood
BL 40 (Weizhong)	removes pathogenic factors from blood, is pricked for bleeding
SP 10 (Xuehai)	removes Heat from the blood and stops the blood loss

b) The Deficiency of Qi

Therapeutic principle: tone Qi, support the Kidney

Prescription:

ST 36 (Zusanli)	is the He point of the Stomach channel, tones the Spleen and Stomach, supports Qi, regulates Qi and blood, has a general fortifying effect
BL 23 (Shenshu)	is the Back-Shu point of the Kidney, strengthens the Kidney, tones the Yang and nourishes the Yin, strengthens the lumbar region
DM 4 (Mingmen)	regulates Qi, strengthens the Kidney Yang, preserves the Essence, strengthens the lumbar region
K 8 (Jiaoxin)	strengthens the Kidney Qi
BL 52 (Zhishi)	strengthens the Kidney and supports the Essence

In cases with associated blood deficiency, the following points can be used:

BL 17 (Geshu)	is the Influential point of the blood, supports the blood, strengthens the Spleen and promotes Qi circulation
SP 4 (Gongsun)	is the Luo point of the Spleen channel, strengthens the Spleen and Stomach, sources of blood, regulates the functions of the Spleen, regulates Qi
SP 1 (Yinbai)	is the Jing Well point of the Spleen channel, strengthens the Spleen, tones the Qi and stops the blood loss

c) The Deficiency of Blood

Therapeutic principle: tone blood, tone Yin

Prescription:

SP 6 (Sanyinjiao)	is the Crossing point of the three Yin channels of the foot, strengthens the Spleen, supports the formation of blood, regulates Qi and blood circulation
BL 20 (Pishu)	is the Back-Shu point of the Spleen, strengthens the Spleen, regulates the Stomach, supports the blood
BL 17 (Geshu)	is the Influential point of blood, supports the blood, promotes Qi circulation
ST 36 (Zusanli)	is the He point of the Stomach, regulates the Stomach, tones the Spleen, regulates Qi and blood
BL 18 (Ganshu)	is the Back-Shu point of the Liver, strengthens the Liver functions, where the blood is stored

The selected points are stimulated with the reinforcing method, using acupuncture or moxibustion for ST 36. For the other points, moxibustion on the abdominal and lumbar sacral region should be avoided during pregnancy.

In cases where a deficiency of the Kidney exists, other points can be added to nourish the Kidney Yin:

K 2 (Rangu) is the Ying point of the Kidney channel, nourishes the Yin of the Kidney, warms Lower Jiao

K 5 (Shuiquan) is the Xi point of the Kidney channel, strengthens the Kidney, promotes Qi and blood circulation, tones the Chong Mai and Ren Mai vessels

K 1 (Yongquan) is the Jing-Well point of the Kidney channel, nourishes the Kidney Yin

d) The Injury of Chong Mai and Ren Mai Vessels

Therapeutic principle: strengthen the Kidney, regulate Chong Mai and Ren Mai vessels

Prescription:

BL 23 (Shenshu) is the Back-Shu point of the Kidney, strengthens the Kidney, tones the lumbar region

K 5 (Shuiquan) is the Xi point of the Kidney channel, regulates Qi and blood, regulates Chong Mai and Ren Mai vessels

K 14 (Siman) is the Crossing point of the Kidney channel and the Chong Mai Vessel, tones Kidney Qi, regulates Chong Mai and Ren Mai vessels, promotes Qi and blood circulation

RM 4 (Guanyuan) is the Crossing point of the Ren Mai Vessel with the three Yin channels of the foot, the Kidney, Spleen and Liver, tones Qi, strengthens the Kidney, regulates the Chong Mai and Ren Mai vessels, regulates Qi and blood

Other points can also be used in alternative prescriptions:

K 3 (Taixi) is the Yuan-Source point of the Kidney channel, nourishes the Lower Jiao, regulates the Chong Mai and Ren Mai vessels

K 13 (Qixue) is the Crossing point of the Kidney channel with the Chong Mai Vessel, tones Kidney Qi, regulates the Chong Mai and Ren Mai vessels.

Acupuncture is given with the reinforcing method.

THREATENED ABORTION

Threatened abortion refers to vaginal bleeding before 20 weeks of gestational age, usually accompanied by uterine contractions, but no cervical dilatation. Ultrasound examination is useful to confirm signs of fetal life. With bedrest and medication to treat symptoms (e.g. sedatives, tocolytics), the pregnancy is usually preserved. From the perspective of Chinese traditional medicine, threatened abortion represents the aggravated condition following abdominal pain and vaginal bleeding during pregnancy. It is called "abnormal movements of the fetus" (Tai Chong Bu An). Treatment usually is achieved with pharmacotherapy but different prescriptions of acupoints can be tried. Typically acupuncture is performed as prophylactic therapy, before conception if possible, in cases with a history of miscarriages.

Etiopathogenesis

There are several conditions that can cause threatened abortion or miscarriage. Without treatment the following conditions will present at each pregnancy:

a) Deficiency of Qi and blood

b) Deficiency of Kidney Qi

c) Heat in the blood

d) Stagnation of Liver Qi

e) Dysfunction of the Chong Mai and Ren Mai Vessels

The common result of all these conditions is the imbalance of Qi and blood in favor of Qi. But the nidation and development of the pregnancy are closely related to blood, which should be plentiful within the uterus; otherwise, the placenta "overturns," resulting in abortion and restoration of menstruation.

Clinical Manifestations

The main symptom of threatened abortion is the sensation of abnormal movement of the fetus, perceived as a "falling down of the fetus." Abdominal pain and vaginal bleeding can be associated, together with other symptoms according to the etiopathogenic type.

a) The Deficiency of Qi and Blood

Associated symptoms include asthenia; palpitations; dizziness; insomnia; numbness of the limbs, with a sensation of cold; a pale complexion; lack of taste and appetite; polyuria; and leukorrhea. The patient may have a pale tongue with a thin coating and a weak pulse.

b) The Deficiency of Kidney Qi

Associated symptoms include a sensation of weakness in the lumbar region and limbs, dizziness, insomnia, frequent urination with a clear stream. A pale tongue with a thin, white coating and a weak, thready pulse may be noted.

c) Heat in the Blood

Associated symptoms include vaginal bleeding with light red blood, a flushed complexion, dizziness, irritability, dry mouth, thirst, constipation, and a yellowish and scanty urine. A dark, red tongue with a yellow coating and a rapid, slippery pulse may be observed.

d) The Stagnation of Liver Qi

Associated symptoms include abdominal pain and distension, a sensation of fullness in the thorax, belching, lack of appetite, acid taste, and irritability. The patient may have a thin, white tongue coating and a wiry, string-taut pulse.

e) The Dysfunction of the Chong Mai and Ren Mai Vessels

Associated symptoms include asthenia, lumbar weakness and pain, and leukorrhea. The patient may present with a pale tongue and a weak, sliding pulse.

Treatment

a) The Deficiency of Qi and Blood

Therapeutic principle: tone Qi and blood

Prescription:

RM 6 (Qihai)   strengths the Essence, tones and promotes Qi circulation

ST 36 (Zusanli)   is one of the four Dominant points and the He point of the Stomach channel, restores the Qi

	of Middle Jiao, tones the Spleen and Stomach, has a generally fortifying effect
SP 6 (Sanyinjiao)	is the Crossing point of the three Yin channels of the foot, strengthens the Spleen and Stomach, regulates Qi and blood, regulates the channels
BL 17 (Geshu)	is the Influential point of the blood, regulates blood and promotes the circulation of Qi
BL 20 (Pishu)	is the Back-Shu point of the Spleen, tones the Spleen and Stomach, a source of blood
H 7 (Shenmen)	is the Yuan-Source point of the Heart channel, calms the Heart and mind, has a sedative effect

b) The Deficiency of Kidney Qi

Therapeutic principle: tone the Kidney

Prescription:

RM 4 (Guanyuan)	is the Crossing point of the Ren Mai Vessel with the three Yin channels of the foot, the Kidney, Spleen and Liver, tones Qi, regulates the Chong Mai and Ren Mai Vessels, has an important action upon the blood balance of the uterus
BL 23 (Shenshu)	is the Back-Shu point of the Kidney, strengthens the Yang of the Kidney, tones the Kidney and the lumbar region
BL 28 (Pangguangshu)	is the Back-Shu point of the Urinary Bladder, strengthens the Urinary Bladder and Kidney, tones the Yuan Qi
K 3 (Taixi)	is the Yuan-Source point of the Kidney channel, tones the Kidney, nourishes the Lower Jiao, regulates the Chong Mai and Ren Mai vessels
DM 4 (Mingmen)	restores Qi and Essence, tones the Kidney and strengthens Yang

ST 36 (Zusanli)   has a generally fortifying effect

Strong stimulation can be given by using moxibustion at points ST 36, RM 4 and DM 4 and acupuncture with the reinforcing method for the rest of the points.

c) Heat in the Blood

Therapeutic principle: cool the blood, remove Heat

Prescription:

RM 3 (Zhongji)	is the Crossing point of the Ren Mai Vessel with the Spleen, Kidney, Liver; regulates Lower Jiao, removes pathogenic Heat
BL 15 (Xinshu)	is the Back-Shu point of the Heart, nourishes the Heart and blood, sedates the mind
BL 18 (Ganshu)	is the Back-Shu point of the Liver, removes Liver stagnation and clears the pathogenic Heat
BL 20 (Pishu)	is the Back-Shu point of the Spleen, strengthens the Spleen and blood, regulates the Spleen Qi and blood
SP 9 (Yinlingquan)	is the He point of the Spleen channel, removes the Heat from Middle Jiao, tones the Spleen, removes Heat from the blood
SP 10 (Xuehai)	cools the blood, removes the Heat

d) The Stagnation of Liver Qi

Therapeutic principle: remove Liver stagnation, drain the channels

Prescription:

BL 18 (Ganshu)	is the Back-Shu point of the Liver, removes Liver Qi stagnation
LV 3 (Taichong)	is the Yuan-Source point of the Liver channel, promotes Qi and blood circulation, removes Liver stagnation
LV 5 (Ligou)	is the Luo point of the Liver channel, removes Liver Qi stagnation
LV 6 (Zhongdu)	is the Xi point of the Liver channel, removes

	Liver Qi stagnation, stimulates blood circulation
RM 4 (Guanyuan)	is the Crossing point of the Ren Mai Vessel with the Kidney, Liver and Spleen channels; promotes Qi and blood circulation
PC 6 (Neiguan)	is the Luo point of the Pericardium channel, sedates the mind

e) The Dysfunction of Chong Mai and Ren Mai Vessels

Therapeutic principle: regulate Chong Mai and Ren Mai

Prescription:

SP 4 (Gongsun)	is the Confluent point of the Chong Mai Vessel and the Luo point of the Spleen channel, regulates the Qi functions and circulation within the Chong Mai Vessel
L 7 (Lieque)	is the Confluent point of the Ren Mai Vessel and the Luo point of the Lung channel, regulates Qi and blood circulation in the channels, strengthens Qi
RM 7 (Yinjiao)	is the Crossing point of the Chong Mai with the Ren Mai Vessel, regulates the circulation within the two vessels
K 5 (Shuiquan)	is the Xi point of the Kidney channel, regulates the Chong Mai and Ren Mai vessels, regulates Qi and blood
K 13 (Qixue)	is the Crossing point of the Kidney channel with the Chong Mai Vessel, regulates Chong Mai and Ren Mai, tones the Kidney

INDUCED ABORTION

From the perspective of Chinese traditional medicine, an unexpected and severe disturbance of Qi/blood balance may cause abortion.

Using the following points during pregnancy may induce abortion.

Prescription:

| **LI 4** (Hegu) | is the Yuan-Source point of the Large Intestine channel, regulates Qi and blood |

| **SP 6** (Sanyinjiao) | is the Crossing point of the three Yin channels of the foot, the Kidney, Spleen and Liver, strengthens the Spleen; nourishes blood; regulates Qi and blood circulation |
| **BL 67** (Zhiyin) | is the Jing-Well point of the Urinary Bladder channel, together with the Kidney channel and Kidney Qi governs the pregnancy |

Acupuncture is given with the reinforcing method and strong stimulation of the point LI 4. When stimulation using the reducing method is given to point SP 6, it causes a sudden deficiency of blood which then becomes insufficient to nourish the fetus and to assure continuation of the pregnancy. BL 67 is an empirical point used to correct the fetal position.

Associated points can also be stimulated if needed: **BL 60** (Kunlun), **RM 3** (Zhongji) or **GB 21** (Jianjing).

Acupuncture is given twice daily and needles are retained for approximately 20 minutes, for 2 to 3 sessions.

MUSCULOSKELETAL PATHOLOGY IN PREGNANCY

Among the most frequent complaints during pregnancy are musculoskeletal disorders such as backache, lower limb cramps and carpal tunnel syndrome.

a) Backache

Lumbar backache can be the result of postural back strain, muscle spasm, or relaxation of the pelvic joints due to action of the steroid sex hormones.

Therapy involves proper posture, back exercises, and massage. Neurologic signs and symptoms should also be assessed.

Acupuncture can offer an alternative therapy that may relieve or alleviate the lower back discomfort.

Prescription:

Points are selected after considering the course of the channels in the affected area and the possible etiology.

| **BL 40** (Weizhong) | is the Dominant point, used to treat lumbar pain, relaxes the muscles and tendons |
| **BL 57** (Chengshan) | relaxes the muscles and tendons |

BL 23 (Shenshu)   is the Back-Shu point of the Kidney that dominates the bones

GB 30 (Huantiao)   is the Crossing point of the Gall Bladder and Urinary Bladder channels, strengthens the sacrolumbar region and has a relaxing effect

GB 34 (Yanglingquan) is the Influential point of the tendons, relaxes the tendons

SP 5 (Shangqiu)   is the Crossing point of joints

E.P. Yaotongxue   is an empirical point used to treat lumbar sprain

Auricular Therapy: points Sciatic, Lumbar, Shenmen, can also be used alone or in other prescriptions:

b) Carpal Tunnel Syndrome

This syndrome is more frequent in late pregnancy and is caused by an excessive retention of water and sodium.

Clinical Manifestations

Carpal tunnel syndrome is evidenced by chronic pains of the hands and fingers, aggravated during the night and accompanied by numbness and edema. Usually there is a spontaneous healing after childbirth.

Treatment

Therapeutic principle: stimulate blood circulation, promote circulation within the channels.

Prescription:

SJ 5 (Waiguan)   is the Luo point of the San Jiao channel, stimulates circulation in the channels and invigorates the collaterals

PC 7 (Daling)   is the Yuan-Source point of the Pericardium channel, has local action

LI 4 (Hegu)   regulates Qi and blood and has an analgesic effect

After each session it is useful to use the plum-blossom needle for taping the wrist region.

c) *Lower Limbs Cramps*

Leg cramps are also a frequent complaint during pregnancy. They can be caused by a reduced level of serum calcium or an increased level of serum phosphorus relative to excessive intake of phosphorus in dairy products; diminished circulation can also be involved. Western therapy calls for adequate diet and treatment of symptoms. Acupuncture can be easily performed; its prescription depends upon the pathological conditions and the involved organs: Liver, Spleen, etc.

Prescription:

Main Points:

ST 36 (Zusanli)	is one of the four Dominant points, regulates Qi and blood, has a general fortifying effect
GB 41 (Zulinqi)	is the Shu-Stream point of the Gall Bladder channel and one of the eight Confluent points, regulates circulation
K 6 (Zhaohai)	is one of the eight Confluent points

Other points can be added, depending upon the location of the cramps.

Calf

-The lateral aspect: the Urinary Bladder channel.

BL 57 (Chengshan)

BL 58 (Feiyang)

- The medial aspect: the Kidney channel

E.P. located midway between K 9 (Zhubin) and K 10 (Yingu)

Toes

- In extension: the Gall Bladder channel

On extensor digitorum brevis muscle:

GB 40 (Qiuxu)	is the Yuan-Source point of the Gall Bladder channel, improves mobility of the toes

On extensor digitorum longus muscle:

GB 34 (Yanglingquan)	is the He point of the Gall Bladder channel and the Influential point of the tendons

-In flexion

Plantaris muscle:

K 1 (Yongquan)

Calf

The peroneus longus muscle relates to a point located 1 cun below GB 34 (Yanglingquan). The sensation produced by the needle should spread along the course of the Gall Bladder channel.

Thigh

- The posterior aspect, the biceps femoris muscle: the Urinary Bladder channel

An extraordinary point is used, located midway between BL 37 (Yinmen) and BL 40 (Weizhong).

GB 34 (Yanglingquan)

- The medial aspect, the adductor muscles: the Liver channel

LV 10 (Zuwuli)   relaxes the muscles and tendons

LV 11 (Yinlian)   relaxes the muscles and tendons

- The anterior aspect, the rectus femoris muscle: the Stomach channel

ST 32 (Futu)   promotes circulation within the channels

Other prescriptions can also be used:

BL 38 (Fuxi) + **BL 57** (Chengshan)

BL 39 (Weiyang) + **GB 34** (Yanglingquan) + **BL 57** (Chengshan) + **LV 3** (Taichong)

BL 55 (Heyang) + **BL 57** (Chengshan) + **GB 34** (Yanglingquan)

BL 56 (Chengjin) + **BL 61** (Pushen) + **LV 6** (Zhongdu)

BL 61 (Pushen) + **BL 57** (Chengshan) + **BL 40** (Weizhong)

BL 63 (Jinmen) + **GB 40** (Qiuxu)

EDEMA DURING PREGNANCY

Increased water retention during pregnancy, with the appearance of edema, is considered to be a physiologic change. Different factors are involved: increasing of the venous pressure due to the development of the uterus and decreasing of the colloid osmotic pressure. Edema is aggravated in the upright position, with swelling of the hands, ankles and feet possibly indicating that it has become generalized. The persistence or aggravation of the edema, when associated with proteinuria and/or hypertension, is a sign that preeclampsia may develop.

From the perspective of Chinese traditional medicine, the subcutaneous fluid retention is due to the dysfunction of water metabolism. The Lung, Spleen, Kidney and San Jiao functions govern the circulation and distribution of fluids in the body. Different etiopathogenic types are caused by the dysfunction of a specific organ. The edema are of Yin and Yang type.

Etiopathogenesis

Three types of edema are most frequent during pregnancy as a result of::

a) The Deficiency of Spleen

The weakness of the Spleen Qi can be caused by inadequate food intake, overstrain and stress which impair the functions of fluid transportation and transformation. The water is not controlled, the Yin is in excess and edema appears. The source of Qi and blood is also insufficient.

b) The Deficiency of Kidney

The deficiency of Kidney may be caused by overstrain, stress or insufficiency of the Kidney in childhood. Kidney deficiency causes an edema of the Yin type. Water retention results from the dysfunction of the Kidney and Urinary Bladder, with symptoms that mainly affect the lower part of the body.

c) The Stagnation of Damp

The stagnation of Damp is a consequence of Damp attack—an exogenous pathogenic factor of Yin type. It is characterized by heaviness, viscosity and stagnation and can impair the circulation of Qi and Spleen Yang. It is an edema of Yang type, with sudden onset, initially in the upper part of the body caused by inadequate body fluids. In cases with prolonged edema of Yang type, weakness of the body may appear, increasing the retention of water and leading to a Yin type edema.

Clinical Manifestations

a) The Deficiency of Spleen

Main symptoms include insidious onset of the edema in early pregnancy, initially on the dorsal aspect of the foot, then towards the face and eyelids. Associated signs of deficiency are a dark yellowish complexion, asthenia, vertigo, depression, lack of desire to speak, lack of appetite, cold body and limbs, a sensation of fullness in the thorax, watery stools, oliguria, and leukorrhea. A pale tongue with a thin, white, moist coating and a deep, slow and slippery pulse may be noted.

b) The Deficiency of Kidney

Main symptoms include insidious onset of edema, later in pregnancy and extending over the entire body, particularly in the lumbar region and the lower limbs. Associated symptoms include a pale, bright complexion; palpitations; aversion to cold; lack of appetite; asthenia; lack of desire to speak; a lower tone of voice; oliguria; and loose stools. A pale, thick tongue with a thin, white, slippery coating and a deep, retarded pulse may be observed.

c) The Stagnation of Damp

Main symptoms include edema of Yang type, extended over the entire body. Associated symptoms are a pale complexion, vertigo, a sensation of head inflation described as "having the head in a bag," asthenia, a sensation of bodily heaviness, a sensation of fullness in the thorax, abdominal distention, lack of appetite, nausea, oliguria, and loose stools. The patient may have a thick, white, greasy tongue coating and a soft, slippery pulse.

Treatment

a) The Deficiency of Spleen

Therapeutic principle: strengthen the Spleen and remove water.

Prescription:

BL 20 (Pishu)   is the Back-Shu point of the Spleen, strengthens the Spleen and regulates the Stomach, removes water

LV 13 (Zhangmen)   is the Front-Mu point of the Spleen, promotes the Spleen functions

ST 36 (Zusanli)   is the He point of the Stomach channel, tones Qi, supports the Spleen function of transportion

SP 5 (Shangqiu)   is the Jing-River point of the Spleen channel, supports water distribution, is indicated in edema of the dorsal aspect of the foot

SP 9 (Yinlingquan)   is the He point of the Spleen channel, strength-

	ens the Spleen and removes Damp, regulates the excretion of the water, favors circulation within San Jiao
RM 9 (Shuifen)	strengthens the Spleen and regulates the Stomach, removes water retention
GB 41 (Zulinqi)	is the Shu-Stream point of the Gall Bladder channel and the Confluent point of the Dai Mai Vessel, transforms retention, is indicated in edema of the dorsal aspect of the foot

Acupuncture is given with the reinforcing method. To stimulate the point RM 9, moxibustion is considered very effective in the treatment of edema.

b) The Deficiency of Kidney

Therapeutic principle: tone Yang of Kidney, support the circulation of water

Prescription:

RM 4 (Guanyuan)	is the Crossing point of the Ren Mai Vessel with the Kidney, Spleen and Liver channels; tones Qi and Kidney, favors the Yang, warms the Kidney and regulates blood
BL 23 (Shenshu)	is the Back-Shu point of the Kidney, warms the Kidney, removes Damp
BL 20 (Pishu)	is the Back-Shu point of the Spleen, strengthens the Spleen, promotes the circulation of water
K 3 (Taixi)	is the Yuan-Source point of the Kidney channel, nourishes and strengthens the Kidney, regulates the Chong Mai and Ren Mai vessels
K 7 (Fuliu)	is the Jing-River point of the Kidney channel, nourishes the Kidney, favors the drainage of Lower Jiao, tones the lumbar region
DM 4 (Mingmen)	tones the Essence and Kidney Qi, strengthens the Yang, regulates Qi, tones the lumbar region

Stimulation of the selected points uses acupuncture with the reinforcing method or moxibustion.

c) The Stagnation of Damp

Therapeutic principle: remove Damp, promote the circulation of water

Prescription:

RM 9 (Shuifen)   strengthens the Spleen and regulates the Stomach, removes the pathogenic Damp

RM 11 (Jianli)   strengthens the Spleen, dispels Damp, supports food transformation

ST 36 (Zusanli)   promotes the transportation and transformation functions of the Spleen and Stomach, redistributing the body fluids

SP 9 (Yinlingquan)   is the He point of the Spleen channel, strengthens the Spleen and removes Damp, regulates water excretion

SP 12 (Chongmen)   is the Crossing point of the Spleen and Liver channels with Yin Wei Mai Vessel, regulates Qi circulation, removes Damp

GB 39 (Weiyang)   regulates the functions of San Jiao, regulates the metabolism of water

BL 28 (Pangguangshu) is the Back-Shu point of the Urinary Bladder, strengthens the Urinary Bladder, regulates circulation in the Lower Jiao

Acupuncture is given with the reinforcing method and even movement for points located on the Spleen channel.

HYPERTENSION AND PREGNANCY

From the perspective of Chinese traditional medicine the progress of pregnancy is especially under the control of the Kidney, Spleen and Liver.

There is an adjustment of the Qi/blood balance in the pregnant woman, with a prevalence of Yin in early pregnancy and an increase of Yang in late pregnancy through delivery which is considered to be a Yang manifestation. Hypertension is also a manifestation of Yang.

Etiopathogenesis

Many factors may be involved in the elevation of blood pressure, but a primary one is the ascent of Liver Yang resulting from a deficiency of Kidney and Spleen.

The deficiency of Zang organs, located in the lower part of the body, will cause a pathogenic excess in the upper part. Hypertension disorders are a consequence of the dysfunction of Qi and blood circulation.

Clinical Manifestations

Main symptoms include blood pressure values exceeding 140/90 mm Hg. Associated symptoms are morning headache, vision disturbances, tinnitus, insomnia, palpitations, numbness of the limbs, edema, and abdominal distension. A string-taut pulse may be palpated.

Treatment

Acupuncture may be used as adjuvant therapy together with bedrest (with placement in a left lateral position to increase placental blood flow), reduced sodium intake according to individual needs, and hypotensor drugs when necessary.

The hypertensive gravida is considered a high-risk pregnancy. Clinical and biological maternal evaluation is mandatory and the following parameters should be assessed: blood pressure values, weight gain, red cell count, uric acid levels, serum creatinine, and proteinuria.

Dynamic evaluation of fetal growth should entail repeated maternal clinical evaluation, and measurement of fetal heart rate, intrauterine growth, and placental blood flow (mainly by ultrasonography).

In cases of obvious symptomatology and/or pathologic changes of the evaluated parameters, hospital admission is necessary and appropriate therapy should be started immediately.

a) Prophylactic Therapy of Yin Deficiency of the Kidney and Spleen

Therapeutic principle: strengthen the Kidney and Spleen

BL 23 (Shenshu)	is the Back-Shu point of the Kidney, nourishes the Yin and strengthens the Yang of the Kidney
BL 20 (Pishu)	is the Back-Shu point of the Spleen, strengthens the Spleen, regulates the Stomach
RM 4 (Guanyuan)	tones Qi, strengthens the Kidney and Spleen, regulates blood
ST 36 (Zusanli)	is one of the four Dominant points, restores Qi of the Middle Jiao, strengthens the Spleen,

	supports the transportation of body fluids, has a reinforcing effect
SP 4 (Gongsun)	is the Luo point of the Spleen channel and the Confluent point of Chong Mai Vessel, strengthens the Spleen and regulates Qi
SP 6 (Sanyinjiao)	is the Crossing point of the Yin channels of the foot, tones the Kidney and Spleen, regulates Qi and blood circulation
LV 13 (Zhangmen)	is the Front-Mu point of the Spleen and the Influential point of Zang organs, regulates the organs, tones the Spleen

Acupuncture is given with the reinforcing method at the selected acupoints, in bimonthly sessions, starting in early pregnancy, if necessary.

b) Therapy of the Yang Excess of the Liver

Therapeutic principle: remove Heat, regulate Qi and blood circulation

LV 2 (Xingjian)	is the Ying point of the Liver channel, removes pathogenic Heat from the Liver, cools the blood
LV 3 (Taichong)	is the Yuan-Source point of the Liver channel, dispels pathogenic Fire of the Liver, supports Qi and blood circulation
PC 6 (Neiguan)	is the Luo point of the Pericardium channel and the Confluential point of the Yin Wei Mai Vessel, removes pathogenic Heat and stimulates Qi circulation, calms the mind
H 7 (Shenmen)	is the Yuan-Source point of the Heart channel, calms the Heart and mind
ST 36 (Zusanli)	supports Qi circulation in the channels, regulates blood
LI 11 (Quchi)	is the He point of the Large Intestine channel, removes Heat, regulates Qi and blood circulation
LV 13 (Zhangmen)	is the Front-Mu point of the Spleen, strengthens the Spleen, controls blood

GB 34 (Yanglingquan) is the He point of the Gall Bladder channel, removes the Heat, cools the blood, supports the channels

BL 23 (Shenshu) is the Back-Shu point of the Kidney, tones the Kidney, nourishes Yin

The selected acupoints can be used in alternative prescriptions, based upon individual needs.

a) In cases with chronic hypertension, acupuncture treatment can be given prophylactically in early and middle pregnancy.

Therapeutic principle: strengthen the Kidney and Spleen

Prescription:

BL 23 (Shenshu) + **K 3** (Taixi) + **RM 6** (Qihai) + **ST 36** (Zusanli) + **LI 11** (Quchi)

RM 4 (Guanyuan) + **ST 36** (Zusanli) + **BL 20** (Pishu) + **LI 11** (Quchi) + **SP 4** (Gongsun)

Acupuncture is given with the reinforcing method, in bimonthly sessions.

When hypertension is found to have existed during previous pregnancies, the use of the acupoint K 9 (Zhubin) as the "marvelous point of pregnancy" should be considered among the selected points.

b) Hypertension treatment in late pregnancy

In late pregnancy there is a physiologic increasing of Yang until childbirth. In this circumstance the prevalent etiologic feature is the excess of Liver Yang and the deficiency of the Kidney and Spleen, with impaired circulation of Qi.

Prescription:

LV 3 (Taichong) + **LI 11** (Quchi) + **PC 6** (Neiguan) + **BL 23** (Shenshu)

LV 3 (Taichong) + **LI 11** (Quchi) + **LV 13** (Zhangmen) + **ST 36** (Zusanli)

RM 6 (Qihai) + **ST 36** (Zusanli).

Alternative prescriptions can be used in weekly sessions, when necessary.

Auricular Therapy: Points Shenmen, Subcortex, Lower of blood pressure, Sympathetic nervous system, Helix 1-6. Two or three points are selected and mild stimulation is given. Sessions are scheduled every second day, then bimonthly, when the values of blood pressure are stable and close to normal.

PREECLAMPSIA

Preeclampsia is characterized by hypertension, generalized edema and proteinuria occurring after the 20th week of pregnancy through the 6th week of postpartum, in the absence of vascular and renal pathology.

The precise etiology is unknown and preeclampsia remains the "disease of theories." Vasospasm is considered to be its main component.

Maternal and fetal complications explain the poor prognosis in the absence of an early diagnosis and proper therapy.

Etiopathogenesis

From the perspective of Chinese traditional medicine, the following circumstances can be involved in the onset of preeclampsia:

- A deficiency of blood
- A deficiency of the Kidney Qi
- An excess of Liver Yang

The energetic imbalances mentioned above—mainly the deficiency of Yin and the resulting excess of Yang—are the same as those involved in the etiopathogenesis of edema, hypertension during pregnancy and, when prolonged, eclampsia.

Clinical Manifestations

Main symptoms include hypertension, edema, possible headache with painful distension in the flank and epigastric regions, irritability, nervousness, insomnia, and oliguria. The patient may present with a pale tongue with a white coating or a red tongue with a yellow coating, if Yang is excessive. A pulse of the deficiency type may be noted.

Treatment

Early diagnosis of the energetic imbalances involved in the etio-pathogenesis allows a precocious treatment. If the deficiency of blood and Yin of the Kidney is discovered before conception, prophylactic treatment may be administered.

If there are obvious clinical manifestations, hospital admission and careful evaluation and monitoring are necessary.

Acupuncture treatment, if performed at all, should only be adjuvant and only in close collaboration with the obstetrician.

Therapeutic principle: nourish the Yin of the Kidney, remove the excess of Yang

Prescription:

BL 23 (Shenshu)   is the Back-Shu point of the Kidney, strengthens the Kidney, nourishes the Yin of the Kidney

K 3 (Taixi)   is the Yuan-Source point of the Kidney channel, nourishes the Kidney

K 1 (Yongquan)   is the Jing-Well point of the Kidney channel, nourishes the Kidney Yin, cools Heat, calms the spirit

GB 25 (Jingmen)   is the Front-Mu point of the Kidney, warms the Yang and removes Qi stagnation, regulates the elimination of fluids

ST 36 (Zusanli)   tones the Qi of Middle Jiao, clears the channels, has a reinforcing effect

LI 11 (Quchi)   is the He point of the Large Intestine channel, regulates Qi and blood and clears the channels

LV 3 (Taichong)   is the Yuan-Source point of the Liver channel, supports Qi and blood circulation

Other points can also be used to reduce the excess of Yang and the high values of blood pressure:

GB 20 (Fengchi)   is the Crossing point of the Gall Bladder channel with the Yang Qiao Mai Vessel, removes pathogenic Heat, clears the channels

LV 2 (Xingjian)   is the Ying point of the Liver channel, removes pathogenic Heat and cools the blood

H 7 (Shenmen)   is the Yuan-Source point of the Heart channel, calms the Heart and mind

PC 6 (Neiguan)   is the Luo point of the Pericardium channel, removes pathogenic Heat, sedates the mind

GB 34 (Yanglingquan) is the He point of the Gall Bladder channel, supports Liver function, removes pathogenic Heat and Damp

Few points are selected considering the deficiency involved, and acupuncture is given with mild stimulation.

ECLAMPSIA

Eclampsia is a major complication of preeclampsia, still of unknown etiology, the vasospasm being the main physiopathologic element involved. An increased frequency has been observed in primiparas. The symptomatology consists of: headache, dizziness, vision disturbances, high values of blood pressure, convulsive seizures, coma, proteinuria and anuria. Eclampsia is an obstetrical emergency with increased maternal and fetal mortality.

The treatment consists of resuscitation maneuvers, intensive care and termination of the pregnancy.

From the perspective of Chinese traditional medicine, this condition is correlated with the internal movement of Wind. The energetic circumstances of the onset of eclampsia are represented by Qi deficiency of the Liver and Kidney which are consumed to provide for the development of the fetus. This deficiency is more severe if there is a Qi deficiency previous to pregnancy. The deficiency of Yin will cause an excess of Yang with obstruction of the channels and collaterals.

Etiopathogenesis

a) The Deficiency of Blood

Constitutional deficiency of blood can be aggravated by pregnancy, as blood is used to nourish the fetus. The deficient Yin from the lower part of the body cannot hold the Yang, which ascends with possible generation of Wind. Given the relationship of Qi to blood (i.e., blood is the "mother of Qi"), the deficient blood will damage the circulation of Qi, resulting in its stagnation and the stagnation of Phlegm.

b) Heat in the Liver

During a pregnancy with known deficiency of Yin and prevalence of Yang (a characteristic feature of late pregnancy), an accumulation of Heat in the interior of the body is possible. Excessive Heat turns into Fire that stirs the Wind and disturbs blood. Fire as a pathogen factor of Yang type can consume the body fluids and worsen the deficiency of Yin.

c) The Attack of Wind-Cold

Previous energy deficiency can favor the attack of the exogenous pathogenic factors. Wind is a Yang pathogenic factor characterized by upward dispersion, rapid changes and unceasing movement. If the pathogenic attack injures the Spleen channel, the Yin, the blood and the body fluids will be more damaged and characteristic clinical manifestations will appear.

Clinical Manifestations

a) The Deficiency of Blood

Main symptoms include dizziness, palpitations, dyspnea, edema of lower limbs and face, convulsive seizures and coma during the attack. A pale tongue with a thin coating and a rapid, thready or slippery pulse may be noted.

b) Heat in the Liver

Main symptoms include vertigo, flushed complexion and conjunctivae, red lips, vision disturbances, palpitations, restlessness, irritability, anger, constipation, dry stools, and oliguria. This condition has a sudden onset. A red tongue with a yellowish coating and a rapid, wiry pulse may be observed.

c) The Attack of Wind-Cold

Main symptoms include fever, aversion to cold, painful limbs, headache, and a sensation of oppression in the thorax. During the eclamptic attack the associated symptoms that may occur include convulsive seizures, opisthotonus, and coma. The patient may evidence a pale tongue with a white coating and a superficial, slippery and wiry pulse.

Treatment

Acupuncture treatment can be effective when prophylactic, given, if possible, before conception in order to correct an already known Qi and blood deficiency.

Precocious diagnosis of preeclampsia and adequate monitoring during pregnancy are very important, allowing the physician to detect the worsening of symptoms and signs (see hypertension and preeclampsia on pages 90-95).

The eclamptic attack is a major obstetrical emergency and a matter of intensive care.

Acupuncture treatment should be considered as adjuvant, only in close cooperation with the obstetrician and intensive care therapist. When giving acupuncture, strong manual or electrostimulation is needed to resuscitate the patient and to calm the Wind.

a) The Deficiency of Blood

Therapeutic principle: nourish the blood, calm Wind

Prescription:

BL 17 (Geshu)   is the Influential point of blood, strengthens the Spleen, regulates blood, stimulates Qi circulation

BL 20 (Pishu)   is the Back-Shu point of the Spleen, tones the Spleen, supports blood formation

BL 23 (Shenshu)   is the Back-Shu point of the Kidney, nourishes the Yin and strengthens the Yang of the Kidney, stimulates the cerebral activities

SP 10 (Xuehai)   nourishes and stimulates blood circulation, removes Wind from blood

ST 36 (Zusanli)   is the He point of the Stomach channel and the Dominant point, regulates the Stomach and tones Spleen, supports blood formation, has a generally reinforcing effect

DM 26 (Renzhong)   sedates spasm, is an important point for resuscitation

GB 20 (Fengchi)   regulates the channels, revives the sense organs from unconsciousness

E.P. Yintang has a tranquilizing effect

b) Heat in the Liver

Therapeutic principle: remove Heat, cool the Liver, calm the Wind

Prescription:

LV 3 (Taichong)   is the Yuan-Source point of the Liver channel, removes Liver Fire, stimulates Qi and blood circulation

SP 6 (Sanyinjiao)   regulates the channels, regulates Qi and blood
                           circulation, nourishes blood

GB 34 (Yanglingquan) is the He point of the Gall Bladder channel and
                           the Influential point of the tendons, nourishes
                           and relaxes tendons, removes spasms

DM 26 (Renzhong)   is a resuscitation point

LI 11 (Quchi)   is the He point of the Large Intestine channel,
                           removes pathogenic Heat, regulates Qi and
                           blood, drains the channels

PC 6 (Neiguan)   is the Luo point of the Pericardium channel,
                           calms the Heart and mind

Pricked for bleeding, the twelve Jing-Well points can also remove
Heat from the channels.

c) The Attack of Wind-Cold

Therapeutic principle: nourish blood, calm the Wind, remove Cold.

Prescription:

DM 26 (Renzhong)   is the Crossing point of the Du Mai Vessel
                           with the Large Intestine and Stomach chan-
                           nels, removes pathogenic Wind, sedates
                           spasm, is an important point for resuscitation

DM 14 (Dazhui)   is the Crossing point of the Yang channels
                           with the Du Mai Vessel, stimulates the circu-
                           lation of Yang, removes Wind

DM 16 (Fengfu)   is the Crossing point of the Du Mai with Yang
                           Wei Mai Vessels, indicated for mental disor-
                           ders

GB 20 (Fengchi)   is the Crossing point of the Gall Bladder and San
                           Jiao channels with the Yang Wei Mai Vessel,
                           dispels pathogenic Wind, tones the channels,
                           revives the sense organs from unconsciousness

SP 6 (Sanjinjiao)   nourishes blood, regulates Qi and blood cir-
                           culation

SP 10 (Xuehai)   stimulates blood circulation, removes Wind
                           from blood

PC 6 (Neiguan)   is the Luo point of the Pericardium channel,
                          calms the Wind and mind

Auricular Therapy: points Lower blood pressure, Shenmen, Subcortex, Liver, Kidney, Helix 1-6. Needles are retained for approximately
20 minutes.

INTRAUTERINE DEMISE OF THE FETUS

In Chinese traditional medicine the intrauterine demise of the fetus
is called "Tai Si Bu Xai" and is considered to be caused by:
- maternal deficiency of Qi and blood
- exogenous pathogenic factors such as Wind, Cold, and Heat
  that may injure the fetus
- infectious diseases
- traumas
- umbilical cord compression

Etiopathogenesis

In cases of intrauterine demise of the fetus, the lack of spontaneous
expulsion is caused by two pathogenic conditions of deficiency and
excess type:

a) The Deficiency of Qi and Blood

Maternal deficiency of Qi and blood will cause the inability of the
uterus to eject the dead fetus.

b) The Stagnation of Blood

The stagnation of blood may have various causes such as the invasion
of pathogenic factors, traumas, deficiency of Qi or disturbances of Qi
circulation etc. As blood is "the mother of Qi," this stagnation can also
affect the circulation of Qi.

If Qi and blood are adequate and balanced, the spontaneous expulsion of the fetus is accomplished without any difficulty.

Clinical Manifestations

a) The Deficiency of Qi and Blood

Main symptoms include depression, asthenia, lack of appetite, a
sensation of cold, a pale complexion, palpitations, and lack of uterine
growth with possible blood loss. The patient may evidence a pale tongue
with a thin coating and a weak, slippery pulse.

b) The Stagnation of Blood

Main symptoms include bluish lips and face, abdominal and lumbar pains, and vaginal loss of dark blood . A dark red tongue, possibly with purplish spots on the borders, and a deep, wiry pulse may be present.

If stagnation of Qi coexists, other symptoms appear including a sensation of distension in the thoracic, epigastric and abdominal regions, belching, and abdominal pain.

Treatment

Before starting any treatment, it is mandatory to establish with certainty the intrauterine death of the fetus: absence of fetal heart beats and an absence of fetal movements which may be felt by the mother and confirmed by ultrasonography.

a) The Deficiency of Qi and Blood

Therapeutic principle: tone Qi and blood, strengthen the Yang.

Prescription:

SP 6 (SanyinJiao)	is the Crossing point of the three Yin channels of the foot, tones the Spleen and supports blood, regulates Qi and blood circulation
LI 4 (Hegu)	is the Yuan-Source point of the Large Intestine channel, regulates Qi and blood

Acupuncture is given with the reducing method for SP 6 and with the reinforcing method for LI 4. This may promote uterine contractions and may have an abortive effect.

LV 3 (Taichong)	is the Yuan-Source point of the Liver channel, supports Qi and blood circulation
ST 30 (Qichong)	regulates the uterus

b) The Stagnation of Blood

Therapeutic principle: promote blood and Qi

Prescription:

SP 6 (Sanyinjiao)	supports blood, regulates Qi and blood circulation
RM 4 (Guanyuan)	is the Crossing point of the Ren Mai Vessel with the three Yin channels of the foot,

	strengthens Yuan Qi, stimulates Qi and blood circulation, tones Qi and harmonizes blood
SP 10 (Xuehai)	regulates blood and the uterus
GB 26 (Daimai)	is the Crossing point of the Dai Mai Vessel with the Gall Bladder channel, drains and tones the channels
GB 41 (Zulinqi)	is the Shu-Stream point of the Gall Bladder channel and the Confluent point of Dai Mai Vessel
BL 37 (Yinmen)	strengthens the spine, tones the collaterals, sedates pain

In cases with stagnation of Qi, other points that can regulate Qi circulation need to be used:

ST 29 (Guilai)	regulates Qi, regulates the Lower Jiao
LI 4 (Hegu)	regulates Qi and blood
GB 20 (Fengshi)	tones the channels and collaterals, promotes Qi circulation
LV 3 (Taichong)	is the Yuan-Source point of the Liver channel, removes stagnation, stimulates the circulation of Qi
LV 14 (Qimen)	is the Front-Mu point of the Liver, removes Liver Qi stagnation, stimulates the circulation of blood

Acupuncture is given with the reducing or reinforcing method according to the selected points.

ABNORMAL PRESENTATION OF THE FETUS

Abnormal presentation of the fetus occurs in approximately 5% of all deliveries. The most common types are the breech and transverse presentations. Several circumstances can be involved: grand multiparity, prematurity, multiple pregnancy, abnormal placental implantation, contracted pelvis, and praevia tumors etc.

The diagnosis is made by vaginal examination. In many cases Caesarean section may be necessary for delivery.

From the perspective of Chinese traditional medicine, a presentation is abnormal when after 30 weeks of gestation, the fetal presentation in utero is unfavorable to delivery.

Acupuncture is regarded as effective in changing the fetal position, especially in multiparous women. Precautions should be taken to rule out possible surgical cases in which acupuncture is contraindicated: transverse position, contracted pelvis, and praevia tumors.

Etiopathogenesis

a) The Deficiency of Qi and Blood

Maternal Qi and blood deficiency, previous to pregnancy or aggravated by it, will cause a deficiency of Qi in the fetus that can make the Du Mai Vessel inactive and cause an abnormal positioning of the fetus in utero.

b) The Deficiency of Kidney Qi

This condition, associated with imbalance of the Kidney and Urinary Bladder channels, is compatible with the notion of polyhydramnios in western medicine, which is considered a possible cause of abnormal presentation.

c) The Stagnation of Qi and Blood

As Qi is the commander of blood, the stagnation of Qi impairs blood circulation and causes the fetus to permanently change its position.

Clinical Manifestations

There are no characteristic symptoms. The diagnosis is established upon clinical and, if necessary, ultrasound examination.

Treatment

Therapeutic principle: regulate Qi circulation in the Kidney and Urinary Bladder channels

Prescription:

BL 67 (Zhiyin)   is the Jing-Well point of the Urinary Bladder channel related to the Kidney channel, stimulates Qi and blood circulation

It is an empirical point used to treat the abnormal positioning of the fetus. Stimulation with moxa is preferred. Two to three applications of moxa daily are performed until the fetus changes its position. Good results are reported in up to 80 % of cases.

Other points that can promote the descent of the fetus can be added:

BL 60 (Kunlun)

GB 21 (Jianjing)

LABOR

PREPARATION OF LABOR

Preparation of labor should be systematic for those women who wish to benefit from acupuncture management of both labor and delivery.

Several aspects are to be considered when performing acupuncture, which is given in 1 to 3 sessions during the 9th month of pregnancy:

- increasing the woman's confidence in acupuncture as a therapeutic method
- increasing the woman's confidence in the acupuncture practitioner who will be present during labor
- assessing the acupuncture sensation and subsequent therapeutic response
- diagnosing the possible energetic imbalances that may become manifest during labor or puerperium

The acupuncture prescriptions aim to:

- correct major energetic imbalances
- maintain emotional balance
- increase body resistance

Few points should be selected, without any fixed prescription:

ST 36 (Zusanli)	with the reinforcing method, using moderate stimulation; regulates Qi and blood; has a generally reinforcing effect
H 7 (Shenmen)	regulates the Heart, sedates the mind
PC 6 (Neiguan)	sedates the mind
K 9 (Zhubin)	the "marvellous point of pregnancy"

ELEMENTS OF PHYSIOPATHOLOGY

The experience of labor is determined by many factors, including mechanical, nervous, hormonal and biochemical crcumstances all of which are not entirely understood.

The onset of labor is said to have occurred when uterine contractions are systematized in frequency and intensity, causing cervical effacement and progression of dilatation.

Several phenomena take place as labor progresses and these have been categorized as the stages of labor:
- the first stage of labor consists of cervical effacement and dilatation, ending in full dilatation (about 10 cm).
- the second stage of labor is characterized by the expulsion of the fetus
- the third stage of labor involves the separation and expulsion of placenta
- the fourth stage of labor is the early postpartum (the first 24 hours), uterine hemostasis being the essential element

The following parameters are to be observed during the evolution of labor:
- the uterine contractions and the progression of cervical dilatation
- the condition of fetal heart rate (FHR)
- the evolution of presentation
- the condition of membranes
- the aspect of the amniotic fluid

The dynamic follow-up of these parameters allows assessment of the evolution of labor. The management of labor is accomplished by vaginal examination every four hours, monitoring of FHR (fetal heart rate) every 30 minutes, and follow-up monitoring of the uterine contractions (i.e., rhythm, frequency, duration and intensity) for 10 minutes.

Diagnosis can be completed by ultrasound examination (presentation, FHR, somatometry etc.), amnioscopy, cardiotocography etc.

From the perspective of Chinese traditional medicine, labor is considered to be a movement of the uterus. The onset of labor is the moment of maximum Yang (Tai Yang = Great Yang) and concurs with an increase of parasympathetic nervous system activity. The main trigger is the development of the fetus as it undergoes major changes before birth, through the manifest function of San Jiao and the definement of its own energetic system (channels and organs).

As the pregnancy concludes, the energetic condition is changing as follows:

- the Yang is increasing and exceeding the Yin (that had been dominant), because childbirth is a Yang manifestation
- Qi/blood balance is changing. Qi increases, exceeding blood (that had been excessive) in order to nourish the uterus and to assure fetal development
- the uterus opens and its movement allows the expulsion of the fetus

In the above mentioned circumstances Qi and blood are well balanced and labor is physiologic. Any disturbance of the Qi/blood balance resulting from affected Zang-Fu organs or emotional factors can cause an abnormal evolution of labor. The main Zang-Fu organs involved are the Kidney, Liver and Spleen-Stomach couple.

The deficiency of Kidney Qi will cause a prolonged labor with weak, irregular contractions and lumbar pains. The stagnation of Qi and blood causes frequent and painful uterine contractions, often with a lack of labor progression.

When Liver is the involved organ, excessive lumbar and sacral pains appear and the cervical dilatation is affected: the cervix becomes spastic with onset of dilatation dystocia. In these circumstances, stagnation results in a lack of presentation of the fetus, which remains oriented upward.

The fetus, with its own functional energetic system, reacts as an autonomous individual and so is subject to the same injuries as the mother. The disturbance of fetal balance is referred to as fetal jeopardy.

An important element in determining the progress of labor is the condition of membranes. During a eutocic labor the rupture of membranes causes sudden dispersion of blood, thus favouring Qi and regulating the uterine contractions.

In cases with dystocic labor, the artificial amniotomy at 4 to 5 cm of cervical dilatation allows a reduction in the stagnation of Qi and blood which is usually the cause of dystocia. In this way, the circulation of Qi and blood is stimulated.

Premature rupture of the membranes, usually before the onset of labor, will cause a sudden dispersion of Qi and blood which become deficient, causing dystocic labor.

NORMAL LABOR

From the perspective of Chinese traditional medicine, when Qi/ blood balance is maintained, the progression of labor is normal. This ensures that the woman will experience normal, tolerable uterine contractions and emotional balance.

Acupuncture treatment can be an effective intervention when the progression of labor leads to excessive pain, fear, restlessness and anxiety or when management of labor is desired.

Sedative Therapy

Points located on the Heart and Pericardial channels are selected to calm the Heart and sedate the mind:

H 3 (Shaohai)	is the He point of the Heart channel, stimulates Qi and blood circulation and calms the mind
H 5 (Tongli)	is the Luo point of the Heart channel, regulates the Heart and mind, strengthens the channel
H 7 (Shenmen)	is the Yuan-Source point of the Heart channel, regulates and calms the Heart and mind
H 9 (Shaochong)	is the Jing-Well point of the Heart channel, calms the Heart and mind, removes pathogenic Heat from blood
PC 6 (Neiguan)	is the Luo point of the Pericardium channel, cools the Heart and calms the mind, alleviates pain
PC 7 (Daling)	is the Yuan-Source point of the Pericardium channel, removes pathogenic Heat from the Heart, cools blood, sedates the mind

Other points that can be used are:

LV 3 (Taichong)	is the Yuan-Source point of the Liver channel, removes Liver stagnation, is used in depressive conditions
BL 13 (Feishu)	is the Back-Shu point of the Lung, useful in emotional conditions

E.P. Anmian 1 and 2

E.P. Yintang

Management of Labor

Acupuncture can promote normal physiological childbirth serving to shorten the duration of labor and to provide pain relief.

The effectiveness of acupuncture treatment is determined by the precocity of acupoint stimulation, the optimum moment being at cervical dilatation of 4 to 5 cm, after amniotomy.

Acupoints are selected to strengthen and concentrate Qi toward the pelvis and stimulate uterine contractions, cervical effacement and dilatation.

SP 6 (Sanyinjiao)	is the Crossing point of the Yin channels of the foot, the Spleen, Liver and Kidney; strengthens the Spleen; regulates Qi and blood
LI 4 (Hegu)	is the Yuan-Source point of the Large Intestine channel, regulates blood and Qi circulation
ST 36 (Zusanli)	is the He point of the Stomach channel, regulates the Stomach, tones the Qi of the Middle Jiao, drains the channels, has a generally reinforcing effect

When used in alternative prescriptions, with the reducing method for SP 6 and the reinforcing method for LI 4 and ST 36, these points regulate uterine contractions and reduce labor duration.

BL 31 (Shangliao)

BL 32 (Celiao)

BL 33 (Zhongliao)

BL 34 (Xialiao)

The four points mentioned above can regulate Qi and blood and relieve lumbar and sacral pains. Strong stimulation, either manual or electrostimulation is necessary.

BL 23 (Shenshu)	is the Back-Shu point of the Kidney, strengthens the Yang and tones the Yin, tones and regulates the Kidney Qi
BL 57 (Chengshan)	alleviates lumbar and sacral pain

Auricular Therapy: points Uterus, Endocrine, Subcortex, Kidney, and Shenmen. The needles can be left in place and continuous stimulation is necessary during contractions.

UTERINE DYSTOCIA

Uterine dystocia refers to abnormal or difficult labor caused by abnormal labor patterns. Two types of uterine dystocia can be defined, which may appear at any stage of labor: hypotonic and hypertonic uterine dysfunction.

Careful evaluation of the fetal position, of pelvic contractions as well as fetal well-being is mandatory.

Ongoing evaluation of uterine contractions allows early recognition of abnormal patterns and proper intervention to decrease perinatal risk.

The abnormal progress of labor has certain signs:
- disturbances of emotional balance: anxiety, irritability, an increase in the perceived pain associated with uterine contractions, excessive lumbar and sacral pains
- abnormal uterine contractions - evaluation of the uterine contractions should consider fundal dominance, uterine relaxation between contractions, intensity, frequency, and duration of effective contractions
- cervical dysfunction involving effacement and dilatation (e.g., too rigid to dilate)

These circumstances influence fetal presentation and, in time, may cause fetal distress as a result of mechanical and chemical injury.

From the perspective of Chinese traditional medicine, uterine dystocia is determined by the imbalance of Qi/blood.

This pathology is called lack of progression, "Zhichan," or difficult labor, "Nanchan."

Etiopathogenesis

Two different etiopathogenic types are described:

a) The Deficiency of Qi and Blood

The deficiency of Qi and blood can be a constitutional deficiency of Zheng Qi (Normal Qi) or may be caused by overstrain, multiparity, excessive sexual life, or a history of miscarriages. Premature rupture of the membranes with sudden dispersion of Qi and blood or exhausting labor (especially in primiparas) with consumption of maternal energetic resources can cause deficiency of Qi and blood.

Of the Zang organs involved, the Kidney and Spleen are most affected by this deficiency.

b) The Stagnation of Qi and Blood

A variety of circumstances can cause the stagnation of Qi and blood, among which are disorders of the seven emotional factors, especially in young primiparas (e.g. fear of childbirth, anxiety about unwanted pregnancies or the maternity condition etc.) The stagnation of the Liver Qi is most frequently involved.

Another possible cause of the stagnation of Qi and blood is the exposure to Cold during labor. As Cold is a Yin pathogenic factor, it is characterized by constriction and stagnation and thus affects free circulation of Qi and blood.

The stagnation of Qi and blood can also appear in pregnant women who remain in recumbent or sitting positions during labor, thus obstructing Qi and blood circulation.

Clinical Manifestations

a) The Deficiency of Qi and Blood

Main symptoms include rare, weak, irregular uterine contractions associated with continuous lumbar pain and lower abdominal pain of moderate intensity. The labor is prolonged and sometimes vaginal bleeding occurs because the deficient Qi can no longer control blood, which escapes from blood vessels and exteriorizes. Associated signs are asthenia, lack of desire to speak, palpitations, a pale complexion, spontaneous sweating, and dyspnea. A pale, dry tongue with a thin coating and a deep and thready pulse may also be present.

The deficiency of Qi and blood can be correlated with different entities of western obstetrics as follows:

- false labor
- multiple pregnancy or polyhydramnios
- hypotonic uterine dysfunction
- lack of labor progression due to protracted dilatation

- prolonged delivery due to maternal exhaustion, especially in primiparas, after long and exhausting labor
- therapeutically induced dystocia (e.g., sedative abuse, early peridural anesthesia etc).

Lack of maternal nutritive support and adequate hydration can be involved in the appearance of fetal distress.

b) The Stagnation of Qi and Blood

Main symptoms include frequent, painful uterine contractions, of high intensity, associated with lumbar and sacral pains which are exacerbated during contractions. A spastic, rigid cervix that fails to dilate properly is also characteristic of this condition. The presentation is mobile and the fetus remains oriented upward. There is an increased risk of fetal distress. Vaginal bleeding with dark colored blood can sometimes appear.

Associated symptoms are a bluish or dark complexion, irritability or depression with easy crying, a sensation of fullness in the thorax, belching, nausea or vomiting. A dark red tongue, possibly with purplish spots on borders, and a thick, greasy coating may be observed. A deep, string-taut and wiry pulse may be palpated.

The stagnation of Qi and blood can be correlated with different entities of western obstetrics as follows:

- cervical dystocia with spastic cervix caused by congenital anomalies; older age of primiparas; maternal anxiety; abnormal presentation of the fetus; or iatrogenic causes (e.g., inadequate therapy)
- hypertonic uterine dysfunction
- precipitant labor and delivery

Treatment

Use of any therapeutic method requires careful evaluation and establishment of a precise diagnosis. Dystocia caused by contracted pelvis, cephalopelvic disproportion,inability of the birth canal to accommodate fetal size (necessitating cesarean section), fetal abnormalities (e.g. congenital anomalies or multiple gestation) or cervical pathology (e.g. post scar stenosis, malignant injury, congenital malformations etc.) needs to be excluded.

A careful evaluation of the progression of labor is necessary in order to institute early and proper therapy as signs of abnormal patterns are recognized.

It is well known that once dysfunctional uterine contractions begin, they tend to worsen, thus increasing the risk of therapeutic failure for both the mother and fetus.

When implemented in a timely manner, acupuncture treatment can help to remove possible causes of fetal distress, when it may otherwise be necessary to end the labor through cesarean section or application of forceps.

The two major aspects of deficiency and excess are to be considered when selecting acupoints:

a) The Deficiency of Qi and Blood

Therapeutic principle: tone Qi and blood

Prescription:

SP 6 (Sanyinjiao)	is the Crossing point of the three Yin channels of the foot, the Kidney, Liver and Spleen that govern the uterus; strengthens the Spleen that controls blood; stimulates Qi and blood circulation; supports the Kidney and promotes uterine movement
LI 4 (Hegu)	is the Yuan-Source point of the Large Intestine channel, regulates Qi and blood, drains the channels, moves the uterus
Bl 67 (Zhiyin)	is the Jing-Well point of the Urinary Bladder channel and empirical ocitocic point, supports the descending of the fetus

Acupuncture is given with the reinforcing method and strong stimulation is necessary, using manual or electrostimulation. Moxibustion can also be used for approximately 15 to 20 minutes.

To tone the Qi and move the uterus other points can also selected:

RM 4 (Guanyuan)	is an important point of Yin reunion of the Ren Mai Vessel with the three Yin channels of the foot, nourishes Kidney Qi, restores Yang, stimulates circulation of Qi and blood, regu-

	lates circulation in the Chong Mai and Ren Mai vessels
RM 6 (Qihai)	tones the Yang and regulates the circulation of Qi
BL 23 (Shenshu)	is the Back-Shu point of the Kidney, tones and regulates Kidney Qi
DM 4 (Mingmen)	tones Kidney Qi, drains the channels, supports the lumbar region

In cases of deficiency resulting from the weakness of the Spleen-Stomach couple caused by prolonged labor with lack of food intake, other points can be added in alternative prescriptions, if necessary:

ST 36 (Zusanli)	is the He point of the Stomach channel, restores the Qi of Middle Jiao, regulates the Spleen and Stomach, regulates the Qi and blood
RM 12 (Zhongwan)	is the Front-Mu point of the Stomach and the Influential point of Fu organs, strengthens the Spleen and regulates the Stomach
BL 32 (Ciliao)	regulates the Lower Jiao and sedates pain, concentrates Qi in the pelvis
BL 54 (Zhibian)	as local point
E.P. Duyin	is located on the interphalangeal distal fold on the plantar aspect of the second toe, tones uterine contractions. Moxibustion can be used after needle insertion.

b) The Stagnation of Qi and Blood

Therapeutic principle: regulate Qi, promote blood circulation, remove stagnation

Prescription:

SP 6 (Sanyinjiao)	regulates Qi and blood circulation, promotes uterine movement
LI 4 (Hegu)	regulates Qi and blood, drains the channels, moves the uterus
BL 31 (Shangliao)	stimulates blood, alleviates pains

BL 32 (Ciliao)   stimulates blood and regulates Qi, has analgesic effect

BL 67 (Zhinyin)   is an empirical ocitocic point, stimulates the descending of the fetus

Acupuncture is given with the reinforcing method for LI 4 and the reducing method for SP 6. BL 67 is needled and then moxibustion is applied. Strong stimulation is needed.

Other points can be used to remove stagnation:

ST 30 (Qichong)   is the Crossing point of the Stomach channel with the Chong Mai Vessel, regulates Chong Mai, removes stagnation and has a major energetic effect

LV 2 (Xingjian)   is the Ying point of the Liver channel, removes Liver Qi stagnation, cools the Liver and blood, drains Lower Jiao

LV 3 (Taichong)   is the Yuan-Source point of the Liver channel, calms Liver Yang, regulates and stimulates Qi and blood circulation, removes channels obstruction

LV 14 (Qimen)   is the Front-Mu point of the Liver, removes Liver stagnation, stimulates Qi and blood circulation, soothes the hypochondriac region

GB 28 (Weidao)   transforms stagnation, is indicated in cases of hypertonic uterine dysfunction, alleviates pain

GB 34 (Yanglingquan)   is the He point of the Gall Bladder channel and the Influential point of tendons, stimulates Liver function, removes the Heat, removes obstruction

In cases where descent of the fetus is needed, one of the following points can be selected:

BL 60 (Kunlun)   is the Jing-River point of the Urinary Bladder channel, regulates blood, clears the channels

GB 21 (Jianjing)   stimulates Qi circulation within the channels

E.P. Duyin

INDUCTION OF LABOR

Induction of labor is indicated in the following circumstances:
- post-term pregnancy
- premature rupture of membranes
- diabetes mellitus with mature fetus
- preeclampsia/eclampsia
- placental insufficiency
- isoimmunization
- renal insufficiency of different causes etc.

Several methods can be used to induce labor. Among them the most effective are amniotomy and parenteral administration of a dilute solution of oxytocin. Previous ripening of the cervix can be attended using prostaglandins.

In modern obstetrical practice, induction of labor remains a problem. It continues to pose maternal and fetal risks and the possibility of failure for which a surgical approach is needed.

Acupuncture can facilitate the action of oxytocin and prostaglandins upon the parasympathetic nervous system and, consequently, is able to promote and support uterine contractions, inducing normal, physiologic labor.

From the perspective of Chinese traditional medicine, there are two main indications for induction of labor:
- post-term pregnancy
- premature rupture of membranes

Etiopathogenesis

a) The Deficiency of Qi and Blood

The rupture of membranes either prematurely or at the onset of labor causes a sudden and excessive dispersion of both Qi and blood, resulting in a deficiency condition. Without adequate energetic support, labor can not start.

b) The Stagnation of Blood

The stagnation of blood is a characteristic circumstance of post-term pregnancy, a situation in which blood circulation is affected. The blood stasis can be caused by the deficiency of Qi, which can be constitutional or the result of overstrain or stress. As "Qi is the commander of blood," the deficient Qi is unable to maintain blood circulation and blood stasis occurs.

Another factor that can be involved is Cold in the blood. Because Cold is a Yin pathogenic factor, it is characterized by stagnation and blood circulation is obstructed.

Clinical Manifestations

The major sign is the absence of the uterine contractions. Depending upon the etiopathogenic type, other signs and symptoms can be associated:

a) The Deficiency of Qi and Blood

Main symptoms include asthenia, a pale complexion, palpitations, and dyspnea. A pale tongue with a thin coating and a deep, weak and thready pulse may be noted.

b) The Stagnation of Blood

Main symptoms include a dark, bluish complexion, depression, a sensation of fullness in the thorax, epigastric distension, and nausea. A dark red tongue, possibly with purplish spots, and a thick coating may be observed and a deep, forceful pulse may be recorded.

In cases of Cold in the blood, the symptoms are a pale complexion and lips, an aversion to cold, and a cold body and limbs. The patient may evidence a pale tongue with a thin, white coating and a deep, weak and delayed pulse.

Treatment

Several factors should be taken into account when induction of labor is intended.

Establishment of the gestational age, assessment of fetal wellbeing, and completion of maternal evaluation are mandatory. Ultrasonographic measurements, biophysical profile testing, and amnioscopy can be used.

The obstetric examination will evaluate the cervical condition, measured by using the Bishop score (dilatation, effacement in %, consistency, position, station of vertex) and the condition of membranes.

Possible contraindications to induction of labor should be ruled out: cephalopelvic disproportion, previous uterine surgery, unfavourable obstetrical circumstances, fetal distress present before starting labor induction, placental praevia, multiparity etc.

Considering all of these parameters permits evaluation of the available time and affords the individual the opportunity of acupuncture treatment, thus minimizing complications that may need cesarean section to end the labor.

If there is not adequate time and induction of labor is necessary, acupuncture can be used as adjuvant therapy to specific obstetrical methods.

The most frequently used prescriptions are:

LI 4 (Hegu)   with reinforcing method

SP 6 (Sanyinjiao)   with reducing method

BL 31 (Shangliao)

BL 32 (Ciliao)

Strong stimulation of the acupoints is necessary, either manually or by electrostimulation, with duration of approximately 15 to 20 minutes.

When maternal and fetal conditions allow, acupuncture can be given to support cervical ripening and an increase in the Bishop score before promoting uterine contractions.

RM 4 (Guanyuan)   is the Crossing point of the Ren Mai Vessel with the Yin channels of the foot, the Kidney, Spleen and Liver that command the uterus; this point is considered effective in opening the lower uterine pole

SJ 6 (Zhigou)   regulates the uterus, favors cervical ripening

Other points can be added, depending upon the etiopathogenic type:

a) The Deficiency of Qi and Blood

Therapeutic principle: tone Qi and blood, promote the movement of the uterus

Prescription:

SP 6 (Sanyinjiao)   tones the Spleen and Stomach, supports Qi and blood, regulates Qi and blood circulation

LI 4 (Hegu)   is the Yuan-Source point of the Large Intestine channel, regulates Qi and blood

RM 3 (Zhongji)	is the Crossing point of the Ren Mai Vessel with the Spleen, Liver and Kidney channels, strengthens Yang Qi, regulates Lower Jiao
GB 34 (Yanglingquan)	is the He point of the Gall Bladder channel and the Influential point of tendons, regulates the Liver functions, relaxes the tendons, stimulates the channels
ST 30 (Qichong)	is the Crossing point of the Stomach channel with the Chong Mai Vessel, tones Qi, regulates blood, regulates the uterus, is a major energetic point
ST 36 (Zusanli)	strengthens the Spleen, tones Qi and blood
SP 12 (Chongmen)	regulates the functions of Qi
RM 6 (Qihai)	strengthens the Yang and Essence, tones Qi and regulates Qi circulation

One to two acupoints are selected from the above mentioned ones and acupuncture is given with the reinforcing method during a period of up to 30 minutes.

b) The Stagnation of Blood

- When due to the deficiency of Qi

Therapeutic principle: tone Qi, regulate blood

Prescription:

ST 36 (Zusanli)	strengthens the Spleen, tones Qi and regulates blood
RM 6 (Qihai)	supports the Kidney, tones Qi, preserves the Essence
BL 20 (Pishu)	is the Back-Shu point of the Spleen, strengthens the Spleen and regulates the Stomach
BL 23 (Shenshu)	is the Back-Shu point of the Kidney, tones Kidney Qi
BL 21 (Weishu)	is the Back-Shu point of the Stomach, regulates the Stomach and strengthens the Spleen
LI 11 (Quchi)	regulates Qi and blood, regulates the circulation within the channels

- When it is due to Cold in the blood

Therapeutic principle: dispel Cold, regulate the Chong Mai and Ren Mai vessels

Prescription:

SP 4 (Gongsun)   is the Luo point of the Spleen channel and the Confluent point of Chong Mai Vessel, regulates the Spleen and the functions of Qi, promotes circulation in the Chong Mai Vessel

L 7 (Lieque)   is the Luo point of the Lung channel and the Confluent point of the Ren Mai Vessel, strengthens Qi, regulates Qi and blood circulation in the channels

LV 3 (Taichong)   is the Yuan-Source point of the Liver channel, regulates Liver function of maintaining free circulation of Qi and blood, opens the channels

LV 2 (Xingjian)   is the Ying point of the Liver channel, promotes Qi and blood circulation, is indicated in conditions of Cold

LV 8 (Ququan)   is the He point of the Liver channel, regulates Qi and blood, relaxes the tendons and the channels

GB 34 (Yanglingquan) is the He point of the Gall Bladder channel, drains the Liver, promotes the circulation within the channels

GB 27 (Wushu)   is the Crossing point of the Gall Bladder channel with the Dai Mai Vessel, reduces Liver stagnation

K 3 (Taixi)   is the Yuan-Source point of the Kidney channel, nourishes the Kidney and Liver, regulates Chong Mai and Ren Mai

K 5 (Shuiquan)   is the Xi point of the Kidney channel, tones the Chong Mai and Ren Mai vessels, regulates Qi and blood

K 13 (Qixue)   is the Crossing point of the Kidney channel with the Ren Mai Vessel, tones Kidney Qi, regulates the Chong Mai and Ren Mai vessels

K 14 (Siman)   is the Crossing point of the Kidney channel with the Chong Mai Vessel, has the same functions as K 13

Needles are retained for approximately 30 minutes and intermittent stimulation is given. Usually one session is sufficient.

After the cervix is prepared, the delivery can be spontaneous or, if the Bishop score has not risen, induction of uterine contractions may be needed.

Therapeutic principle: favor Qi, reduce blood

Prescription:

LI 4 (Hegu)   with the reinforcing method

SP 6 (Sanyinjiao)   with the reducing method

ST 36 (Zusanli)   with the reinforcing method

Other points known to influence descent of the fetus can be added:

BL 67 (Zhiyin)

BL 60 (Kunlun)

GB 21 (Jiangjing)

RM 3 (Zhongji)

E.P. Duyin

Stimulation is given with the reinforcing method and acupuncture or moxibustion is used.

Data from the literature reveal effectiveness of approximately 70% with no maternal or fetal side effects.

Auricular Therapy: points Uterus, Shenmen, Sympathetic nervous system can be added, in cases of either deficiency or excess.

MANAGEMENT OF DELIVERY

The second stage of labor starts with full dilatation of the cervix and concludes with delivery. The average duration is 30 to 45 minutes in nulliparas and 15 to 20 minutes in multiparas.

The management of the second stage of labor involves several aspects:

- facilitating the efficiency of the uterine contractions

- providing perineal relaxation
- providing relief of pain
- reducing the duration of the second stage of labor

Several maneuvers can be used but should always take account of individual circumstances: parenteral oxytocin infusion, if there is hypotonic uterine dysfunction; episiotomy; local or loco-regional anesthesia; and forceps application, if needed.

Acupuncture can help to stimulate the uterine contractions, reducing the duration of second stage of labor and relaxing the soft parts of the birth canal with reducing perineal resistance to expulsion.

a) Stimulate the Delivery

Prescription:

LI 4   (Hegu)   on both sides, with the reinforcing method and strong stimulation during the delivery of the fetus; supports uterine contractions and decreases the duration of delivery. Hemorrhage is minimal with easy placental extrusion

SP 6   (Sanyinjiao)   with the reducing method

BL 67   (Zhiyin)   favors the descending of the fetus

K 6   (Zhaohai)   regulates blood, drains the Lower Jiao

GB 34   (Yanglingquan) is the He point of the Gall Bladder channel, stimulates Liver function to maintain free circulation of Qi

ST 36   (Zusanli)   has a generally reinforcing effect

b) Relaxing the soft parts of birth canal and reducing perineal resistance

Preparing the perineum for birth:

BL 35   (Huiyang)

LV 9   (Yinbao)

During delivery the following points can be added:

LV 8 (Ququan) + **SP 11** (Jimen) + **DM 1** (Changqiang)

RM 1 (Huiyin) + **RM 3** (Zhongji) + **RM 4** (Guanyuan)

E.P. Longgu + **GB 28** (Weidao)

The point Longgu is located 1 cun beyond RM 2 (Qugu).

NEWBORN RESUSCITATION

The delay or absence of the first breath of air in the newborn is a critical condition. Complex methods of resuscitation and intensive care have priority.

Several simple and helpful exercises that may save a life are presented as follows:

Etiology

The circumstances that most frequently affect the first respiration of the newborn are: inhaling of amniotic fluid, tight loops of umbilical cord around the neck, and exposure to cold after birth etc.

Clinical Manifestations

The absence of a newborn's cry or weak respiration, bluish skin, and obstruction of the nose and mouth with aspirated substances are characteristic signs indicating a need for resuscitation.

Treatment

The first step is clearance of the airway.

Therapeutic principle: strengthen the Qi

Prescription:

DM 26 (Renzhong)

L 9 (Zhongchong)

L 11 (Shaoshang)

ST 36 (Zusanli)

RM 6 (Qihai)

RM 17 (Shanzhong)

DM 4 (Mingmen)

Stimulation of the selected points is given by pinching or strong massage. An adjuvant method of stimulating crying is the gentle beating of the newborn's back while holding him by the feet.

THE DELIVERY OF PLACENTA

The delivery of placenta is a complex phenomenon consisting of placental extrusion and expulsion and uterine hemostasis. During the third stage of labor, postpartum hemorrhages are by far the most severe complications.

From the perspective of Chinese traditional medicine, acupuncture can be useful in stimulating the delivery of placenta and reducing hemorrhage during the third stage of labor.

Etiopathogenesis

Hemorrhage of early postpartum can be due to several conditions:
- the deficiency of Spleen Qi
- Heat in the blood
- damage of the Chong Mai and Ren Mai vessels

Treatment

The lack of energetic balance should be corrected before conception. As emergency treatment, when it is necessary to stop uterine hemorrhage, the following points can be used:

ST 36 (Zusanli)

SP 10 (Xuehai)

SP 9 (Yinlingquan)

LV 1 (Dadun)

According to the etiopathogenic type, different points can be used:

a) The Deficiency of Spleen Qi

Therapeutic principle: strengthen the Spleen, tone Qi.

Prescription:

RM 4 (Guanyuan)	regulates the uterus
SP 1 (Yinbai)	is the Jing-Well point of the Spleen channel, strengthens the Spleen, tones Qi and retains blood
BL 20 (Pishu)	is the Back-Shu point of the Spleen, strengthens the Spleen to support blood

Acupuncture is given with the reinforcing method.

b) Heat in the Blood

Therapeutic principle: cool the blood, disperse Heat

Prescription:

LV 3 (Taichong)   is the Yuan-Source point of the Liver channel, removes Heat, removes stagnation, regulates Liver Qi

K 2 (Rangu)   is the Ying point of the Kidney channel, removes pathogenic Heat, regulates the Chong Mai and Ren Mai vessels

Acupuncture is given with the reducing method.

c) Dysfunction of the Chong Mai and Ren Mai Vessels

Therapeutic principle: regulate Chong Mai and Ren Mai

Prescription:

RM 4 (Guanyuan)   tones Qi, regulates Qi and blood, regulates circulation within the Chong Mai and Ren Mai vessels

K 13 (Qixue)   tones Kidney Qi, regulates the Chong Mai and Ren Mai vessels

K 14 (Siman)   has the same actions as point K 13

If stimulation of placental extrusion and expulsion is desired, the following points can be used:

RM 3 (Zhongji) + **K 6** (Zhaohai) + **SP 4** (Gongsun) + **ST 30** (Qichong)

BL 60 (Kunlun) + **ST 30** (Qichong) + **PC 6** (Neiguan)

RM 6 (Qihai) reduces the amount of blood loss during the third stage of labor.

In cases of deficiency of uterine contractility that may result in insufficient uterine hemostasis, the following prescription can be used:

RM 2 (Qugu) + **SP 5** (Shangqiu) + **K 3** (Taixi) + **K 10** (Yingu)

Acupuncture is given with the reinforcing method.

RETENTION OF PLACENTA

The delay of placental separation during the third stage of labor can be caused by uterine hypotonia or by abnormally adherent placenta. In these circumstances excessive bleeding caused by partial separation of the placenta or the lack of spontaneous expulsion after 35 to 40 minutes makes manual removal of the placenta mandatory. The management of the third stage of labor using drugs such as ergonovine and oxytocin can avoid prolongation of this stage and excessive bleeding.

Acupuncture treatment provides correction of energetic balance, supporting the uterine contractions and reducing the risk of complications and intrauterine maneuvers.

Etiopathogenesis

a) The Deficiency of Yuan (Original) Qi

Labor and delivery can cause an important deficiency of Qi or can aggravate a previous one, such that during the third stage of labor there is asthenia and depression. Under these circumstances, spontaneous expulsion of placenta cannot take place, because of the weak energetic support of the uterus.

b) The Attack of Wind-Cold

The condition of exhaustion caused by the deficiency of the Yuan Qi can favor the attack of the exogenous pathogenic factors: Wind and Cold. As a Yin pathogenic factor, Cold causes constriction and obstruction. Qi and blood circulation is damaged with consequent obstruction of the channels, formation of clots and retention of placenta.

Clinical Manifestations

a) The Deficiency of Yuan Qi

Main symptoms include placenta retention, asthenia, dizziness, vision disturbances, palpitations, dyspnea, and spontaneous sweating. The patient may have a pale tongue with a thin coating and a deep, thready pulse.

b) The Attack of Wind-Cold

Main symptoms include retention of the placenta with scanty vaginal bleeding. Lower abdominal pain, which is dull when caused by Cold and sharp when caused by Wind may be associated. A pale tongue with a white coating and a string-taut pulse may be noted.

Treatment

a) The Deficiency of Yuan Qi

Therapeutic principle: warm and tone Qi

Prescription:

RM 4 (Guanyuan)	strengthens and regulate Yuan Qi, warms the uterus
SP 6 (Sanyinjiao)	is the Crossing point of the Yin channels of the foot, strengthens the Kidney, promotes Qi and blood circulation, moves the uterus
LI 4 (Hegu)	is the Yuan-Source point of the Large Intestine channel, regulates Qi and blood, drains the channels, stimulates the uterine contractions
GB 21 (Jianjing)	stimulates Qi circulation within the uterus

Other points that tone Qi can also be used:

RM 3 (Zhongji)	is the Crossing point of the Ren Mai Vessel with the Kidney, Spleen and Liver channels; tones Qi, regulates the uterus and Lower Jiao
RM 6 (Qihai)	reduces weakness, regulates Qi circulation
RM 17 (Shanzhong)	is the Influential point of Qi, strengthens Qi and regulates Qi circulation

Acupuncture is given with the reinforcing method.

b) The Attack of Wind-Cold

Therapeutic principle: warm Cold, promote Qi and blood circulation, dissolve clots

Prescription:

LI 4 (Hegu)	regulates Qi and blood circulation, drains the channels
SP 6 (Sanyinjiao)	promotes Qi and blood circulation
RM 4 (Guanyuan)	warms the uterus
SP 8 (Diji)	is the Xi point of the Spleen channel, regulates blood
SP 10 (Xuehai)	regulates Qi and blood circulation, dispels Wind
BL 60 (Kunlun)	is the Jing-River point of the Urinary Bladder, stimulates Qi circulation, promotes blood, removes Wind

GB 21 (Jianjing)   stimulates the circulation of Qi in the uterus
LV 14 (Qimen)   stimulates blood, dissolves stasis

ANALGESIA DURING CHILDBIRTH

For more than 85% of women, childbirth is associated with pains, causing labor and delivery to be extremely uncomfortable and exhausting. Usually primiparas are more affected, their onset of pain corresponding to first uterine contractions. The intensity of pain is variable and influenced, in great measure, by emotional balance.

Pain in childbirth is a multifactorial phenomenon that normally depends upon:

- traction upon adnexa, uterus; pressure upon ureters, bladder, urethra
- dilatation of the soft parts of birth canal
- accumulation of catabolites in the myometrium
- release of prostaglandins, endorphins etc.
- the function of the "gate control" system, dependent on the activity of thick A beta fibers from the sensitive branch of the spinal nerve. It is believed that acupuncture, in obtaining an analgesic effect, acts upon the A beta fibers.
- the integration of pain in the cerebral cortex. It has been demonstrated that the excitement state of the brain has direct influence upon the analgesic effect of acupuncture. Thus emotions such as fear, anxiety can intensify pain.

Obstetrical analgesia should respect three main conditions: simplicity, safeness and maintaining fetal homeostasis. Different types of pain relief can be used: psychoprophylaxis, hypnotics and amnestics, and analgesics in local, regional or general anesthesia.

Relief of pain during childbirth should always be adapted for the individual patient.

In China there are two schools of thought regarding the use of analgesics during childbirth: pain during childbirth is considered to be physiological, so there is no need for relief; others consider the suppression of pain to be a nonfacilitative intervention. Acupuncture treatment can offer a simple therapeutic alternative with neither maternal nor fetal side effects.

The character and location of pain depends upon the stage of labor and the eutocic or dystocic progression of labor.

Anterior Located Pain

Anterior located pain is an abdominal or pelvic pain that increases in intensity with the progression of labor during a eutocic labor. The pain is primarily located above the pubis symphysis. It spreads toward the flanks, the lumbar region and thighs, and the buttocks.

In terms of a physiological labor, characterized by the balance of Qi and blood and a bearable pain, intervention helps to maintain a psychical balance and to improve the efficiency of uterine contractions toward increased dilatation.

In cases with a high intensity of pain, hardly bearable by the woman, different methods can be used to stimulate the points :

a) Electrostimulation

Local points and points located at a distance are selected and strong stimulation is given in order to obtain an analgesic effect.

The selected local points can treat disorders within their immediate area as well as those of the neighboring organs:

RM 2 (Qugu), **RM 6** (Qihai), **ST 25** (Tianshu), **ST 26** (Wailing), **ST 29** (Guilai), **ST 30** (Qichong), **GB 26** (Daimai), **GB 27** (Wushu), **GB 28** (Weidao), **GB 29** (Juliao), **SP 13** (Fushe), and **SP 14** (Fujie).

Points located at a distance that increase uterine contractions and increase the sedative effect can be used:

ST 36 (Zusanli), **LI 4** (Hegu) , **SP 6** (Sanjinjiao)

LV 3 (Taichong) + **LV 2** (Xingjian) + **BL 60** (Kunlun) + **ST 30** (Qichong) + **SP 6** (Sanyinjiao)

GB 26 (Daimai) + **ST 25** (Tianshu) + **SJ 5** (Weiguan) + **PC 6** (Neiguan)

RM 3 (Zhongji) + **RM 4** (Guanyuan)

Auricular Therapy: points Shenmen, Sympathetic nervous system, Uterus, Kidney, Endocrine, and Subcortical can be selected and added, if necessary.

Stimulation should be started early during labor at 3 to 4 cm of cervical dilatation, if possible, with intact amniotic membranes.

Low frequencies are used (1-3 Hz) for points located at a distance and higher frequencies (at least 5 Hz) for local points, maintaining a level of low intensity and increasing to the maximum bearable with each contraction.

One disadvantage is that patients may have difficulty tolerating the strong stimulation that is needed. Two or three acupoints are selected. The stimulation can also be manual, but strong stimulation is necessary for approximately 20 minutes.

b) The Technique of Blocking the Points

The therapeutic effect is based upon the longlasting stimulation of the point or the pharmacologic action of the injected drug upon the surrounding tissues. After inserting the needle and obtaining the acupuncture sensation, the drug is injected into the point.

In order to obtain analgesia during childbirth, the following points are selected:

LI 4 (Hegu)

SP 6 (Sanyinjiao)

Saline solution with 1% Procaine is injected at both sides, after previously testing the sensibility of the involved drug. 0,5 to 2,5 ml are injected in the point LI 4 and 5 ml in the point SP 6 after which the sensation of fullness at those points will increase, especially in point LI 4.

In this way a shorter duration of labor can be obtained by regulating the uterine contractions and maintaining an emotional balance. In cases of hypertonic uterine dysfunction, the increased intensity and frequency of uterine contractions causes an exacerbation of pain. Other points useful to treat uterine dystocia can be added if needed.

Posterior Located Pain

Posterior pain has a lumbar sacral location and settles, in proportion, as the cervical dilatation increases. The pain is of high intensity in abnormal presentations or at the onset of a uterine dystocia.

Pain is located primarily in the lumbar area in uterine dystocia because of Qi and blood deficiency. It is continuous and the intensity is correlated with the uterine contractions.

Treatment aims to correct the uterine contractions by restoring Qi/ blood balance and to relieve the posterior pain.

Prescription:

ST 30 (Qichong) + **BL 31** (Shangliao) + **BL 32** (Ciliao) + **BL 33** (Zhongliao)+ **GB 41** (Zulinqi)

BL 23 (Shenshu) + **BL 25** (Dachangshu) + **BL 47** (Hunmen)

BL 32 (Ciliao) + **DM 2** (Yaoshu)

The main point used for relieving the lumbar-sacral pain is **BL 32** (Ciliao) which has the following actions:

- drains the channels and stimulates Qi circulation

- promotes blood circulation, sedates pain

- has a favorable effect upon cervical dilatation

Different methods of stimulating the point **BL 32** (Ciliao) can be used:

- perpendicular insertion of the needle, on both sides at 1,5-3 cun depth, waiting for the acupuncture sensation and then retaining the needles for approximately 15 to 20 minutes, with strong stimulation during each uterine contraction. The patient remains in a lateral recumbent position.

- blocking the point with 10 ml of analgesic drug injected on both sides with a long needle

- electrostimulation

Ashi points can also be associated.

Auricular Therapy: points Shenmen, Uterus, Endocrine, Kidney can be selected and added in different prescriptions.

Another possible and easy-to-use method is lumbar reflexotherapy, which consists of the infiltration of the local regional points.

Prescription:

BL 52 (Zhishi)

BL 26 (Guanyuanshu)

BL 32 (Ciliao)

One or two points are selected and an intradermal injection of approximately 2 ml of saline solution with 1% Procaine is given.

The above mentioned points can also be stimulated manually for approximately 15 to 20 minutes during a session which may be repeated to provide further relief of pain.

Also an extraordinary vessel point, located at 1,5 cun of RM 6 (Qihai) can be used. Deep insertion is necessary.

Data from the literature show positive results. In 35% to 50% of cases analgesia is obtained, and in 30% to 40% of cases, the pain is alleviated.

THE PUERPERIUM

The puerperium is the period of approximately 6 to 8 weeks after childbirth characterized by lactation and physiologic changes that restore the woman's body to the nonpregnant state.

From the perspective of Chinese traditional medicine, there is an important loss of blood and Qi during labor. This causes a deficiency of blood and Qi during puerperium and, thus, an energetic imbalance that increases the body's vulnerability.

This deficiency primarily affects the Kidney and the Chong Mai and Ren Mai vessels. Associated exogenous or endogenous factors, that support or aggravate this physiologic deficiency may be present: inadequate food intake of the mother, interruption of Qi circulation within Chong Mai and Ren Mai due to scars after surgery (Pfannenstiel incision in cesarean section or episiotomy), or the attack of exogenous pathogenic factors.

There is a spontaneous tendency toward restoration of the blood, body fluids and Yin. Blood is restored before Qi, which explains the tendency to anxiety and depression, but also the lack of ovulation in the circumstances of incompletely restored Yin that cannot support Qi.

This particular energetic context is reflected in puerperal pathology.

Treatment aims to tone the Yin and blood. As acupuncture may help to prevent the appearance of a future obstetrical or gynecological pathology, the benefit of this type of therapy should not be overlooked.

UTERINE INVOLUTION

Some authors believe that strong stimulation of the point **RM 8** (Shenque) stimulates uterine involution.

RM 8 (Shenque) has the following functions: strengthens the Spleen and regulates the Stomach, warms the Yang, and supports the sensitive organs.

Acupuncture stimulation is contraindicated in the treatment of uterine involution. Moxibustion with salt is used. Good results can be obtained in approximately 80% of cases. Allopathic treatment using ergotine or oxytocin can also be employed.

POSTPARTUM HEMORRHAGE

Postpartum hemorrhage can be an emergency condition. Possible causes of bleeding, the amount of blood loss and the possible complications need to be seriously considered. Proper clinical assessment is mandatory and the retention of placental tissue should be ruled out.

Chinese traditional medicine refers to postpartum hemorrhage as "Chan Hou Xue Geng"; postpartum faint is called "Chan Xue Yun."

Etiopathogenesis

a) The Deficiency of Qi and Blood

Qi and blood loss during labor, and afterward during puerperium, causes the weakness of the channels, with the exhaustion of the Chong Mai and Ren Mai Vessels. These vessels can no longer retain the Qi and thus blood loss continues and the physiologic deficiency of both Qi and blood is aggravated.

Zang-Fu organs lack nourishment, the Liver and Heart being most affected, and symptoms of deficiency appear.

b) The Stagnation of Blood

The existence of lacerations of the birth canal or of the uterus can cause the stagnation of blood and the formation of clots. Vessel obstruction by the stagnant blood impairs normal circulation, causing hemorrhage and other symptoms of excess.

Clinical Manifestations

a) The Deficiency of Qi and Blood

Main symptoms include excessive blood loss, major pallor, spontaneous sweating, cold limbs, palpitations, vertigo, vision disturbances, dyspnea, nausea, and vomiting. A pale tongue with a thin coating and a deep, weak and thready pulse may also be present.

b) The Stagnation of Blood

Main symptoms include vaginal bleeding with blood clots, lower abdominal pain and distension aggravated on pressure, and nausea. The patient may evidence a red tongue, possibly with purplish spots, and a string-taut, wiry pulse.

Treatment

a) The Deficiency of Qi and Blood

Therapeutic principle: tone Qi, nourish blood and stop blood loss

Prescription:

RM 4 (Guanyuan)	is the Crossing point of the Ren Mai with the three Yin channels of the foot, the Kidney, Spleen and Liver; strengthens Qi; stimulates Yang; stimulates Qi and blood circulation; regulates the Chong Mai and Ren Mai vessels
RM 6 (Qihai)	strengthens the Yang and Essence, tones Qi, regulates the Qi of the Chong Mai and Ren Mai vessels, regulates the channels system
RM 12 (Zhongwan)	is the Influential point of the Fu organs, regulates the Stomach and strengthens the Spleen, sources of blood
SP 6 (Sanyinjiao)	strengthens the Kidney and Spleen, regulates Qi and blood, regulates the channels, has a fortifying effect when associated with other points
SP 1 (Yinbai)	is the Jing-Well point of the Spleen channel, strengthens Qi and promotes blood circulation, soothes the mind
ST 36 (Zusanli)	is one of the four Dominant points and the He point of the Stomach channel, restores the Qi of the Middle Jiao, tones the Stomach and Spleen, has a generally fortifying effect
BL 17 (Geshu)	is the Influential point of blood, regulates blood, stimulates Qi circulation
BL 20 (Pishu)	is the Back-Shu point of the Spleen, tones the Spleen, regulates blood
BL 23 (Shenshu)	is the Back-Shu point of the Kidney, regulates Kidney Qi, tones Yang

Different points can be selected in alternative prescriptions. Stimulation is given using acupuncture with the reinforcing method and moxibustion, usually a session daily.

b) The Stagnation of Blood

Therapeutic principle: promote blood, stimulate the circulation of Qi

Prescription:

RM 4 (Guanyuan)	stimulates Qi and blood circulation, regulates Chong Mai and Ren Mai
ST 36 (Zusanli)	is one of the four Dominant points in the abdominal area, stimulates Qi and blood circulation, has a generally fortifying effect
LV 1 (Dadun)	is the Jing-Well point of the Liver channel, stimulates Liver Qi, regulates the Chong Mai and Ren Mai vessels
LV 3 (Taichong)	is the Yuan-Source point of the Liver channel, regulates Liver function, removes stagnation, stimulates Qi and blood circulation
SP 10 (Xuehai)	regulates blood circulation
SJ 6 (Zhigou)	is the Jing-River point of the San Jiao channel, regulates Qi and blood circulation within the channels
PC 6 (Neiguan)	is the Luo point of the Pericardium channel, regulates Qi circulation, calms the Heart and mind, regulates Lower Jiao
GB 28 (Weidao)	is the Crossing point of the Gall Bladder channel with the Dai Mai Vessel, regulates Qi and blood circulation in the Dai Mai Vessel

Acupuncture is given with the reducing method.

AFTERPAINS

In early postpartum, lumbar and abdominal pains similar in character to colic can create a real discomfort for the mother. Afterpains have a higher incidence in multiparas and appear to be related to the particularities of uterine tonus and contractions. Duration varies from hours to several days. Suckling can cause an increase of the pain's intensity. The treatment is analgesic and sedative.

From the perspective of Chinese traditional medicine, postpartum pains are described as manifestations both of excess and of deficiency.

Etiopathogenesis

a) The Syndrome of Excess Type

The syndrome of excess type is caused by:

- the stagnation of blood and retention of lochia within the uterus
- retention of food in the Stomach caused by inadequate food intake

b) The Syndrome of Deficiency Type

The syndrome of deficiency type is caused by:

- the attack of Cold after exposure to exogenous pathogenic factors during labor and puerperium
- the deficiency of blood caused by the excessive blood loss during labor that may worsen a constitutional deficiency of blood

Clinical Manifestations

a) The Syndrome of Excess Type

Main symptoms include abdominal pain and distension, aggravated by pressure; belching; nausea; acid regurgitation; intermittent fever; constipation; and oliguria. A thick, clammy and yellowish tongue coating and a string-taut, rapid pulse may be noted.

b) The Syndrome of Deficiency Type

Main symptoms include abdominal pain alleviated by pressure and heat, a pale complexion, cold body and limbs, and a lack of appetite. A thin, white tongue coating and a weak, slow pulse may be present.

Treatment

a) The Syndrome of Excess Type

Therapeutic principle: stimulate Qi circulation, remove blood stagnation

Prescription:

RM 4 (Guanyuan)	tones Qi, regulates blood, stimulates circulation in the Chong Mai and Ren Mai vessels, removes stagnation
RM 3 (Zhongji)	tones Qi, regulates Lower Jiao
SP 6 (Sanyinjiao)	is the Crossing point of the Yin channels of the foot, the Kidney, Spleen and Liver that

	command the uterus; tones Qi; removes stagnation
SP 10 (Xuehai)	cools the blood, stimulates blood circulation and removes stagnation
ST 25 (Tianshu)	is the Front-Mu point of the Large Intestine, regulates the Spleen and Stomach, regulates the circulation of Qi within the channels
LV 14 (Qimen)	is the Front-Mu point of the Liver, tones the Spleen, regulates the Stomach, promotes blood, removes stagnation

b) The Syndrome of Deficiency Type

Therapeutic principle: regulate Qi and blood, disperse the Cold

Prescription:

ST 36 (Zusanli)	is the Dominant point with abdominal action and the He point of the Stomach channel, strengthens and regulates the Stomach, restores Qi of Middle Jiao, has a generally fortifying effect
RM 4 (Guanyuan)	tones Qi and regulates blood, warms the Kidney
RM 7 (YinJiao)	warms the Yang of the Kidney
RM 12 (Zhongwan)	is the Influential point of the Fu organs and the Front-Mu point of the Stomach, regulates the Stomach and the circulation of Qi
SP 6 (Sanyinjiao)	tones Qi, regulates Qi and blood
BL 23 (Shenshu)	is the Back-Shu point of the Kidney, tones Kidney Qi
ST 29 (Guilai)	regulates Lower Jiao, warms the uterus, regulates Qi

The already mentioned points can be used in alternative prescriptions. Stimulation of the selected points is with the reducing method in cases of excess type and with the reinforcing method using acupuncture or moxibustion in cases of deficiency type.

Another prescription may select Ashi points from those mentioned below and insert the needles intradermally:

SP 6 (Sanyinjiao)   regulates Qi and blood

DM 3 (Yaoyangguan) regulates Qi and blood circulation in the Chong Mai and Ren Mai vessels, removes pathogenic Fire

E.P. Shangxian   is located between the L 5 and S 1 vertebrae

Usually the needles are left in place for approximately 30 minutes or, considering the severity of the pain, until relief is obtained. Two sessions, on the average, are usually sufficient. Good results, with relief or alleviation of pain are obtained in 70% to 85% of cases.

PATHOLOGY OF LOCHIA

The term "lochia rubra" refers to the bloody discharge that follows delivery and is a physiologic event of puerperium.

Retention of lochia in the uterus can be caused by prolonged urinary retention, uterine anteflexion, or rapid cervical involution etc.

Lochiorrhea refers to heavy lochia. When heavy or persistent, examination and treatment may be required.

Acupuncture can be a useful alternative therapy, but puerperal septic and hemorrhagic complications need to have been ruled out.

RETENTION OF LOCHIA

Etiopathogenesis

a) The Stagnation of Blood

The exhaustion of Zang-Fu organs after childbirth can favor the attack of exogenous pathogenic factors: Cold and Wind. As Yin pathogenic factors, they can cause constriction and blood stagnation. Because "blood is the mother of Qi," the circulation of Qi will be impaired and stagnation of Qi may develop.

b) The Deficiency of Blood

The deficiency of blood is physiologic during puerperium but can be aggravated by an excessive blood loss. If the amount of blood is insufficient to exteriorize, lochia will be retained.

Clinical Manifestations

a) The Stagnation of blood

Main symptoms include scant bloody discharge, painful distension and a sensation of fullness in the lower abdomen, pain that worsens with pressure, and nausea or vomiting. The patient may have a dark red tongue, possibly with purplish spots, a little coating and a string-taut pulse.

b) The Deficiency of Blood

Main symptoms include scanty, light red discharge; a soft, usually painless, abdomen; dizziness; vertigo; insomnia; palpitations; a pale complexion; and asthenia. A pale tongue with a thin coating and a weak pulse may be noted.

Treatment

a) The Stagnation of Blood

Therapeutic principle: remove stagnation, tone Qi

Prescription:

RM 4 (Guanyuan)	is the Crossing point of the Ren Mai with the Yin channels of the foot, tones and regulates Qi, regulates circulation in the Chong Mai and Ren Mai vessels
RM 3 (Zhongji)	tones the Yang Kidney and regulates Lower Jiao, drains the Urinary Bladder
SP 6 (Sanyinjiao)	is the Crossing point of the three Yin channels of the foot, strengthens the Spleen and Kidney, regulates Qi and blood
SP 10 (Xuehai)	promotes blood circulation and removes stagnation
LV 8 (Ququan)	is the He point of the Liver channel, regulates Qi and blood
BL 25 (Dachangshu)	is the Back-Shu point of the Large Intestine, regulates the Qi of the Fu organs, disperses stasis
BL 32 (Ciliao)	regulates Qi and promotes blood

b) The Deficiency of Blood

Therapeutic principle: nourish blood, tone Yin

Prescription:

RM 4 (Guanyuan)	regulates Qi and blood, regulates circulation in the Chong Mai and Ren Mai vessels
RM 6 (Qihai)	strengthens the Yang and Qi, stimulates circulation in the channels
ST 36 (Zusanli)	is the He point of the Stomach channel, tones the Spleen and Stomach, regulates Qi and blood, has a generally fortifying effect
SP 6 (Sanyinjiao)	nourishes the Spleen and Stomach, strengthens the Yin, regulates Qi and blood
BL 17 (Geshu)	is the Influential point of blood, nourishes and regulates blood
BL 23 (Shenshu)	is the Back-Shu point of the Kidney, nourishes Yin and strengthens Yang, tones the lumbar region and marrow

Acupuncture is given with the reinforcing method and strong stimulation of the selected points is usually necessary. Moxibustion can be useful.

LOCHIORRHEA

Etiopathogenesis

a) Heat in the blood

As childbirth is considered to be a Yang manifestation, the accumulation of Heat is possible during labor. During postpartum period, the weakened Qi is restored more slowly than blood and, consequently, Heat is not dispersed.

b) The Dysfunction of Chong Mai and Ren Mai Vessels

The puerperal deficiency of Qi and blood may cause weakness and dysfunction of Chong Mai and Ren Mai. The recently produced blood is not maintained in the vessels and a heavy bloody discharge appears.

Clinical Manifestations

Main symptoms, caused by blood deficiency, include heavy lochia; a painless, soft abdomen; a pale complexion; asthenia; palpitations; and vision disturbances. A pale tongue with a little, sometimes yellowish, coating and a thready pulse may be observed.

Treatment

Therapeutic principle: nourish blood, tone Qi

Prescription:

RM 4 (Guanyuan)	tones Qi, regulates Qi and blood, regulates the circulation in the Chong Mai and Ren Mai vessels
RM 6 (Qihai)	strengthens Qi, tones the Yang, stimulates circulation in the channels
SP 6 (Sanyinjiao)	is the Crossing point of the Yin channels of the foot, nourishes the Kidney and strengthens the Spleen and Stomach, regulates Qi and blood
SP 1 (Yinbai)	is the Jing-Well point of the Spleen channel, strengthens the Spleen, regulates the Stomach, tones Qi and retains blood, sedates the mind
SP 9 (Yinlingquan)	is the He point of the Spleen channel, strengthens the Spleen, regulates the circulation in San Jiao

POSTPARTUM URINARY RETENTION

Urinary retention with vesical overdistension is a common complication during postpartum. It can be caused by a large episiotomy, traumatic injuries of the birth canal, hematoma or anesthesia. Lack of spontaneous urination after four hours in postpartum may need draining of the bladder with a catheter, with subsequent risk of urinary tract infections and a need for antibiotherapy.

From the perspective of Chinese traditional medicine, good results can be obtained using acupuncture or moxibustion.

Several prescriptions can be used:

a) RM 4 + ST 36

RM 4 (Guanyuan)	is the Crossing point of the Ren Mai Vessel with the Yin channels of the foot, the Kidney, Liver and Spleen; tones Qi; regulates the Chong Mai and Ren Mai vessels
ST 36 (Zusanli)	is the Dominant point and the He point of the Stomach, has a generally reinforcing effect and restores Qi of the Middle Jiao

RM 2 (Qugu) can also be used in alternative prescriptions.

Moderate stimulation is given during a session of approximately 15 to 20 minutes. Usually the effect appears within a few minutes after the needles are withdrawn.

b) ST 28 + BL 54 + SP 6

ST 28 (Shuidao)	removes pathogenic Damp and regulates fluids excretion
BL 54 (Zhibian)	regulates the Lower Jiao and removes Damp-Heat
SP 6 (Sanyinjiao)	is the Crossing point of the Yin channels of the foot, regulates Qi and blood circulation, supports blood

The point that is painful on palpation is selected. It is necessary to obtain the acupuncture sensation, which should spread towards the perineum for ST 28, onward to the lower abdomen for BL 54, and upward to the knees and thigh for SP 6.

Strong stimulation for approximately 10 to 15 minutes is necessary. Moxibustion can be added and repeated as often as 2 or 3 times a day. Usually few sessions are needed to obtain good results.

Other points can also be used in alternative prescriptions:

RM 3 (Zhongji)	is the Front-Mu point of the Urinary Bladder and the Crossing point of the Ren Mai with the Kidney, Liver and Spleen channels; tones the Kidney Yang
K 5 (Shuiquan)	is the Xi point of the Kidney channel, drains and regulates the Urinary Bladder functions

RM 6 (Qihai)   strengthens the Yang and Essence; regulates Qi circulation

BL 28 (Pangguangshu) is the Back-Shu point of the Urinary Bladder, tones Qi, regulates the excretion of fluids

DM 20 (Baihui)   is the Crossing point of the Du Mai Vessel with the Yang channels, removes pathogenic Heat and opens the orifices

SP 6 (Sanyinjiao)   regulates Qi and blood

E.P. Weibao   is located at 1 cun lower and lateral to GB 28 (Weidao)

Strong stimulation is necessary until the sensation of cramps or urination appears. Moxibustion can also be used.

POSTPARTUM URINARY INCONTINENCE

Postpartum urinary incontinence is usually due to the weakness of Qi that affects the Kidney, which is no longer able to command the Urinary Bladder and its functions.

When acupuncture treatment is desired, different prescriptions can be used and the following points can be added:

BL 23 (Shenshu)   is the Back-Shu point of the Kidney, strengthens the Kidney Qi, supports the Urinary Bladder functions

BL 28 (Pangguangshu) is the Back-Shu point of the Urinary Bladder, regulates fluid excretion, strengthens Qi of the Urinary Bladder

RM 3 (Zhongji)   is the Front-Mu point of the Urinary Bladder, tones Kidney Yang, supports the Urinary Bladder function

RM 4 (Guanyuan)   tones the Kidney, regulates the Chong Mai and Ren Mai vessels

RM 6 (Qihai)   strengthens the Yang and Essence, tones Kidney Yang

ST 36 (Zusanli)   regulates Qi and blood, has a generally reinforcing effect

ST 25 (Tianshu)   regulates Qi and tones the Spleen

K 3 (Taixi)   is the Yuan-Source point of the Kidney chan-
                                   nel, supports and regulates the Lower Jiao,
                                   regulates the Chong Mai and Ren Mai vessels

BL 23 or BL 28 is used, as one of the two main points, to which a few points located on the lower limbs or abdomen should be added. Moxibustion can also be used when strong stimulation is desired. Good results are usually obtained after a few minutes of stimulation, two sessions are given daily.

INSUFFICIENT LACTATION

The notion of hypogalactia refers to an insufficient secretion of milk, in any period of suckling, that demands the addition of milk or other food in order to assure the eutrophic development of the newborn. Insufficient lactation can be primary or secondary and both maternal and fetal causes can be involved. Allopathic treatment is, in large measure, prophylactic; attempts to cure the condition produce few results.

From the perspective of Chinese traditional medicine, milk is formed from Qi and blood. It is believed that insufficient lactation appears 48 to 72 hours following childbirth and the secretion of milk can be completely missing.

Etiopathogenesis

a) The Deficiency of Qi and Blood

The deficiency of Qi and blood, while considered physiologic after childbirth can, when constitutional, be increased by inadequate food intake, by weakness of the Spleen and Stomach or by excessive loss of Qi and blood during labor or delivery.

Another possible cause is the obstruction of circulation within the Chong Mai and Ren Mai vessels due to the existence of a surgical scar (Pfannenstiel incision in cesarean section or episiotomy). Chong Mai is unable to make the fluids ascend, to spread Qi to the thoracic capillary network and to the Stomach vessels, causing the mammary gland to be unable to produce and secrete milk. A deficiency of Yin fluids results with an exhaustion of the milk source and insufficient lactation.

b) The Stagnation of Liver Qi

The psychoemotional instability of postpartum, frequently expressed by anxiety and depression can negatively alter the Liver function of maintaining the free circulation of Qi. The spreading of Liver Qi is impeded with disturbance of Qi and blood circulation, the channels are blocked and the secretion of milk is obstructed.

Clinical Manifestations

The insufficient secretion of milk or its progressive decrease is associated with other symptoms of deficiency or excess:

a) The Deficiency of Qi and Blood

Main symptoms include lack of breast milk, painful distention, a pale complexion, dry skin, palpitations, asthenia, lack of appetite, vertigo, tinnitus, scanty lochia, vision disturbances, nausea, and cold limbs. A pale tongue with a thin coating and a weak, thready pulse may be present.

b) The Stagnation of Liver Qi

Main symptoms include stretched, hard and painful breasts; a sensation of discomfort in the thoracic and epigastric regions, hypochondriac pain, depression, anxiety, irascibility, difficulty with food intake, constipation, and, in severe cases, fever. A pink or purplish tongue with a thick, white or yellow coating and a string-taut, wiry pulse may be noted.

Treatment

An adequate food and fluid intake and establishing a relaxing climate at home are important adjuvant components of the therapy.

Main points prescription:

SI 1 (Shaoze)	is the Jing-Well point of the Small Intestine channel related to the Heart channel, regulates and nourishes the Heart Qi, stimulates the circulation in the channels. Is an empirical point for promoting lactation.
RM 17 (Shanzhong)	is the Influential point of Qi and the Crossing point of the Ren Mai Vessel with the Stomach, Kidney, Small Intestine and San Jiao channels; regulates the Qi of the entire body and stimulates blood formation
ST 18 (Rugen)	is located on the Stomach channel, rich in Qi and blood and also located in the breast area, stimulates Qi and blood formation, promotes lactation

According to the clinical manifestations of excess or deficiency type, other points can be added:

a) The Deficiency of Qi and Blood

Therapeutic principle: nourish and tone Qi and blood

Prescription:

ST 36 (Zusanli)	is a Dominant point and the He point of the Stomach channel, nourishes and tones the Spleen and Stomach, sources of blood, has a generally reinforcing effect
BL 20 (Pishu)	is the Back-Shu point of the Spleen, tones the Spleen
BL 17 (Geshu)	is the Influential point of blood, strengthens the Spleen and regulates the Stomach, regulates blood, stimulates Qi circulation

In cases with interrupted circulation due to Pfannenstiel incision, e.g. Ren Mai, Spleen, Liver, Stomach and Chong Mai Channels, acupoints located immediately above and below the scar can be included.

b) The Stagnation of Liver Qi

Therapeutic principle: drain the Liver, remove stagnation, promote blood circulation

Prescription:

LV 3 (Taichong)	is the Yuan-Source point of the Liver channel, stimulates Qi circulation, regulates blood, removes pathogenic Heat, drains the channels
LV 14 (Qimen)	is the Front-Mu point of the Liver and the Crossing point of the Liver and Spleen channels with Yin Wei Mai Vessel, removes Liver Qi stagnation, stimulates blood circulation, strengthens the Spleen and Stomach
PC 6 (Neiguan)	is the Confluent point of the Yin Wei Mai Vessel, stimulates Qi spreading and circulation of the stagnant Liver Qi, soothes the Heart and mind, regulates Middle Jiao, regulates the Spleen and Stomach

Other points can be used in alternative prescriptions:

SP 4 (Gongsun)   is the Confluent point of the Chong Mai Vessel, regulates the circulation in Chong Mai, tones the Spleen

ST 30 (Qichong)   is the Crossing point of the Stomach channel with Chong Mai, warms the Middle Jiao and uterus, tones Qi

H 7 (Shenmen)   is the Yuan-Source point of the Heart channel, regulates the Heart and calms the mind

LI 4 (Hegu)   is the Yuan-Source point of the Large Intestine channel, regulates Qi and blood

RM 4 (Guanyuan)   is the Crossing point of the Ren Mai Vessel with the Yin channels of the foot, the Kidney, Spleen and Liver; stimulates Qi and blood circulation; regulates the Chong Mai and Ren Mai vessels

RM 6 (Qihai)   strengthens the Kidney, tones Qi

RM 12 (Zhongwan)   is the Front-Mu point of the Stomach and the Influential point of the Fu organs, regulates the Stomach, regulates Spleen

SP 6 (Sanyinjiao)   nourishes the Kidney and strengthens the Spleen and Stomach, regulates Qi and blood

LV 2 (Xingjian)   is the Ying point of the Liver channel, removes pathogenic Heat from Liver, sedates fear

E.P. Ruquan   is located on the anterior extremity of the axillar fold, 5 cun in front of H 1, on the tendon of the great pectoral muscle

Stimulation is given with the reinforcing method in cases of deficiency type and moxibustion is indicated for stimulation of RM 17, ST 18 and ST 36. The reducing method is used in cases of excess type. Needles are retained for approximately 15 to 20 minutes and, initially, stimulation is given daily. After the onset of lactation, a session every 2 to 3 days is conducted if needed. An average of 2 to 5 sessions is necessary, with positive results in 75% to 82% of cases.

SUPPRESSION OF LACTATION

When the newborn cannot be nursed or the mother does not choose to nurse her child, the suppression of lactation becomes necessary.

In western medicine different therapeutic methods can be used. Each method (e.g., mechanical inhibition, administration of estrogen or bromocriptine) has its advantages and side effects, but most also have a high failure rate.

Acupuncture can control the secretion of milk.

Prescription:

GB 41 (Zulinqi)   is the Shu-Stream point of the Gall Bladder channel and the Confluent point of the Dai Mai Vessel, removes Liver Qi stagnation, disperses Qi and blood

GB 37 (Guanming)   is the Luo point of the Gall Bladder channel, removes pathogenic Heat from Liver, regulates the channels

GB 21 (Jianjing)   is the Crossing point of the Gall Bladder, San Jiao and Stomach channels with the Yang Wei Mai Vessel, stimulates Qi circulation and removes thoracic obstruction

ST 36 (Zusanli)   is the He point of the Stomach channel, regulates the Stomach and drains the channels, descends Qi, stimulates the suppression of lactation as the breast is in the distribution area of the Stomach channel

Other points can be added in alternative prescriptions if necessary.

E.P. Huinai 1,2 and 3 located under the apophysis of the T 4, T 5 and T 6 vertebrae.

L 1 (Zhongfu)   is the Front-Mu point of the Lung and the Crossing point of the Lung and Spleen channels, which are involved in the onset of lactation

BL 15 (Xinshu)   is the Back-Shu point of the Heart, relaxes the chest, stimulates Qi circulation

H 3 (Shaohai)   is the He point of the Heart channel, regulates

	Qi and blood circulation, sedates the mind
K 7 (Fuliu)	is the Jing-River point of the Kidney channel, regulates the circulation of fluids in the body
K 23 (Shenfeng)	regulates the Stomach and descends the perverse Qi
K 24 (Lingxu)	descends the perverse Qi, relaxes the chest, is indicated in pain and fullness of the chest, reduces tumefaction

Acupuncture is given with the reducing method and stimulation is performed every 10 minutes. Needles are retained for approximately 30 minutes and slow extraction of the needles is necessary, leaving open the orifice of acupuncture. Usually 1 to 3 sessions are enough, one session daily.

POSTPARTUM HEMORRHOIDS

Hemorrhoids are anorectal varicosities. Internal hemorrhoids are derived from the superior and middle hemorrhoidal veins, while the external ones are derived from the inferior hemorrhoidal vein. Their degree of protrusion and reductibility makes a three-stage differentiation. The second stage is more frequently seen in practice: spontaneous reductible prolapse. Western medical treatment includes treatment of symptoms (using hemorrhoidal preparations, mild laxatives), hygienic means of reestablishing the normal intestinal transit, adjustment of food and ample fluids, and avoidance of sedentary life and straining. Surgical procedures rarely are indicated until after the puerperium.

Because of hormonal changes, pregnancy can stimulate constipation and can cause the development or aggravation of hemorrhoids, primarily during puerperium when they can become clinically manifest.

From the perspective of Chinese traditional medicine, hemorrhoids can benefit from acupuncture treatment because it reduces hemorrhoidal tumefaction and pain and acts upon etiologic conditions.

Etiopathogenesis

Hemorrhoids appear as the result of two etiologic conditions:

a) Consumption of Large Intestine Fluids

This condition can be caused by an excess of Heat of alimentary origin. It is more frequent during postpartum because of the loss of Yin fluids that is physiologic during childbirth. Loss of Yin fluids will cause dryness of intestinal mucosa, the stools are dry, with constipation. The excess of Heat can injure the blood vessels causing blood loss during defecating.

b) The Deficiency of Qi

There is a physiologic deficiency of Qi during puerperium and also Qi restores later than blood. The deficiency of Qi leads to deficiency of the Spleen and Large Intestine Qi, and thus to the appearance of hemorrhoids and an increase of blood deficiency with the characteristic symptoms.

Clinical Manifestations

Based upon the location of the hemorrhoids, the following symptoms and signs can be found:

- external hemorrhoids: usually of bluish color, painful anorectal sensation, sensitivity, moderate pruritus, possible bleeding if ulceration of the lesion occurs
- internal hemorrhoids: often may prolapse during defecation, can be associated with sensation of anal tension, pain, bleeding, and anal pruritus

Acute hemorrhoidal thrombosis is more frequent during puerperium, mostly in cases with perineotomy.

Other associated symptoms may be present, depending on the etiopathogenic conditions:

a) Consumption of Large Intestine Fluids

Main symptoms include dry mouth, thirst, possible abdominal pain, and an anal burning sensation. A red tongue with little coating or a dry, yellow coating and a rapid, thready pulse may be noted.

b) The Deficiency of Qi

Main symptoms include dizziness, vision disturbances, palpitations, asthenia, a pale complexion, and spontaneous sweating. The patient may evidence a pale tongue with a thin coating and a weak, thready pulse.

Treatment

The following main points are used:

BL 57 (Chengshan)   drains the Intestine and removes stagnation

BL 17 (Geshu)   is the Influential point of blood, regulates blood and removes stagnation

According to etiopathogenesis, other points can be used:

a) Consumption of Large Intestine Fluids

Therapeutic principle: remove Heat from Large Intestine, restore Qi and blood circulation, moisten the intestines

Prescription:

ST 37 (Shangjuxu)   is the Lower He point of the Large Intestine channel, removes Heat from the channel, moistens the intestines

SP 5 (Shangqiu)   is the Jing-River point of the Spleen channel, strengthens the Spleen and removes pathogenic Heat and Damp, moistens the intestines, reduces stagnation

DM 1 (Changqiang)   is the Luo point of the Du Mai Vessel and the Crossing point of the Kidney and Gall Bladder channels, strengthens the rectum against prolapse, is selected as local point

BL 25 (Dachangshu)   is the Back-Shu point of the Large Intestine, strengthens the Large Intestine and restores circulation

BL 35 (Huiyang)   cools the Heat from the Large Intestine

LI 4 (Hegu)   is the Yuan-Source point of the Large Intestine channel, cools the Heat, regulates Qi and blood

b) The Deficiency of Qi

Therapeutic principle: restore Qi, strengthen the Spleen

Prescription:

RM 4 (Guanyuan)   tones Qi, regulates Qi and blood

RM 6 (Qihai)   stimulates the ascent of Yang, tones Qi

DM 1 (Changqiang)   is the Luo point of the Du Mai Vessel, strengthens the rectum against prolapse, is selected as local point

DM 20 (Baihui)   is the Crossing point of the Du Mai Vessel with the Yang channels of the hand and foot, tones the Yang

BL 20 (Pishu)   is the Back-Shu point of the Spleen; strengthens the Spleen and regulates the Stomach

ST 36 *(Zusanli)*   is the He point of the Stomach channel, restores the Qi of the Middle Jiao, tones the Stomach, regulates the Intestine, regulates Qi and blood, has a generally fortifying effect

SP 4 (Gongsun)   is the Luo point of the Spleen channel and the Confluent point of the Chong Mai Vessel, regulates Qi functions

Acupuncture is given with the reducing or reinforcing method according to the etiopathogenic type. Moxibustion is used to stimulate RM 4, RM 6, DM 1, DM 20. Usually a session is performed daily and the needles are retained for approximately 15 to 20 minutes.

Acupuncture should be avoided in cases with previous surgical procedures, anal fissure or systemic diseases with rectal manifestations (e.g. Crohn's disease, ulcerative colitis etc.).

PSYCHICAL DISORDERS IN PUERPERIUM

The specialty literature refers to these disorders as "postpartum blues" or the third day syndrome.

Relatively frequent, in up to 12% of women these psychological disorders are usually transient, benign and self-limited. Several factors can be involved: discomfort of early puerperium, emotional letdown following the excitement of delivery, fatigue from lack of sleep during labor and postpartum, anxiety concerning future abilities to assume maternal role etc. In almost 10% of all cases the evolution may be severe with subsequent risk of a major depressive pathology. Women with unwanted pregnancies and major marital problems are most susceptible to develop this pathology.

Clinical manifestations from the 3rd up to 10th day of postpartum include the following: asthenia, emotional letdown with frequent crying, anxiety, irritability or a state of indifference, insomnia or dream-disturbed sleep, difficult concentration and recall, and insufficient lactation.

From the perspective of Chinese traditional medicine there is an asthenic condition after childbirth, maintained by the physiologic deficiency of Qi and blood. The excessive excitement of mental Shen is based upon the separation of the mother from the others around her and her exclusive concentration upon her infant. Confused feelings concerning the maternal condition can cause disorders of the seven emotional factors and can directly affect the Zang-Fu organs, especially the Liver. The Heart and Kidney can also be involved.

Etiopathogenesis

a) The Deficiency of Heart and Spleen

The deficiency of both Heart and Spleen can be due to slow, difficult recovery after birth, overstrain and stress. The blood of the Heart is consumed and the Spleen Qi becomes weak. The Spleen becomes a less capable source of blood and Qi production, thus increasing the Heart deficiency of blood. The deficiency of Qi and blood can weaken the Chong Mai and Ren Mai vessels and the weakened Spleen can no longer control blood. Blood is insufficient to house the mind and psychical disorders can develop.

b) The Yin Deficiency of the Liver and Kidney

After childbirth there is a physiologic deficiency of Yin caused by excessive blood loss to which are added overstrain and stress. As a consequence the Yin of the Liver and Kidney is consumed, producing internal Heat and affecting normal circulation within the Chong Mai and Ren Mai Vessels. The Heart Fire is no longer checked, leading to disturbance of the mind.

c) The Stagnation of Liver Qi

The disordered emotional factors affect the Liver's function of maintaining free circulation of Qi and cause stagnation and retardation of Qi circulation. The persistence of this stagnation of Qi can cause the Spleen and Stomach to be subject to digestive problems. Damp stagnation and Phlegm formation occur. Blood circulation is retarded and the Chong Mai and Ren Mai vessels are affected. Stagnant Liver Qi and Phlegm move upward and invade the mind.

d) The Deficiency of Blood

The Yin deficiency, in the absence of any treatment and the persistence of causal factors, will result in an excess of Yang that turns into Fire. The internal agitation of Fire, a Yang pathogenic factor characterized by ascending movement, will disturb the Shen. In this condition, the clinical manifestations can evolve toward a major disorder—depressive psychosis.

Clinical Manifestations

a) The Deficiency of Heart and Spleen

Main symptoms include a sallow complexion, asthenia, lack of appetite, lack of desire to speak, fearfulness, insomnia or dream-disturbed sleep, decrease of memory, palpitations, and loose stools. A pale tongue with a thin coating and a deep, weak and thready pulse may also be present.

b) The Yin Deficiency of the Liver and Kidney

Main symptoms include irritability, insomnia, palpitations, vision disturbances, and tinnitus. Associated symptoms include lumbar pain and weakness; spontaneous nocturnal sweating; a sensation of heat in the thorax, palms and feet; and vertigo. A red tongue with a thin coating and a rapid, thready pulse may be noted.

c) The Stagnation of Liver Qi

Main symptoms include depression, irritability, anger, vision disturbances, and tinnitus. Lack of appetite, nausea, belching, dry mouth, a sensation of distension in the flank and hypochondriac regions, breast distension, and insufficient lactation may also be reported. The patient may have a dark red tongue, or one with bluish spots, and a sticky tongue coating. A rapid, string-taut pulse may be palpated.

d) The Deficiency of Blood

Main symptoms include sadness, depression or mood lability, irritability, a sensation of thoracic fullness, nausea, belching, vomiting, and body trembling with a possible loss of consciousness.

Treatment

The treatment aims to tone the Yin, fluids and blood.

The use of the acupoint BL 43 is considered to be extremely effective in the first week of postpartum.

BL 43 (Gaohuang) has the following functions:

- strengthens the Spleen and regulates the Stomach, stimulates Qi
  functions and tones the Kidney, calms the Heart and mind
- instantaneous formation of red cells (Soulie de Morant)
- increases body resistance with a fortifying effect at least equal to
  acupoint **ST 36** (Auteroche)

The addition of acupoint SI 1 in early postpartum is useful, depending upon changes observed by the 3rd day of puerperium.

SI 1 (Shaoze) is the Jing-Well point of the Small Intestine channel and has the following functions:

- regulates and nourishes the Heart Qi
- tones Middle Jiao
- cools the Heart and removes Heat from the channels
- opens the orifices
- favors Qi and blood circulation
- strengthens the state of consciousness
- acts upon the excretion-secretion balance (Soulie de Morant)
- empirical point for the onset of lactation

Other points can be added according to the etiopathogenic type:

a) The deficiency of Heart and Spleen

Therapeutic principle: tone the Spleen and Heart, stimulate Qi, tone blood

Prescription:

BL 15 (Xinshu)   is the Back-Shu point of the Heart, strengthens the Heart, nourishes blood, cools the Heart, sedates the mind, opens the thorax, stimulates Qi circulation

BL 20 (Pishu)   is the Back-Shu point of the Spleen, regulates Spleen Qi, stimulates Spleen function of transforming and transporting blood, tones blood, regulates the Stomach, removes Damp

H 7 (Shenmen)   is the Yuan-Source point of the Heart channel, removes the channels obstruction, has sedative function, calming the Heart and mind

SP 6 (Sanyinjiao)	is the Crossing point of the three Yin channels of the foot, the Kidney, Liver and Spleen; tones Yin; tones the Spleen and Stomach; regulates Qi and blood; regulates the channels
SP 1 (Yinbai)	is the Jing-Well point of the Spleen channel, strengthens the Spleen, regulates the Stomach, tones Qi, supports blood, calms the mind
RM 6 (Qihai)	tones Qi, stimulates ascent of Yang, regulates Chong Mai and Ren Mai

Acupuncture is given with the reinforcing method, aiming to obtain the acupuncture sensation, mainly for the acupoint RM 6 which should be perceived as heat spreading into the lower abdomen.

b) The Yin Deficiency of the Liver and Kidney

Therapeutic principle: tone the Liver and Kidney, stimulate the Heart and calm the mind

Prescription:

BL 15 (Xinshu)	is the Back-Shu point of the Heart, cools the Heart, sedates the mind
BL 18 (Ganshu)	is the Back-Shu point of the Liver, cools the Liver and removes pathogenic Heat, regulates blood, comforts Liver Wind, sedates the mind
BL 23 (Shenshu)	is the Back-Shu point of the Kidney, tones Yang Kidney, tones the lumbar region, removes water and Damp
K 3 (Taixi)	is the Yuan-Source point of the Kidney channel, nourishes and fortifies Lower Jiao, tones and regulates the Kidney, regulates circulation in Chong Mai and Ren Mai vessels
DM 4 (Mingmen)	strengthens the Yang Kidney, tones Jing Qi, regulates Qi, strengthens the lumbar region
SP 6 (Sanyinjiao)	is the Crossing point of the Yin channels of the foot, tones the Kidney and Liver, strengthens the Yin

| H 7 (Shenmen) | is the Yuan-Source point of the Heart channel, calms the Heart and mind |
| PC 6 (Neiguan) | is the Luo point of the Pericardium channel, cools the Heart and calms the mind, regulates the Stomach and sedates vomiting, alleviates pain |

Acupuncture is given with the reinforcing method. For acupoints located on the abdomen and lower limbs, moxibustion can also be used when strong stimulation is needed.

c) The Stagnation of Liver Qi

Therapeutic principle: regulate Liver Qi, cool the Heat

Prescription:

PC 6 (Neiguan)	stimulates the circulation of stagnant Liver Qi, calms the mind
H 7 (Shenmen)	removes the obstruction of the channels, calms the Heart and mind
RM 17 (Shanzhong)	is the Influential point of Qi, regulates the functions and circulation of Qi
LV 14 (Qimen)	is the Front-Mu point of the Liver, spreads Qi stagnation, regulates Qi circulation, stimulates blood, transforms clots, tones the Spleen and regulates the Stomach, resolves stasis

The acupoint LV 14 is considered to be effective in "all disorders after childbirth" (Soulie de Morant).

GB 20 (Fengchi)	is the Crossing point of the Gall Bladder and San Jiao channels with the Yang Wei Mai Vessel, removes pathogenic Heat, drains the channels
GB 21 (Jianjing)	is the Crossing point of the Gall Bladder, Stomach, and San Jiao channels and the Yang Wei Mai, drains the Liver and Gall Bladder, cools the Stomach Heat, acts upon body fluids, opens the orifices
LV 2 (Xingjian)	is the Ying point of the Liver channel, cools Heat from blood, cools the Lower Jiao

LV 3 (Taichong)   is the Yuan-Source point of the Liver chan-
                            nel, calms Liver Yang, cools and sedates the
                            mind

Acupuncture is given with the reducing method.

d) The Deficiency of Blood with Agitation of Internal Fire

In severe cases tending towards depressive psychosis, some of the following points can be used, depending upon the clinical manifestations:

DM 16 (Fengfu)   and

DM 26 (Renzhong)   both indicated in mental disorders

H 7 (Shenmen)   calms the Heart and mind

BL 15 (Xinshu)   is the Back-Shu point of the Heart, cools the
                            Heart, sedates the mind

BL 20 (Pishu)   is the Back-Shu point of the Spleen, regulates
                            Spleen, tones blood

PC 7 (Daling)   is the Yuan-Source point of the Pericardium
                            channel, removes pathogenic Heat from the
                            Heart, sedates the mind, cools the blood

PC 9 (Zhongchong)   is the Jing-Well point of the Pericardium
                            channel, removes pathogenic Heat, cools the
                            blood, sedates the mind

SI 3 (Houxi)   is the Yuan-Source point of the small Intes-
                            tine channel, removes pathogenic Heat, tones
                            the collaterals

LI 11 (Quchi)   is the He point of the Large Intestine channel,
                            cools the Heat, supports Qi circulation, regu-
                            lates the channels, regulates Qi and blood

L 11 (Shaoshang)   is the Jing-Well point of the Lung channel,
                            restores the Yang and the conscious state, is
                            useful in cases of mood lability

ST 40 (Fenglong)   is the Luo point of the Stomach channel,
                            regulates the Stomach and reduces Phlegm,
                            sedates the mind

LV 3 (Taichong)   cools and sedates the mind

Acupuncture is given with the even movement and reducing method.

ACUPUNCTURE TREATMENT AND PREGNANCY

The essential element upon which the physiologic evolution of a pregnancy depends is maintaining of the Qi/blood balance. This objectives forms the main focus of any acupuncture treatment during pregnancy.

It is known that women have a relative excess of Qi because of the loss of menstrual blood. During pregnancy there is a physiologic shifting of this balance in favor of blood, in order to provide for the development of the uterus, placenta and fetus. Thus prescriptions that tone Qi and reduce blood will cause the disturbance of the Qi/blood balance with real danger to the health of the pregnancy.

It is forbidden to use methods for acupoint LI 4 (Hegu) that tone Qi and reducing methods with acupoint SP 6 (Sanyinjiao) that weaken blood.

In *Chinese Acupuncture and Moxibustion* it is specified: "It is contraindicated to puncture points on the lower abdomen and lumbosacral region for women less than three months pregnant. After three months of pregnancy it is contraindicated to needle the points on the upper abdomen and lumbosacral region and those points causing strong sensations such as LI 4 (Hegu), SP 6 (Sanyinjiao), BL 60 (Kunlun) and BL 67 (Zhiyin)."

"Moxibustion of abdominal region and lumbosacral region of the pregnant women is not allowed."

Other contraindicated points are: GB 21 (Jianjing), LV 3 (Taichong), and LV 1 (Dadun) for which moxibustion should be avoided.

The contraindications are relative, applied with an appreciation for the individual's circumstances. In fact many of the acupoints located in areas that should not be punctured during pregnancy are found in several prescriptions for treatment of pregnancy pathology .

As an example RM 5 (Shimen) is believed to cause definitive infertility (mentioned in *Compendium of Acupuncture and Moxibustion*) and is contraindicated during pregnancy. However, it is one of the points prescribed for treating threatened abortion.

For treating morning sickness, ST 36 (Zusanli) and RM 12 (Zhongwan) are indicated. Many other examples can prove the effectiveness of these acupoints for treating the pathology of pregnancy, but adequate prescription and selection of patients is mandatory.

The needle stimulation is also important, and it is suggested that the acupoints LI 4 (Hegu) and SP 6 (Sanyinjiao) not be needled during pregnancy. Even so there are different classic prescriptions that use these precise acupoints to treat fainting during pregnancy.

In practice the using of contraindicated points should be avoided and other points with similar action should be used. Prescriptions known to be capable of inducing labor should also be avoided:

LI 4 (Hegu) + **SP 6** (Sanyinjiao)

RM 3 (Zhongji) + **BL 67** (Zhiyin)

BL 60 (Kunlun) + **SP 6** (Sanyinjiao)

LV 3 (Taichong) + **SP 6** (Sanyinjiao)

or prescriptions for the retention of the placenta:

RM 3 (Zhongji) + **SP 6** (Sanyinjiao)

RM3 (Zhongji) + **GB 21** (Jianjing)

RM 3 (Zhongji) + **SP 6** (Sanyinjiao) + **BL 60** (Kunlun)

K 6 (Zhaohai) + **SJ 5** (Weiguan)

An important therapeutic principle that should always be respected is the avoidance of blood dispersion; toning Qi or stimulation is given with extreme precaution, only when really necessary.

CHAPTER 3

GYNECOLOGY

PREMENSTRUAL SYNDROME

The premenstrual syndrome is an aggregate of benign clinical manifestations that can affect all the systems of the body, their only common point being a cyclic, premenstrual character. The symptoms disappear at the onset of, or during, menstruation.

The syndrome is believed to affect approximately 35% to 40% of women.

The main symptoms are as follows:
- a sensation of breast tenderness, preceding by 5 to 7 or more days the onset of menstruation and with progressive intensity.
- painful abdominal distension, with no exact location, to which can be added constipation, increased appetite for sweets and salty food, and continuous thirst
- edema of the extremities, with capricious evolution, aggravated by standing
- neuropsychological disorders of variable intensity
- headache, sometimes severe, progressive, and persistent

Other symptoms may be associated including cardiovascular, respiratory, urinary, neurovegetative, and allergic disorders or recurrence of the already existing pathologies (e.g. urticaria, genital pruritus, recurrent herpes, asthma, tetany attacks or epilepsy etc.).

The etiopathogenesis of the syndrome remains unclear. Different theories have been proposed as far back as Hippocrates, who noted "the moving of blood looking for a way to come out from the uterus." The following circumstances may be factors in the syndrome: increasing of the capillary permeability, luteal deficiency, the lack of balance between progesterone and aldosterone in the second part of the menstrual cycle, the adrenals, the deficiency of vitamins (B 6 and A), or a decrease in the serotonin level.

Western medical treatment is usually symptomatic, while in severe cases, hormonal therapy, diuretics and vitamins are prescribed.

From the perspective of Chinese traditional medicine, the functional manifestations of the premenstrual syndrome are considered to be consequences of the Liver, Spleen and Kidney disturbances.

Etiopathogenesis

a) The Stagnation of the Liver Qi

Disorders of the emotional factors affect the Liver function of maintaining the free circulation of Qi. As a result there is Qi stagnation with retarded Qi circulation and, as "Qi is the commander of blood," this will also cause blood stagnation.

In these conditions Liver Qi can damage the Spleen-Stomach couple, thus explaining the presence of digestive symptoms. The deficient circulation of Qi and blood affects the Chong Mai and Ren Mai vessels, leading to irregular menstrual cycles and dysmenorrhea. Persistent Liver Qi obstruction with Qi and blood stagnation can cause the appearance of abdominal tumoral masses.

b) Yang Deficiency of the Spleen and Kidney

Chronic diseases can cause consumption of Qi, with injury of Yang, thus affecting the Spleen. The deficient Spleen will, in turn, damage the Kidney. The Yang deficiency of the Spleen may be caused by raw and cold, greasy or sweet food. The deficiency of the Kidney Yang can also cause the syndrome. Yang deficiency affects digestion, food transport and transformation, and the ability to transport body fluids, with accumulation of water and Damp and the onset of edema.

c) The Deficiency of the Spleen and Heart

This type of deficiency can be the result of overstrain, stress, anger, chronic hemorrhage or chronic diseases. These factors cause the consumption of the Heart blood and weakness of the Spleen Qi. The deficient Spleen is no longer able to produce enough blood, aggravating the Heart deficiency and producing a lack of adequate nutritive support for the heart and brain. The Spleen function of transporting can damage the Chong Mai Vessel, causing the decrease of menstrual flow or amenorrhea. When the deficient Spleen can no longer control the blood, excessive menstrual flows appears.

Clinical Manifestations

a) The Stagnation of the Liver Qi

Main symptoms include irritability, insomnia, headache, painful distension of the breasts, painful abdominal distension (mostly in the hypochondriac region, aggravated with pressure and warmth), and a sensation of fullness in the chest. The menstrual cycle is irregular with scanty flow, dark colored blood, and possible clots; dysmenorrhea may occur. Associated symptoms may include a loss of appetite, belching, nausea or vomiting, a foreign body sensation in the throat or mobile tumoral masses in the lower abdomen. A red dark colored tongue, or one with purplish spots on borders, and a string-taut pulse may be present.

b) Yang Deficiency of the Spleen and Kidney

Main symptoms include asthenia, tendency to sleep, edema of the limbs and face, premenstrual increase of weight, and lack of appetite. Delayed menstruation and a scanty menstrual flow with fluid, bright blood are characteristic. A sensation of weakness in the lumbar area and in the knees; cold extremities; pallor; loose stools; and a fluid, white, excessive leukorrhea are associated with this condition. A pale tongue, thick with a white, thin coating and a deep, weak pulse may be noted.

c) The Deficiency of the Spleen and Heart

Main symptoms include pallor, weakness, palpitations, insomnia, lack of appetite, and abdominal distension. An irregular menstrual cycle with scanty flow, bright blood or with excessive flow and loose stools are also characteristic. The patient may have a pale tongue with a thin, white coating and a weak, thready pulse.

Treatment

a) The Stagnation of the Liver Qi

Therapeutic principle: regulate Qi to remove stagnation

Prescription:

LV 2 (Xingjian)	is the Ying point of the Liver channel, removes pathogenic heat from the Liver, removes stagnation
LV 3 (Taichong)	is the Yuan-Source point of the Liver channel, stimulates Liver Qi circulation, regulates Qi and blood circulation
LV 14 (Qimen)	is the Front-Mu point of the Liver, stimulates blood circulation and removes stagnation, strengthens the Spleen

SP 6 (Sanyinjiao)	tones the Spleen and Liver, regulates Qi and blood circulation
RM 4 (Guanyuan)	tones Qi, regulates the Chong Mai and Ren Mai vessels
BL 18 (Ganshu)	is the Back-Shu point of the Liver, removes Liver Qi stagnation and regulates the Gall Bladder, stimulates the brain and improves vision
BL 19 (Danshu)	is the Back-Shu point of the Gall Bladder, removes pathogenic Heat from the Liver and Gall Bladder, stimulates Qi circulation, strengthens the Spleen and regulates the Stomach
SJ 6 (Zhigou)	is the Jing-River point of the San Jiao channel, regulates Zang-Fu organs, drains the channels and tones the collaterals
GB 34 (Yanglingquan)	is the He point of the Gall Bladder, stimulates the functions of the Liver and Gall Bladder

Adding the acupoints SJ 6 and GB 34 is indicated when the pain is mainly in the hypochondriac region and the breasts.

PC 6 (Neiguan)	is the Yuan-Source point of the Pericardium channel, nourishes and calms the mind

b) Yang Deficiency of the Spleen and Kidney

Therapeutic principle: strengthen the Yang, tone the Spleen and Kidney

Prescription:

DM 4 (Mingmen)	tones Yang, strengthens the Kidney, drains the channels, regulates menstruation
RM 4 (Guanyuan)	is the Crossing point of the Ren Mai Vessel with the Yin channels of the foot (Kidney, Liver and Spleen), tones Qi and favors the ascending of Yang, tones the Kidney, regulates Qi and blood, regulates the Chong Mai and Ren Mai vessels
BL 23 (Shenshu)	is the Back-Shu point of the Kidney, nourishes the Yin and tones the Kidney and lumbar

	region, increases the activity of brain
BL 20 (Pishu)	is the Back-Shu point of the Spleen, tones the Spleen, regulates the Stomach
RM 9 (Shuifen)	strengthens the Spleen and regulates the Stomach, removes pathogenic Damp, is very effective in the treatment of edema. Moxibustion is indicated
ST 43 (Xiangu)	is the Shu point of the Stomach, regulates the Stomach, strengthens the Spleen and promotes urination
ST 29 (Guilai)	warms and regulates the Lower Jiao
SP 7 (Longu)	tones the Spleen and Stomach, removes pathogenic Damp

Inclusion of the last four acupoints is effective in toning the Spleen and removing edema.

K 5 (Shuiquan)	is the Xi point of the Kidney channel, tones the Ren Mai and Chong Mai vessels, regulates Qi and blood

c) The Deficiency of the Spleen and Heart

Therapeutic principle: tone the Spleen and Heart

Prescription:

BL 15 (Xinshu)	is the Back-Shu point of the Heart, nourishes the Spleen and calms the mind, stimulates Qi circulation
BL 20 (Pishu)	is the Back-Shu point of the Spleen, tones the Spleen and regulates Stomach
SP 6 (Sanyinjiao)	strengthens the Yin, tones Spleen, regulates Qi and blood circulation
RM 6 (Qihai)	regulates Qi circulation, regulates the Chong Mai and Ren Mai vessels
ST 36 (Zusanli)	is the He point of the Stomach channel, regulates the Stomach and tones the Spleen, restores the Qi of Middle Jiao, tones the body
H 7 (Shenmen)	is the Yuan-Source point of the Heart channel,

regulates and calms the Heart and the mind

E.P. Yintang   regulates sleep when dreams are frequent

In cases where it is difficult to determine a certain etiopathogenic type, long-term and symptomatic therapy can be employed, as the clinical manifestations are polymorphous.

Long-Term Therapy

Long-term therapy aims to act upon:

a) The Sacral and Hypogastric Plexus

Prescription:

BL 31 (Shangliao)

BL 32 (Ciliao)

BL 33 (Zhongliao)

BL 34 (Xialiao)

RM 6 (Qihai)

b) Reticulated Substance

Auricular points are used: Uterus, Ovary, Shenmen, Adrenals.

Acupuncture is given in one session every three days, between the 16th and 28th days of the menstrual cycle, for three months. The needles are left in place for approximately 10 to 15 minutes and the stimulation is gentle.

Symptomatic Therapy

Breast Tenderness

a) **SP 1** (Yinbai) + **SP 3** (Taibai) + **SP 21** (Dabao) + **ST 42** (Chongyang)

b) **L 9** (Taiyuan) + **L 7** (Lieque) + **RM 17** (Shanzhong) + **BL 17** (Geshu)

c) **ST 45** (Lidui) + **ST 36** (Zusanli) + **LI 5** (Yangxi) + **LI 11** (Quchi)

d) **ST 12** (Quepen) + **ST 21** (Liangmen) + **ST 36** (Zusanli) + **SI 3** (Houxi) + **K 23** (Shenfeng)

e) **L 7** (Lieque) + **ST 15** (Wuyi) + **ST 23** (Taiyi) + **K 3** (Taixi)

f) **ST 34** (Liangqiu) + **GB 42** (Diwuhui)

Painful Abdominal Distension

a) **ST 25** (Tianshu) + **RM 6** (Qihai) + **RM 4** (Guanyuan) + **K 10** (Yingu)

b) **SJ 3** (Zhongzhu) + **LI 11** (Quchi) + **SP 2** (Dadu) + **PC 9** (Zhongchong)

c) **SP 10** (Xuehai) + **ST 27** (Daju) + **LV 14** (Qimen)

Acupuncture can be given in two sessions weekly during the second phase of the menstrual cycle.

Edema - Premenstrual Increase of Weight

a) **ST 28** (Shuidao) + **K 6** (Zhaohai) + **GB 25** (Jingmen)

b) **K 7** (Fuliu) + **K 4** (Dazhong) + **GB 25** (Jingmen) + **BL 67** (Zhiyin)

c) **GB 43** (Xiaxi) + **SJ 3** (Zhongzhu) + **RM 22** (Tiantu) + **SI 5** (Yanggu)

d) **SP 2** (Dadu) + **SP 3** (Taibai) + **BL 20** (Pishu) + **ST 41** (Juexu) + **RM 12** (Zhongwan)

Headache

Acupuncture treatment is used only in the case of functional disorders, after the possible organic causes have been excluded. Upon such determination, several prescriptions can be used:

- frontal

BL 67 (Zhiyin) + **DM 22** (Xinhui) + **ST 41** (Jiexi)

DM 20 (Baihui) + **BL 60** (Kunlun) + **LV 2** (Xingjian)

- temporal or parietal

GB 20 (Fengchi) + **SJ 5** (Waiguan)

GB 38 (Yangfu) + **GB 20** (Fengchi) + **LV 8** (Ququan)

- occipital

DM 15 (Yamen) + **BL 10** (Tianzhu) + **BL 60** (Kunlun)

GB 38 (Yangfu) + **SI 3** (Houxi) + **BL 11** (Dazhu) + **DM 17** (Naohu)

- global

DM 15 (Yamen) + **LI 4** (Hegu) + **SJ 5** (Waiguan)

Migraine

- acute stage

a) **LV 2** (Xingjian) + **LV 3** (Taichong) + **GB 41** (Zulinqi) + **BL**

10 (Tianzhu)

b) **GB 38** (Yangfu) + **LV 3** (Taichong) + **BL 60** (Kunlun) + **SP 5** (Shangqiu)

c) **PC 6** (Neiguan) + **L 7** (Lieque) + **GB 20** (Fengchi) + **BL 10** (Tianzhu) + **BL 19** (Danshu)

The insertion of the needles is opposite to the pain and needles are left in place for approximately 10 to 15 minutes.

- between crises

a) **GB 24** (Riyue) + **L 19** (Danshu) + **GB 36** (Waiqiu) + **LI 4** (Hegu)

b) **SP 5** (Shangqiu) + **SJ 10** (Tianjing) + **LV 2** (Xingjian) + **GB 37** (Guanming)

c) **GB 38** (Yangfu) + **LV 3** (Taichong) + **LV 8** (Ququan)

Constipation

a) **SP 25** (Tianshu) + **PC 6** (Neiguan) + **RM 4** (Guanyuan) + **LI 11** (Quchi)

b) **BL 19** (Danshu) + **LV 3** (Taichong) + **GB 34** (Yanglingquan) + **H 3** (Shaohai)

c) **ST 36** (Zusanli) + **ST 45** (Lidui) + **RM 12** (Zhongwan) + **SP 5** (Shangqiu)

Auricular points can be added: Sympathetic Nervous System, Gall Bladder, Small Intestine.

Nausea and Vomiting

a) **RM 12** (Zhongwan) + **ST 25** (Tianshu) + **SP 6** (Sanyinjiao)

b) **BL 20** (Pishu) + **BL 23** (Shenshu) + **PC 6** (Neiguan) + **SP 6** (Sanyinjiao)

Auricular points can be included: Stomach, Small Intestine, Gall Bladder.

ALLERGIC MANIFESTATIONS

Urticaria

a) **LV 13** (Zhangmen) + **LV 14** (Qimen) + **LV 2** (Xingjian) + **SP 10** (Xuehai) + **SP 6** (Sanyinjiao) + **ST 36** (Zusanli)

b) **DM 14** (Dazhui) + **LV 11** (Yinlian) + **LI 4** (Hegu) + **SP 6** (Sanyinjiao)

Auricular points can be added: Shenmen, Lung, Liver, Adrenals.
Considering the location, certain points can be used:
- in the upper part of the body
L 7 (Lieque) + **LI 4** (Hegu) + **LI 11** (Quchi) + **SJ 5** (Waiguan)
- in the lower part of the body
SP 6 (Sanyinjiao) + **SP 10** (Xuehai) + **K 6** (Zhaohai) + **ST 36**
(Zusanli) + **GB 31** (Fengshi)

Menstrual Herpes

a) **L 7** (Lieque) + **LI 4** (Hegu) + **LI 11** (Quchi) + **ST 36** (Zusanli)
b) **BL 13** (Feishu) + **BL 20** (Pishu) + **SI 3** (Houxi) + **BL 60** (Kunlun)

Acne

a) **LI 11** (Quchi) + **SP 2** (Dadu) + **BL 40** (Weizhong) + **LV 13**
(Zhangmen) + **LV 5** (Ligou)
b) **K 12** (Dahe) + **LV 8** (Ququan) + **L 7** Lieque) + **ST 36** (Zusanli)

Vaginal Pruritus

a) **RM 3** (Zhongji) + **RM 2** (Qugu) + **SP 6** (Sanyinjiao) + **SP 10**
(Xuehai) + **SP 9** (Yinlingquan)
b) **LI 11** (Quchi) + **K 12** (Dahe) + **SP 8** (Diji) + **ST 29** (Guilai)
c) **LV 2** (Xingjian) + **LV 8** (Ququan) + **H 9** (Shaochong) + **RM 3**
(Zhongji) + **LV 14** (Qimen)

Psychological Disorders

- irritability
a) **LV 6** (Zhongdu) + **PC 9** (Zhongchong) + **RM 17** (Shanzhong)
+ **PC 4** (Ximen)
b) **LV 2** (Xingjian) + **LV 3** (Taichong) + **LV 14** (Qimen) + **BL 20**
(Pishu)
- anxiety
BL 20 (Pishu) + **LV 13** (Zhangmen) + **RM 17** (Shanzhong) + **K 4**
(Dazhong)

DYSMENORRHEA

The painful syndrome that precedes or accompanies menstruation
and in which genito-abdominal pain prevails is called dysmenorrhea.

Dysmenorrhea can be primary, usually functional, or secondary, when it accompanies a genital or extragenital injury.

From the perspective of Chinese traditional medicine, pain always signifies a disorder of Qi and blood circulation. There are two types, the excess type (Shi) and the deficiency type (Xu).

Knowing the character of pain helps to understand the etiopathogenesis. Establishing the location of pain allows identification of the Zang-Fu organs or channels involved.

Pain with a sensation of distension is caused by Qi stagnation. Colic pain is a sign of Qi obstruction resulting from the aggression of pathogenic factors.

Prick pain with a fixed location is a sign of blood stagnation.

Pain accompanied by a sensation of cold and a preference for warmth is due to pathogenic Cold that obstructs the channels.

Pain with a burning sensation and a preference for Cold is caused by the invasion of the Heat.

Etiopathogenesis

a) The Stagnation of Qi

Qi stagnation is frequently the result of emotional factors disturbance. The circulation of Qi is damaged, thus Qi cannot maintain the free circulation of blood. The Chong Mai and Ren Mai vessels are affected and there will be blood stagnation within the uterus, with pain.

b) The Stagnation of Blood

The stagnation of blood can be caused by different conditions.

- The attack of external Cold - due to exposure to Cold or Wind during menstruation, living in a damp and cold climate, drinking cold drinks or ingestion of food that produces cold during menstruation. The Lower Jiao is damaged and Cold is retained within the uterus leading to delayed and painful menstruation.
- The stagnation of blood remaining within the uterus after surgery, abortion or uterine curettage. The clots left interrupt the circulation of blood and impede normal exteriorization of the new menstrual flow. Menstruation becomes painful.

- The accumulation of Damp and Heat, either of external or internal origin, through transformation or by constitutional excess at the uterine level. These factors obstruct blood, the free circulation of blood is impeded and dysmenorrhea appears.

c) The Deficiency of Kidney Yin

This condition is caused by chronic diseases, excessive sexual life, or blood loss that consumes the Yin of the Kidney. The deficient Kidney cannot control the Liver, the Liver Qi ascends and endogenous Heat is produced.

d) The Deficiency of Blood

Blood deficiency can be caused by excessive blood loss, chronic diseases that consume the Qi, or malnutrition. This deficiency affects the Chong Mai and Ren Mai vessels and the uterine vessels, which are no longer nourished and develop pain.

Clinical Manifestations

a) The Stagnation of Qi

Main symptoms include pain which precedes menstruation and is accompanied by painful abdominal distension, breast tenderness, and a sensation of fullness in the chest. Late menstruation with scanty flow is characteristic. Irritability, lack of appetite, and belching are associated symptoms. A pale tongue with a thin coating and a string-taut pulse may be noted.

b) The Stagnation of Blood

- The attack of the exogenous Cold

Main symptoms include pain which precedes or occurs during menstruation and is accompanied by a sensation of cold in the lower abdomen, alleviated by warmth. Delayed menstruation, with clots is possible. Lumbar pains may develop. The patient may have a dark colored tongue with a white, thin coating and a deep, string-taut pulse.

- The Stagnation of Blood

Main symptoms include pain during menstruation, stinging, with a colic-like character, that is aggravated with pressure. A late and difficult menstruation with scanty menstrual flow and dark colored blood or clots is characteristic. The pain decreases after menstruation. On palpation one can feel pelvic tumoral masses. A dark complexion; dry mouth; a red tongue, or bluish tongue with purplish spots; and a deep, string-taut pulse may be observed.

- The Accumulation of Damp and Heat

Main symptoms include pain which precedes menstruation, and is located in the iliac fossa, possibly spreading to the lumbar area and aggravated with pressure. Antedated menstruation with excessive flow and dark menstrual blood, with a strong odor are typical. Associated symptoms include warm skin, fever, a dry mouth, nervousness, insomnia, constipation, and oliguria. The patient may evidence a dark red tongue with a yellowish coating and a rapid, string-taut pulse.

c) The Deficiency of Kidney Yin

Main symptoms include pain during menstruation, located in the lower abdomen and a sensation of lumbar weakness. The menstrual blood is bright red, with scanty flow. Associated symptoms include dizziness, insomnia, memory disorders, dry mouth, nocturnal sweating, oliguria and constipation when there is an excess of Yang. Pale tongue with a thin coating and a deep, weak pulse.

d) The Deficiency of Blood

Main symptoms include pain, usually during menstruation, that is continuous in character, dull and alleviated with application of pressure and warmth. The menstrual flow is scanty with bright colored blood. Pallor, apathy, dizziness, palpitations, dyspnea, insomnia, and numbness may be present. The patient may have a pale tongue with a thin coating and a thready pulse.

Treatment

a) The Stagnation of Qi

Therapeutic principle: regulate Qi to remove stagnation

Prescription:

LV 2 (Xingjian)	is the Reducing point of the Liver channel, stimulates Qi and blood circulation in the Liver and Gall Bladder channels
RM 3 (Zhongji)	stimulates Qi and blood circulation, regulates the uterus, removes stagnation and pain
SP 8 (Diji)	is the Xi point of the Spleen channel, regulates

	blood circulation and menstruation
BL 32 (Ciliao)	is an empirical point effective in treating dysmenorrhea
RM 6 (Qihai)	regulates the whole body Qi

Acupuncture is given with the reducing method.

b) The Stagnation of Blood

Therapeutic principle: stimulate blood to transform clots.

Prescription:

LI 4 (Hegu)	regulates Qi and blood, drains the channels, stimulates blood circulation, cools the Heat
SP 6 (Sanyinjiao)	stimulates Qi and blood circulation
SP 10 (Xuehai)	regulates blood circulation
ST 25 (Tianshu)	regulates the channels and stimulates the circulation of Qi
ST 29 (Guilai)	removes blood and Qi stagnation, especially from the uterus

Acupuncture is given with the reducing method, a session being approximately 15 to 20 minutes.

- When stagnation is due to Cold

Therapeutic principle: reduce Cold and warm the channels

Prescription:

BL 23 (Shenshu)	is the Back-Shu point of the Kidney, nourishes the Yin and strengthens Yang, warms the Kidney
BL 20 (Pishu)	is the Back-Shu point of the Spleen, warms and tones the Spleen
DM 4 (Mingmen)	tones the Kidney, strengthens Yang, drains the channels
RM 3 (Zhongji)	regulates the Chong Mai and Ren Mai vessels, regulates the uterus
RM 4 (Guanyuan)	regulates Qi and blood circulation, regulates the Chong Mai and Ren Mai
RM 6 (Qihai)	regulates Qi, regulates the Chong Mai and

	Ren Mai vessels
K 12 (Dahe)	is the Crossing point of the Kidney channel with the Chong Mai Vessel, regulates the Chong Mai and Ren Mai vessels

- Accumulation of Damp and Heat

Therapeutic principle: remove Heat, cool the blood, stimulate blood circulation, remove Damp when necessary

Prescription:

SP 10 (Xuehai)	removes Heat from the blood
SP 9 (Yinlingquan)	is the He point of the Spleen channel, tones the Spleen and removes Damp, favors circulation in San Jiao
LV 2 (Xingjian)	is the Ying point of the Liver channel, cools the Heat and Lower Jiao
BL 30 (Baihuanshu)	drains Lower Jiao, regulates menstruation

c) The Deficiency of Kidney Yin

Therapeutic principle: strengthen and tone the Kidney Yin, nourish the Liver

Prescription:

BL 23 (Shenshu)	nourishes the Yin and strengthens Yang, tones the Kidney
SP 6 (Sanyinjiao)	is the Crossing point of the three Yin channels of the foot—the Kidney, Spleen and Liver, regulates the Yin
LV 8 (Ququan)	is the He point of the Liver channel, nourishes and tones the Liver
SP 10 (Xuehai)	nourishes the blood
RM 4 (Guanyuan)	is the Crossing point of the Ren Mai Vessel with the Kidney, Liver and Spleen channels; strengthens the Qi; regulates Qi and blood circulation and the Chong Mai and Ren Mai vessels

d) The Deficiency of Blood

Therapeutic principle: tone Qi, nourish blood

Prescription:

BL 17 (Geshu)	is the Influential point of blood, strengthens the Spleen and regulates blood
BL 20 (Pishu)	is the Back-Shu point of the Spleen, tones the Spleen, the source of blood
RM 6 (Qihai)	regulates Qi and blood, the Chong Mai and Ren Mai vessels and the uterus

The points can be stimulated using acupuncture or moxa.

MENSTRUAL CYCLE DISORDERS

The disorders of menstrual cycle are disorders of the regular character of menstruation, as menstruation is the only clinical manifestation of the existence of the menstrual cycle.

The term "menstrual cycle disorder" refers to any abnormal change of menstrual cycle, concerning quantity and color, length of menstrual cycle and other associated symptoms.

These disorders may be of deficiency or excess:

Disorders of Deficiency Type

- hypomenorrhea: reduction of the amount of blood and of the menstrual flow to less then 3 days
- oligomenorrhea: is a rhythm disorder in which menstruation appears rarely and at irregular periods that can vary between 35 and 45 days
- spaniomenorrhea: the period between menstrual cycles extends to over 3 - 4 months

Disorders of Excess Type

- menorrhagia: excessive and prolonged menstrual flow, more than 6 days duration
- hypermenorrhea: quantitative excess of menstrual flow
- polymenorrhea: cyclic hemorrhage, of normal amount, at 17 to 21 day intervals

From the perspective of Chinese traditional medicine, the disorders of menstrual cycle can be caused by different circumstances: the aggression of the pathogenic exogenous factors —Heat, Cold, and Damp; prolonged disturbance of emotional factors; sexual excess; multiparity etc.

These factors may cause an imbalance between Qi and blood that affects the functions of the Chong Mai and Ren Mai vessels, the uterus and the Zang-Fu organs involved in a normal menstrual cycle.

The short menstrual cycle, with antedated menstruation that appears 7 to 8 days early, or even twice a month, is caused by Heat. Endogenous Heat can be generated by Liver Fire in cases of prolonged disturbance of emotional factors or when there is Heat in the blood that rushes the blood and stimulates extravasation.

The long menstrual cycle, with delayed menstruation, from 8 to 9 days late (and sometimes occuring after 40 to 45 days) is due to Cold. Cold can be exogenous, by the attack of Cold that stays within the uterus, obstructs the vessels and delays menstruation. Endogenous Cold may be caused by a congenital excess of Yang. Causing stagnation and constriction, it will slow down circulation within the Chong Mai and Ren Mai vessels and delay the menstruation.

Irregular menstruation may be influenced by a variety of different causes: blood deficiency, congenital deficiency of the Spleen-Stomach couple, sexual excess, multiparity that weakens the Kidney Qi, emotional factors disturbance that cause Liver Qi stagnation, or inadequate food intake with an excess of piquant, greasy, cold food, or cold, alcoholic drinks etc. In all these circumstances the damage to the Chong Mai and Ren Mai vessels acts upon the menstrual cycle characteristics.

Etiopathogenesis

The following etiopathogenic types are described:

a) The Deficiency of Qi

This deficiency can be caused by chronic disease, overstrain, stress, or inadequate food intake. Weakness of Qi affects the Zang-Fu organs and the Chong Mai and Ren Mai vessels. If in physiologic conditions Qi is the commander of blood, the deficient Qi can no longer command blood. The menstrual cycle is short, with excessive menstrual flow.

b) The Deficiency of Blood

Blood deficiency is usually because of the weakness of the Spleen-Stomach couple which is the source of blood. Other factors can include an excessive blood loss, disturbance of emotional factors, or multiparity. The "Sea of blood" becomes deficient and the menstrual cycle will be prolonged, with scanty menstrual flow and bright colored blood.

c) The Yin Deficiency of the Liver and Kidney

Severe emotional factors disturbance, overstrain and stress can affect Yin blood or a chronic disease can consume the Yin of the Liver and Kidney. The affected Liver function of preserving blood will cause long menstrual cycles with scanty menstrual flow. The damage of the Kidney function of controlling and preserving will cause short menstrual cycles with excessive flow. The deficiency of the two organs injures the functions of the Chong Mai and Ren Mai vessels that can no longer control the menstrual cycle.

The Yin deficiency causes endogenous Heat that may injure the Liver and Heart with worsening of Chong Mai and Ren Mai damage and the appearance of irregular cycles.

d) The Deficiency of Spleen

The deficient Spleen, either as a result of congenital causes or overstrain, inadequate food intake, or chronic disease, cannot maintain its function of keeping blood within the vessels. Short menstrual cycles appear, with excessive flow and light colored blood.

e) The Stagnation of Qi

The stagnation of Qi is frequently caused by emotional factors disturbance. The delay of Qi circulation will affect blood circulation. Blood stagnation can cause the formation of clots. The menstrual cycle will be irregular in rhythm and amount of menstrual flow.

f) The Stagnation of Blood

Blood obstruction can be caused by the aggression of Cold that obstructs the blood vessels and impedes Qi and blood circulation within the uterus. The stagnant blood from the uterus may remain unevacuated after a delivery or abortion. There will be long menstrual cycles and menstrual flow with clots.

g) Heat in the Blood

There are multiple circumstances that generate Heat: aggression of exogenous pathogenic Heat due to excessive intake of piquant, hot food or alcoholic drinks; smoking; congenital deficiency of Yin that causes excessive internal Heat; and persistent disorders of the menstrual cycle transforming the Liver Qi stagnation into Fire etc. Heat stimulates blood circulation and causes a short menstrual cycle, with excessive flow (when due to Heat excess) and with scanty flow (when due to the deficiency of Yin).

h) Cold in the Blood

This condition may be caused by aggression of pathogenic Cold through Cold exposure, by cold food or drink intake, or by virtue of a constitutional excess of Yang. Cold causes constriction and stagnation and the circulation within the uterus vessels is impeded. Menstruation will be delayed with scanty flow.

i) The Stagnation of Phlegm-Damp

When the excess of Phlegm is constitutional in obese patients, this accumulates in the Lower Jiao and obstructs the uterus. Stagnation occurs within the vessels and long menstrual cycles develop, with scanty menstrual flow. Aggravation of obstruction can cause amenorrhea.

If the Qi of the Spleen is damaged, the Spleen cannot perform the function of transforming and Damp turns into Heat. The blood, no longer under the control of Spleen, is stimulated by Heat and has a tendency to extravasation. The menstrual cycle will be short, with excessive flow.

Clinical Manifestations

a) The Deficiency of Qi

Main symptoms include short menstrual cycles with excessive flow and light red blood. Associated symptoms include asthenia, insomnia, palpitations, dyspnea, dizziness, and vision disturbances. The patient may evidence a pale tongue with a thin coating and a hollow, weak pulse.

b) The Deficiency of Blood

Main symptoms include late menstrual cycles with scanty flow and light red blood. A pale, withered complexion with dry skin that exfoliates; palpitations; dizziness; insomnia; and numbness may also be present. A pale tongue with a thin coating and a fine or wiry, thready pulse may be noted.

c) The Yin Deficiency of the Liver and Kidney

Main symptoms include short menstrual cycles with excessive flow or long cycles with scanty menstrual flow. Vision disturbances; tinnitus; dry throat; dizziness; a sensation of heat in the chest, palms and foot; a sensation of weakness in the knees and lumbar area; and nocturnal sweating are associated symptoms. The patient may have a red tongue with a thin coating and a rapid, thready pulse.

d) The Deficiency of the Spleen

Main symptoms include long, irregular menstrual cycles with excessive or scanty menstrual flow and light colored blood. Associated symptoms are a pale, waxy complexion; cold limbs; asthenia; lack of appetite; and abdominal distension. A pale tongue with a thin coating and a weak, thready pulse may also be noted.

e) The Stagnation of Qi

Main symptoms include irregular menstrual cycles, with excessive menstrual flow and dark colored blood with clots. A dark complexion, painful abdominal distension, premenstrual breast tenderness, dysmenorrhea, belching, irritability, and depression may also be present. A pale tongue with a thin coating and a string-taut pulse may be observed.

f) The Stagnation of Blood

Main symptoms include long menstrual cycles, delayed menstruation, and scanty flow with dark blood and clots. Associated symptoms are abdominal pain, aggravated on pressure, and dysmenorrhea. A bluish tongue, possibly with purplish spots on the borders and a deep, wiry pulse may be recorded.

g) Heat in the Blood

Main symptoms include short menstrual cycles with excessive flow and dark red, thick, clammy, malodorous blood with clots. A red flushed face, red lips, aversion to heat, a preference for cold, dry mouth, and restlessness may also be present. The patient may have a red tongue with a yellow coating and a rapid, sliding pulse.

If the excess of Heat is due to a Yin deficiency, the menstrual flow is scanty, with light colored blood and no clots. Asthenia and insomnia may be reported. A red, light tongue with a thin coating, or possibly a yellowish and dry coating, and a fine, rapid pulse may be observed.

h) Cold in the Blood

Main symptoms include long menstrual cycles, with scanty flow and light colored blood or dark blood and dysmenorrhea. A pale complexion; dull, continuous abdominal pain, alleviated by warmth and pressure; an aversion to cold; and a preference for warmth are also characteristic. The patient may have a pale tongue with a thin coating and a deep, slow pulse.

i) The Stagnation of Phlegm-Damp

Main symptoms include long menstrual cycles with variable amounts of blood that is light colored and clammy. A sensation of epigastric distension, fullness in the chest, lack of appetite, vomiting, and loose stools are associated symptoms. A swollen tongue with a white, thick coating and a string-taut, sliding pulse may be noted.

Treatment

a) The Deficiency of Qi

Therapeutic principle: tone Qi, regulate Chong Mai and Ren Mai Vessels

Prescription:

RM 6 (Qihai)	tones Qi, regulates the channels system, regulates the Chong Mai and Ren Mai vessels
SP 4 (Gongsun)	is the Luo point of the Spleen channel and the Confluent point of Chong Mai, regulates the Chong Mai and Ren Mai vessels
ST 36 (Zusanli)	regulates Qi and blood
K 3 (Taixi)	is the Yuan-Source point of the Kidney channel, tones the Kidney regulates the Chong Mai and Ren Mai vessels
SP 1 (Yinbai)	is the Jing-Well point of the Spleen channel, increases Qi and stimulates blood circulation

The acupoints are stimulated with the reinforcing method and moxibustion can be used to stimulate RM 6 and SP 4.

b) The Deficiency of Blood

Therapeutic principle: tone blood to regulate menstruation

Prescription:

ST 36 (Zusanli)   is the He point of the Stomach channel, regulates the Stomach and tones the Spleen, stimulates the production of blood

SP 6 (Sanyinjiao)   tones the Spleen Qi, regulates Qi and blood circulation, stimulates the Kidney

BL 17 (Geshu)   is the Influential point of blood, strengthens the Spleen and regulates the Stomach, regulates blood circulation, removes blood stagnation

SP 10 (Xuehai)   stimulates blood circulation and regulates menstruation

The acupoints are stimulated with the reinforcing method, using acupuncture or moxibustion.

c) The Yin Deficiency of the Liver and Kidney

Therapeutic principle: warm and tone the Kidney, nourish the Yin

Prescription:

BL 23 (Shenshu)   is the Back-Shu point of the Kidney, tones and regulates the Kidney

RM 4 (Guanyuan)   is the Crossing point of the Ren Mai Vessel with the Liver, Spleen and Kidney channels; strengthens Qi; regulates the Chong Mai and Ren Mai vessels; stimulates Qi and blood circulation

DM 4 (Mingmen)   strengthens the Kidney Yang, regulates the Qi, regulates menstruation

d) The Deficiency of the Spleen

Therapeutic principle: tone the Spleen to regulate menstruation

Prescription:

BL 20 (Pishu)   is the Back-Shu point of the Spleen, tones Spleen Qi, regulates the Stomach

BL 21 (Weishu)   is the Back-Shu point of the Stomach, strengthens the Spleen, regulates Stomach

SP 6 (Sanyinjiao)	is the Crossing point of the three Yin channels of the foot, tones the Qi of the Spleen, regulates the circulation of Qi and blood
ST 36 (Zusanli)	restores Qi of the Middle Jiao, strengthens the Spleen, regulates the Stomach
SP 8 (Diji)	is the Xi point of the Spleen channel, tones the Spleen and Stomach, regulates menstruation, stops leukorrhea

e) The Stagnation of Qi

Therapeutic principle: regulate Qi, remove stagnation

Prescription:

LV 3 (Taichong)	is the Yuan-Source point of the Liver channel, stimulates the free circulation of Qi
RM 12 (Zhongwan)	is the Front-Mu point of the Stomach, the Influential point of the Fu organs, and the Crossing point of the Ren Mai Vessel with the Short Intestine, San Jiao and Stomach channels, strengthens the Stomach, regulates the Qi of the Ren Mai Vessel
RM 6 (Qihai)	regulates Qi and blood circulation, regulates the Chong Mai and Ren Mai
PC 6 (Neiguan)	is the Luo point of the Pericardium channel, spreads the chest fullness, calms the mind

f) Heat in the Blood

Therapeutic principle: cool blood, disperse the Heat

Prescription:

SP 10 (Xuehai)	cools the blood, spreads the Heat
LV 2 (Xingjian)	is the Ying point of the Liver channel, disperses the Liver Fire, cools the Heat from blood and Lower Jiao
SP 6 (Sanyinjiao)	cools the Heat in the three Yin channels of the foot, stimulates Qi and blood circulation, nourishes the Yin
K 8 (Jiaoxin)	is the Confluent point of Yin Qiao Mai Ves-

sel, disperses pathogenic Heat, regulates Qi and blood, regulates the Chong Mai and Ren Mai vessels

- When the excess of Heat is due to Yin deficiency

Therapeutic principle: nourish Yin to cool the Heat

Prescription:

K 2 (Rangu)	is the Ying point of the Kidney channel, nourishes the Yin, reduces Heat, regulates menstruation
BL 17 (Geshu)	is the Influential point of blood, nourishes and regulates blood
LV 3 (Taichong)	is the Yuan-Source point of the Liver channel, tones the Liver, removes Heat from the Liver

g) The Stagnation of Blood

Therapeutic principle: stimulate blood and transform the clots.

Prescription:

RM 3 (Zhongji)	regulates the Lower Jiao, regulates Chong Mai and Ren Mai Vessels
LV 2 (Xingjian)	is the Ying point of the Liver channel, regulates Qi and blood
SP 10 (Xuehai)	regulates the circulation of blood, regulates menstruation
BL 17 (Geshu)	is the Influential point of the blood, removes stagnation

h) Cold in the Blood

Therapeutic principle: warm the channels and remove Cold

Prescription:

RM 4 (Guanyuan)	warms the Kidney, tones Kidney Qi, regulates Qi and the Chong Mai and Ren Mai vessels, removes the Cold from the uterus
RM 8 (Shenque)	warms the Yang, tones the Spleen and Stomach, moxibustion is used
SP 6 (Sanyinjiao)	tones the Qi of the Spleen, Liver and Kidney;

regulates Lower Jiao; warms the uterus

i) The Stagnation of Phlegm-Damp

Therapeutic principle: strengthen the Spleen to transform the Phlegm

Prescription:

SP 6 (Sanyinjiao)	tones the Spleen to remove Damp and the obstruction of the channels
BL 20 (Pishu)	is the Back-Shu point of the Spleen, tones the Spleen and spreads pathogenic Damp
ST 40 (Fenglong)	is the Luo point of the Stomach channel, regulates the Stomach and reduces the Phlegm
ST 25 (Tianshu)	strengthens the Spleen to transform Damp, regulates menstruation and Qi

ANTEDATED MENSTRUATION

Etiopathogenesis

a) Heat in the Blood

This condition is caused by an excess of endogenous Heat, Yin deficiency and Yang excess, excess of piquant food, or excessive vasodilation that activates the uterus or is produced through the transforming of the Liver Fire. The excessive Heat will damage the Chong Mai and Ren Mai vessels, causing the shortening of the menstrual cycle and excessive menstrual flow.

The classical literature mentions that: "If menstruation extends over 10 days and does not stop, it is Heat in the blood..."

"Usually ... menstruation that does not stop, with weakness and a warm body, is flourishing Fire."

b) The Deficiency of Qi

This deficiency results from overstrain or inadequate food intake that weakens the Spleen Qi and causes Qi deficiency in the Middle Jiao. The Qi can no longer control blood and menstruation, and consequently, the Chong Mai and Ren Mai vessels are injured. The menstrual cycle is short with excessive flow and light colored blood.

In *Chinese Acupuncture and Moxibustion*, it is stated: "If the pulse does not show an excess of internal Heat it means antedated menstruation is caused by the Qi deficiency of the Heart and Spleen which cannot control blood."

Clinical Manifestations

a) Heat in the Blood

Main symptoms include early menstruation with excessive menstrual flow and light colored or dark colored blood in the case of stagnation. Irritability, restlessness, a flushed face, thirst, oliguria, and constipation are associated symptoms. A red tongue with a yellow coating and a rapid, strong or wiry pulse may be present.

b) The Deficiency of Qi

Main symptoms include early menstruation with excessive flow and light red blood. Asthenia, palpitations, vision disturbances, dizziness; spontaneous sweating, and a hollow sensation in the lower abdomen may also be present. The patient may have a pale tongue with a thin coating and a deep, weak pulse.

Treatment

a) Heat in the Blood

Therapeutic principle: remove Heat from the blood, regulate the Chong Mai and Ren Mai vessels

Prescription:

RM 4 (Guanyuan)	regulates Qi and blood, regulates the circulation of Chong Mai and Ren Mai
SP 10 (Xuehai)	removes Heat from the blood
LV 3 (Taichong)	is the Yuan-Source point of the Liver channel, removes Heat and regulates Qi and blood circulation and Liver Fire
LI 11 (Quchi)	is the He point of the Large Intestine channel, removes Heat from the blood
K 5 (Shuiquan)	is the Xi point of the Kidney channel, strengthens the Yin, reduces Heat and regulates menstruation
K 2 (Rangu)	is the Ying point of the Kidney channel, nourishes the Yin, cools the Heat

At the selected points, acupuncture is given with the reducing method.

b) The Deficiency of Qi

Therapeutic principle: tone Qi and restore Qi function of controlling blood

Prescription:

RM 6 (Qihai)	tones Qi, regulates the Chong Mai Vessel and menstruation
SP 6 (Sanyinjiao)	is the Crossing point of the three Yin channels of the foot, tones the Spleen, strengthens the Kidney Qi, regulates Qi and blood
ST 36 (Zusanli)	regulates and balances Qi and blood, has a generally fortifying effect
SP 1 (Yinbai)	is the Jing-Well point of the Spleen channel, strengthens the Spleen, increases Qi
RM 17 (Shanzhong)	is the Influential point of Qi, regulates Qi

POSTDATED MENSTRUATION

Etiopathogenesis

a) The Deficiency of Blood

Several circumstances can cause the deficiency of blood: chronic blood loss, chronic diseases, overstrain, inadequate food intake, or multiparity. Any of these can damage the Spleen-Stomach couple with insufficient production of blood. The Chong Mai and Ren Mai vessels are not adequately nourished or their function of menstruation adjustment is affected, with later onset of menstruation.

b) Cold in the Blood

Cold may be endogenous due to the deficiency of Yang, may be a consequence of exposure to cold and rain during menstruation, or may be caused by ingestion of cold and raw food. Pathogenic cold invades the uterus and the Chong Mai and Ren Mai vessels. Characterized by obstruction and stagnation, Cold will cause the disturbance of the free circulation of blood with slowing of circulation and delaying of menstruation.

c) The Stagnation of Qi

Emotional factors (mainly depression) are primarily involved in the stagnation of Qi, as the activity of Qi is damaged. But as "Qi is the commander of blood" the circulation of Qi supports and promotes blood circulation. Qi stagnation will cause blood stagnation and injure the Chong Mai and Ren Mai vessels. The insufficient blood cannot fill the "Sea of blood" and menstruation is delayed.

Clinical Manifestations

a) The Deficiency of Blood

Main symptoms include postdated menstruation with scanty flow and light colored blood. Weakness, pallor, dizziness, vision disturbances, palpitations, insomnia, lower abdominal pain, cold limbs, and constipation are associated symptoms. The patient may evidence a pale tongue with a thin coating and a weak, thready pulse.

b) Cold in the Blood

Main symptoms include postdated menstruation with scanty flow and dark colored blood, possibly with clots in cases of stagnation. Lower abdominal pain alleviated by warmth, dysmenorrhea, cold limbs, a preference for warmth, and pale lips may also be noted. The patient may reveal a pale tongue with no coating or a thin white coating and a deep, slow pulse.

c) The Stagnation of Qi

Main symptoms include postdated menstruation with scanty flow and dark colored blood with clots. Associated symptoms are painful distension in the hypochondriac and costal regions, fullness in the chest, depression, lack of appetite, belching and dry lips. A white, thin tongue coating and a rapid, string-taut pulse may also be present.

Treatment

a) The Deficiency of Blood

Therapeutic principle: nourish blood and tone Qi

Prescription:

BL 17 (Geshu)   is the Influential point of blood, strengthens the Spleen and regulates the Stomach, regu-

	lates blood, stimulates Qi circulation
ST 36 (Zusanli)	tones the body, regulates the Stomach and tones the Spleen, stimulates blood and Qi circulation
SP 6 (Sanyinjiao)	nourishes the Yin, strengthens and regulates the Spleen, nourishes blood
SP 10 (Xuehai)	tones insufficient, "dry" blood
BL 43 (Gaohuang)	tones the Spleen and Stomach.

The stimulation is given with the reinforcing method.

| H 7 (Shenmen) | is the Yuan-Source point of the Heart channel, calms the mind and is added in cases with insomnia |
| DM 20 (Baihui) | is the Crossing point of the Yang channel, facilitates the ascent of Yang, nourishes the brain |

b) Cold in the Blood

Therapeutic principle: warm the channels and disperse the Cold.

Prescription:

SP 6 (Sanyinjiao)	tones the Spleen and favors the Kidney Qi, regulates Qi and blood circulation
RM 4 (Guanyuan)	nourishes Kidney Qi, favors the Yang, regulates the Chong Mai and Ren Mai vessels, regulates menstruation
ST 29 (Guilai)	disperses Cold, removes Qi and blood stagnation, especially from the uterus
DM 4 (Mingmen)	strengthens the Kidney Yang, restores normal menstruation
RM 8 (Shenque)	warms the channels. The selected acupoints are stimulated with the reinforcing method, using acupuncture or moxibustion. For RM 8, only moxibustion is used.

c) The Stagnation of Qi

Therapeutic principle: promote Qi and blood circulation

Prescription:

RM 6 (Qihai)	regulates Qi and blood circulation
ST 25 (Tianshu)	regulates the channels and stimulates the circulation of Qi
SP 8 (Diji)	is the Xi point of the Spleen channel, regulates Qi and blood circulation
LV 3 (Taichong)	is the Yuan-Source point of the Lower channel, disperses the Liver pathogenic Fire, stimulates Qi and blood circulation
PC 6 (Neiguan)	is the Luo point of the Pericardium channel, relaxes and removes thoracic fullness, stimulates Qi circulation, calms the mind
K 13 (Qixue)	is the Crossing point of the Kidney channel with the Chong Mai Vessel, strengthens the Kidney Qi, regulates the Chong Mai and Ren Mai vessels, regulates Lower Jiao

IRREGULAR MENSTRUAL CYCLE

Etiopathogenesis

a) The Stagnation of the Liver Qi

Persistent depression, as a pathogenic emotional factor, affects the Liver function of maintaining the free circulation of Qi and blood. Liver Qi stagnation reflects upon Liver function and blood circulation. The Chong Mai and Ren Mai vessels and the uterus are damaged and irregular menstrual cycles appear.

b) The Deficiency of the Kidney

This deficiency is mainly caused by excessive sexual activity: sexual excess, early marriage, multiparity etc. that consume the Essence and blood. The deficient Kidney cannot store the Essence and cannot control the Chong Mai and Ren Mai Vessels. The menstrual cycle will be irregular.

Clinical Manifestations

a) The Stagnation of the Liver Qi

Main symptoms include menstrual cycles that are irregular in rhythm, amount and aspect of menstrual flow, usually with dark coloured, thick, clammy blood, and dysmenorrhea. Premenstrual breast tenderness, painful distension in the hypochondriac region, depression, frequent sighing, belching, and a reduced appetite are associated symptoms. A thin, white tongue coating and a string-taut pulse may be noted.

b) The Deficiency of the Kidney

Main symptoms include irregular menstrual cycles with scanty menstrual flow and light red blood. Lumbar and knee weakness may be reported as may pollakiuria, dizziness, tinnitus, and clear leukorrhea. A pale tongue with a thin coating and a deep, weak pulse may be observed.

Treatment

a) The Stagnation of the Liver Qi

Therapeutic principle: drain the Liver, regulate the Chong Mai and Ren Mai vessels

Prescription:

RM 6 (Qihai)	regulates Qi and blood circulation, regulates the Chong Mai and Ren Mai Vessels
LV 5 (Ligou)	is the Luo point of the Liver channel, removes Liver Qi stagnation
LV 14 (Qimen)	is the Front-Mu point of the Liver, removes Liver Qi stagnation, promotes the circulation of blood
PC 5 (Jianshi)	is the Jing-River point of the Pericardium channel, drains the channels, relaxes the chest, nourishes the Heart, sedates the mind
RM 17 (Shanzhong)	is the Front-Mu point of the Pericardium channel and the Influential point of Qi, stimulates Qi circulation

In cases with accompanying depression, the following points can be used:

H 7 (Shenmen)	is the Yuan-Source point of the Heart channel, nourishes the Heart and calms the mind.

The stimulation is given with the even movement method.

b) The Deficiency of the Kidney

Therapeutic principle: tone the Kidney Qi and regulate the Chong Mai and Ren Mai vessels

Prescription:

RM 4 (Guanyuan)	is the Crossing point of the Ren Mai Vessel with the Kidney, Liver and Spleen channels, tones Kidney Qi, strengthens Yang, regulates the Chong Mai and Ren Mai vessels
BL 23 (Shenshu)	is the Back-Shu point of the Kidney, nourishes the Yin and strengthens the Yang, tones the brain and marrow
SP 6 (Sanyinjiao)	regulates and strengthens the three Yin channels of the foot the Kidney, Spleen and Liver, regulates Qi and blood
K 8 (Jiaoxin)	is the Xi point of the Kidney channel, tones the Kidney, regulates the Chong Mai and Ren Mai vessels, supports the uterus

Other points can be added according to circumstances:

E.P. Yaoyan	is indicated in gynecological diseases and lumbar weakness
ST 36 (Zusanli)	regulates Qi and blood, has a generally fortifying effect
DM 20 (Baihui)	is the Crossing point of the Yang channels with the Du Mai Vessel, facilitates ascent of the Yang and nourishes the brain

Acupuncture is given with the reinforcing method, in a session lasting approximately 15 to 20 minutes. A stronger stimulation can be obtained with moxibustion over the points RM 4, ST 36 and DM 20.

ABNORMAL UTERINE BLEEDING

This condition is defined as the abnormal bleeding of the endometrium due to disturbance of the physiological mechanism of the menstrual cycle. The following parameters can be affected: amount, length, frequency, or period of onset of the menstrual cycle. It can manifest as metrorrhagia or menorrhagia. It occurs most frequently at puberty and in perimenopause. In almost 90% of cases the bleeding is anovulatory and bleeding from organic causes due to hematologic diseases must be excluded. The treatment is usually hormonal.

From the perspective of Chinese traditional medicine this pathologic entity is called "Beng Lou." The "Jing Lou" term refers to sudden, excessive, short-term bleeding (metrorrhagia). Although different manifestations, one condition can evolve into the other. Excessive repeated metrorrhagia consumes Qi and blood causing, in time, menometrorrhagia; aggravation of a menometrorrhagia may manifest as excessive metrorrhagia.

"Beng Lou" is caused by damage to the Liver, Spleen and Kidney that, in turn, affects the Extraordinary Vessels Chong Mai and Ren Mai.

The Spleen and Stomach are considered to be the source of Qi and blood. The Spleen Qi controls blood and prevents extravasation. The Liver stores blood and controls its volume. When blood is not consumed it turns into Essence within the Kidney; if the Essence is not spread it turns into blood within the Liver.

Etiopathogenesis

a) The Deficiency of Qi

A variety of circumstances can affect the Spleen Qi: overstrain, stress, inadequate food intake, and worry. The weakened Spleen cannot keep blood in the vessels, the function of Chong Mai and Ren Mai Vessels is damaged, and metrorrhagia appears.

b) Excessive Heat in the Blood

This condition can be caused by exogenous pathogenic Heat invasion, the excess of Yang, abusive consumption of piquant food or the obstruction of Liver Qi that turns into Fire. Frequently the pathogenic Fire consumes the Yin and constrains it outwards, causing an insufficiency of fluids in the body. Being a Yang pathogenic factor, Heat is characterized by ascending movement and can disturb the mind. Excessive Heat accelerates blood circulation and can injure blood vessels, causing hemorrhagia in the genital area.

Clinical Manifestations

a) The Deficiency of Qi

Main symptoms include excessive, sudden metrorrhagia or scanty, continuous, light coloured and thin blood loss. Lower abdominal pain with a sensation of cold, a pale complexion, apathy, lack of appetite, dizziness, and loose stools are associated symptoms. The patient may evidence a pale tongue with a white coating and a weak, thready, slow pulse.

b) Excessive Heat in the Blood

Main symptoms include sudden, excessive metrorrhagia; dark coloured, sometimes malodorous, blood, with clots and scanty, continuous blood loss. Associated symptoms includes restlessness, insomnia, dizziness, a flushed face, dry mouth, thirst with the desire to drink, headache, constipation, and oliguria. A red tongue with a yellowish coating and a rapid, sliding or strained pulse may also be recorded.

Treatment

a) The Deficiency of Qi

Therapeutic principle: tone the Spleen Qi, regulate the Chong Mai and Ren Mai vessels

Prescription:

RM 4 (Guanyuan)	is the Crossing point of the Ren Mai Vessel with the Spleen, Kidney and Liver Channels; regulates Qi and blood; regulates the Chong Mai and Ren Mai vessels
SP 6 (Sanyinjiao)	is the Crossing point of the three Yin channels of the foot, nourishes the Yin, tones the Spleen
SP 1 (Yinbai)	is the Jing-Well point of the Spleen channel, tones and strengthens the Spleen function of controlling blood
BL 20 (Pishu)	is the Back-Shu point of the Spleen, strengthens the Spleen and regulates the Stomach
ST 36 (Zusanli)	tones the Spleen and Qi, which as the commander of blood, maintains the blood within the vessels

DM 20 (Baihui)   is the Crossing point of the Yang channels, facilitates ascent of Qi

Other points can be used according to circumstances:

BL 21 (Weishu)   is the Back-Shu point of the Stomach, strengthens the Spleen and regulates the Stomach

RM 8 (Shenque)   tones the Spleen and regulates the Stomach, warms the Yang

SJ 4 (Yangchi)   is the Yuan-Source of the San Jiao channel which supports the Qi, stimulates the Chong Mai and Ren Mai vessels' function of controlling blood

The stimulation of the selected points is given with acupuncture by the reinforcing method. Moxibustion is used for the points DM 20 and RM 8, with salt for the later, being conducted during one daily session.

The use of cupping glasses is another method of treatment. One to three points located on both sides of the spine (in the lumbar-sacral region, where the patient feels a heavy sensation) are selected. The needles can be left in place for 30 to 60 minutes in cases of bleeding, with stimulation every 10 to 20 minutes until the uterine bleeding either reduces in amount or ceases. After the needles are withdrawn, cupping glasses can be applied, on both sides, for 10 to 15 minutes.

b) Excessive Heat in the Blood

Therapeutic principle: remove Heat and stop bleeding

Prescription:

RM 4 (Guanyuan)   regulates the Chong Mai and Ren Mai Vessels, controlling the blood loss

SP 1 (Yinbai)   is the Jing-Well point of the Spleen channel, and an effective point for uterine bleeding

SP 10 (Xuehai)   removes the Heat from the blood and cools blood, regulates menstruation

LV 8 (Ququan)   is the He point of the Liver channel, removes the Heat and disperses the pathogenic Fire of the Liver

LI 11 (Quchi)   is the He point of the Large Intestine channel, spreads the pathogenic Heat and regulates the channel

Other points can be used:

LV 3 (Taichong)   is the Yuan-Source point of the Liver channel, removes the Heat and spreads the Liver pathogenic Fire, favors the circulation of Qi and blood

K 2 (Rangu)   is the Ying point of the Kidney channel, removes pathogenic Heat, regulates the Chong Mai and Ren Mai vessels

H 8 (Shaofu)   is the Ying point of the Heart channel, disperses the Heart Fire, calms the mind

H 5 (Tongli)   is the Luo point of the Heart channel, regulates the Heart and mind

E.P. Zigong   located at 4 cun inferior to the navel and 3 cun lateral to the median line

Auricular Therapy: points Hormones, Uterus, Ovary, Kidney, Adrenals, and Spleen. The needles are left in place for 20 minutes or more and moderate, intermittent stimulation is used during one session daily.

In emergency with excessive metrorrhagia

Prescription:

RM 5 (Shimen)   for stimulating the point, moxibustion is used to obtain a sensation of warmth in the abdomen

Afterwards the etiopathogenic type can be taken into account or other prescriptions considered such as:

SP 10 (Xuehai) + **SP 1** (Yinbai)

SP 10 (Xuehai) + **SP 6** (Sanyinjiao) + **RM 3** (Zhongji)

VICARIOUS MENSTRUATION

The notion of vicarious menstruation refers to hematemesis or nasal bleeding, sometimes excessive, that appears before, during or after menstruation.

From the perspective of Chinese traditional medicine, it is called menstruation in a reverse way, reversed menstruation or vomiting and nasal bleeding at menstruation.

Etiopathogenesis

Three etiopathogenic types are described:

a) Heat in the Liver

b) Dryness injures the Lung vessels

c) Yin deficiency, Heat in the blood

All these circumstances ultimately cause Heat in the blood. Heat in the blood leads it to exteriorize as hematemesis or nasal bleeding. This may be the result of ingesting hot or piquant food with production of endogenous Heat that may turn into Fire or it may be caused by a congenital excess of Yang.

Clinical Manifestations

a) Heat in the Liver

Main symptoms include short menstrual cycles with scanty menstrual flow or, in severe cases, no blood. Before or during menstruation, hematemesis or nasal bleeding appears. Afternoon fever, tinnitus, painful congestion of the eyes, anxiety, restlessness, red lips, a bitter mouth, and thirst are often associated. A red tongue with a yellow coating and a rapid, string-taut pulse may also be present.

b) Dryness Injures the Lung Vessels

Main symptoms include short menstrual cycles with scanty menstrual flow. Hematemesis or nasal bleeding appears before the onset of menstruation. Associated symptoms are dizziness, vision disturbances, dry lips, and a desire to drink. A red tongue with a yellow coating and a rapid pulse are also characteristic.

c) Yin Deficiency, Heat in the Blood

Main symptoms include long or short menstrual cycles associated with hematemesis or nasal bleeding before or during menstruation. Vision disturbances, dizziness, afternoon fever, dry cough, red lips, a hot sensation in the palms and feet, and a dry mouth are associated symptoms, as are a red tongue with a yellow and dry coating and a rapid, fine pulse.

Treatment

a) Heat in the Liver

Therapeutic principle: cool the Liver, disperse the Heat

Prescription:

RM 6 (Qihai)	tones Qi, favors the ascending of Yang
LI 2 (Erjian)	is the Reducing point of the Large Intestine channel, removes pathogenic Heat
LI 4 (Hegu)	is the Yuan point of the Large Intestine channel, removes pathogenic Heat, regulates Qi and blood
SP 10 (Xuehai)	removes Heat from blood, stimulates blood circulation and regulates menstruation
LV 2 (Xingjian)	is the Reducing point of the Liver channel, removes pathogenic Heat from the Liver and cools the blood
ST 29 (Guilai)	regulates Lower Jiao, regulates the uterus

Acupuncture is given with the reducing method.

b) Dryness Injures the Lung Vessels

Therapeutic principle: cool the Dryness, moistening the Lung

Prescription:

L 10 (Yuji)	is the Ying point of the Lung channel, cools the Heat of the Lung
L 11 (Shaoshang)	is the Jing-Well point of the Lung channel, restores the Yang and moistens the Lung
LI 11 (Quchi)	is the Reinforcing point of the Large Intestine channel, regulates Qi and blood, removes pathogenic Heat
K 3 (Taixi)	is the Yuan-Source point of the Kidney channel, supports the Upper Jiao and removes pathogenic Heat from the Lung
SP 6 (Sanyinjiao)	regulates Qi and blood, regulates the circulation within the channel
BL 42 (Pohu)	regulates Lung Qi and acts against the Dryness of the Lung

Acupuncture is given with the reducing method for the points belonging to the Lung and Large Intestine channels and with the reinforcing method for the other points.

c) Yin Deficiency, Heat in the Blood

Therapeutic principle: tone Yin, remove the Heat from blood and disperse the Fire

Prescription:

SP 6 (Sanyinjiao)	is the Crossing point of the three Yin channels of the foot, the Spleen, Liver and Kidney; nourishes the Yin and removes pathogenic Heat
BL 17 (Geshu)	is the Influential point of the blood, regulates blood and stimulates the formation of the body fluids
K 1 (Yongquan)	is the Jing-Well point of the Kidney channel, nourishes the Yin of the Kidney and cools the Heat
K 5 (Shuiquan)	is the Xi point of the Kidney channel, regulates Qi and blood, regulates the Chong Mai and Ren Mai vessels
LI 11 (Quchi)	regulates Qi and blood, removes the pathogenic Heat and stimulates the circulation within the channels
BL 40 (Weizhong)	is the He point of the Urinary Bladder channel and one of the four dominating points, removes pathogenic Heat

Acupuncture is given with the reducing method for LI 11 and BL 40 which should be pricked for bleeding. The reinforcing method is used for the other points.

AMENORRHEA

Amenorrhea is the absence of menstruation, for a period of more than three months, in women who have achieved pubescence and are not pregnant. Amenorrhea can be primary or secondary. Different etiologic circumstances are described: neurogenic causes, pituitary disturbances, psychogenic causes, nutritional factors, endocrinologic disorders (e.g. thyroid and adrenal dysfunction, diabetes), and gonadal factors etc.

From the perspective of Chinese traditional medicine, the causal factors involve both deficiency and excess. These factors affect the "Sea of blood" either by insufficient production of blood or because of disorders of blood circulation.

Etiopathogenesis

a) The Deficiency of Qi and Blood

The Spleen is the source of Qi and blood that, together with the Stomach, nourishes the entire body. Chronic diseases that consume blood (e.g. hematemesis, melena, hemoptysis etc.), overstrain, stress, inadequate food intake or psychological disorders (e.g. worry) can affect the Spleen function of producing blood, resulting in exhaustion and dryness of the "Sea of blood".

b) The Yin Deficiency of the Liver and Kidney

The blood and body fluids are Yin; they can transform into one another and have the same origin.

The Kidney preserves the body fluids (Jing) and the Yin of the Kidney is the foundation of all fluids of the body. Jing deficiency can be constitutional or may be caused by multiparity, sexual abuses, chronic diseases, overstrain or psychological disorders (especially fear) that consume the Yin of the Liver and Kidney. The production of blood is insufficient and the Liver function of storing blood is damaged. As this condition worsens, the deficiency of Yin can produce endogenous Heat.

c) The Stagnation of Qi and Blood

Blood supports the Qi and Qi is the commander of blood and stimulates blood circulation. One of the possible causes of the Liver Qi stagnation is emotional factors disturbance. The Liver function of maintaining the free circulation of Qi is damaged, causing Qi stagnation, and consequently, blood stagnation. The obstructed blood can no longer be evacuated at menstruation and amenorrhea appears.

The stagnation of blood may be the result of exogenous pathogenic factors — Cold and Damp:

- The aggression of pathogenic Cold due to exposure to Cold or Cold-Damp (rain, bath) or to ingestion of food or drinks that produce Cold is favored in circumstances when the resistance of the body is reduced (e.g. during menstruation, in postpartum or postabortum). Cold causes the constriction and obstruction of the vessels, with subsequent blocking of blood circulation within the uterus, and amenorrhea.

- Heat-Damp in the Spleen and Stomach

Heat-Damp can be caused by exogenous invasion, abusive consumption of greasy and sweet food or alcoholic drinks. The retention of Heat-Damp in the Stomach and Spleen affects their functions of receiving, digestion, transforming and transporting. Damp is characterized by clamminess and stagnation. It causes the obstruction and blocking of the Lower Jiao, with disturbances of circulation within the uterus. It may exist as a congenital excess of Phlegm, mostly in obese patients, that invades the Lower Jiao and blocks the circulation in the Chong Mai and Ren Mai Vessels and in the vessels of the uterus, with subsequent onset of amenorrhea.

Clinical Manifestations

a) The Deficiency of Qi and Blood

Main symptoms include progressive onset of amenorrhea, preceded by oligomenorrhea with hypomenorrhea. A dark, withered complexion, depression, apathy, asthenia, dizziness, palpitations, dyspnea, lack of appetite, abdominal distension, and loose stools are associated symptoms as are a pale tongue with a thin or no coating and a weak, forceless or slow and weak pulse.

b) The Yin Deficiency of the Liver and Kidney

Main symptoms include long menstrual cycles with hypomenorrhea and progressive onset of amenorrhea. Associated symptoms are asthenia, lumbar weakness with a sensation of cold and numbness in the shanks and ankles, dizziness, vision disturbances, tinnitus, and a pale complexion and nails. The patient lacks energy and prefers to lie down. A red tongue with a thin coating and a rapid, string-taut pulse may be noted.

c) The Stagnation of Qi and Blood

Main symptoms include amenorrhea with sudden onset, sometimes with small painful blood loss with clots. Restlessness, irritability, anger, distension in the hypochondriac and thoracic regions, and lower abdominal pain aggravated on pressure are associated symptoms as are a red, bluish tongue, or one with purplish spots on borders, and a string-taut, wiry, deep pulse.

- The aggression of Cold

Main symptoms include sudden amenorrhea with lower abdominal pain and a cold and heavy sensation, alleviated by warmth and aggravated by cold. A dark complexion and cold limbs are also characteristic as are a white tongue coating and a string-taut or slow, deep pulse.

- Heat-Damp in the Spleen and Stomach

Main symptoms include amenorrhea, especially in obese patients. A sensation of fullness in the thorax and epigastrium and "bubbles" in the abdomen, asthenia, desire to sleep, loss of appetite with lack of taste, hypersalivation, and nausea may be present. The patient may have a white, thick and moist tongue coating and a sliding pulse.

Treatment

a) The Deficiency of Qi and Blood

Therapeutic principle: tone the Qi, nourish the blood

Prescription:

RM 4 (Guanyuan)	is the Crossing point of the Ren Mai Vessel with the Yin channels of the foot, nourishes and tones Qi and blood, regulates the functions of the Chong Mai and Ren Mai vessels
SP 6 (Sanyinjiao)	supports the function of the Spleen and Stomach, strengthens the Spleen, stimulates Qi and blood circulation, has a generally fortifying effect
ST 36 (Zusanli)	strengthens the Spleen and Stomach, tones Qi and blood
BL 17 (Geshu)	is the Influential point of blood, nourishes the blood
K 13 (Qixue)	is the Crossing point of the Kidney channel with the Chong Mai Vessel, tones the Kidney Qi, regulates the Chong Mai and Ren Mai vessels

Other acupoints that tone the Spleen and nourish the blood can be used in alternative prescriptions:

LV 13 (Zhangmen)	is the Front-Mu point of the Spleen and the Influential point of Zang organs, regulates the organs, tones the Spleen and Stomach
BL 20 (Pishu)	is the Back-Shu point of the Spleen, tones the Spleen functions, supports blood
BL 21 (Weishu)	is the Back-Shu point of the Stomach, tones the Stomach and Spleen, nourishes the blood
RM 12 (Zhongwan)	is the Front-Mu point of the Stomach and the Influential point of the Fu organs, regulates the Stomach and strengthens the Spleen, regulates the Middle Jiao
LI 4 (Hegu)	is the Yuan-Source point of the Large Intestine channel, regulates Qi and blood

Acupuncture is given with the reinforcing method.

b) The Yin Deficiency of the Liver and Kidney

Therapeutic principle: strengthen the Kidney Essence, nourish and tone the Liver and Kidney

Prescription:

RM 4 (Guanyuan)	strengthens the Yin, nourishes and tones Qi and blood
SP 6 (Sanyinjiao)	is the Crossing point of the three Yin channels of the foot, tones the Liver and Kidney
BL 23 (Shenshu)	is the Back-Shu point of the Kidney, nourishes the Yin and strengthens the Yang, tones Kidney Qi
BL 18 (Ganshu)	is the Back-Shu point of the Liver, tones Liver Qi, regulates blood
RM 7 (YinJiao)	is the Crossing point of the Chong Mai and Ren Mai vessels and the Front-Mu point of Lower Jiao, regulates the circulation within the Chong Mai and Ren Mai vessels and regulates menstruation

Stimulation with the reinforcing method is used, with acupuncture or moxibustion.

In severe cases with Yin deficiency caused by an excess of internal Heat, other points can be added in different prescriptions:

SP 1 (Yinbai)	is the Jing-Well point of the Spleen channel, strengthens the Spleen, supports the Qi and stimulates blood circulation
K 7 (Fuliu)	is the Jing-River point of the Kidney channel, strengthens the Kidney, stimulates the draining of Lower Jiao
K 8 (Jiaoxin)	is the Xi point of the Kidney channel, tones the Kidney, regulates the Chong Mai and Ren Mai vessels, regulates Qi and blood
H 6 (Yinxi)	is the Xi point of the Heart channel, regulates the Heart, removes pathogenic Heat from the blood, cools the blood, reduces sweating
SP 10 (Xuehai)	nourishes the blood and cools the Heat from the blood
L 7 (Lieque)	is the Luo point of the Lung channel, strengthens the Lung function and calms the cough
BL 13 (Feishu)	is the Back-Shu point of the Lung, strengthens the Lung Qi, calms the cough

c) The Stagnation of Qi and Blood

Therapeutic principle: regulate Qi, stimulate blood and remove stagnation

Prescription:

RM 3 (Zhongji)	is the Crossing point of the Ren Mai with the Spleen, Kidney and Liver channels; regulates the uterus and removes the stagnation of blood
SP 6 (Sanyinjiao)	regulates Qi and blood, removes the channels obstruction and stimulates free circulation of Qi
SP 10 (Xuehai)	regulates the circulation of blood, regulates menstruation

LV 3 (Taichong)	is the Yuan-Source point of the Liver channel, regulates the Liver Qi, stimulates Qi and blood circulation, removes stagnation
LV 8 (Ququan)	is the Reinforcing point of the Liver channel, removes Qi stagnation, regulates Qi and blood
ST 30 (Qichong)	is the Crossing point of the Stomach channel with Chong Mai Vessel, restores Qi circulation, regulates the blood removing the stagnation, regulates the uterus
PC 5 (Jianshi)	is the Jing-River point of the Pericardium channel, nourishes the Heart and calms the mind, stimulates Qi circulation. It is especially indicated for this type of amenorrhea

Acupuncture is given with the reducing method, in daily sessions, starting 4 to 5 days before the presumed date of menstruation and lasting until another 4 to 5 days after that date. The duration of a session is of approximately 15 to 20 minutes.

Other supplementary points, related to the symptoms, can be included in alternative prescriptions:

- for distension in the hypogastric region and flanks:

| **LV 14** (Qimen) | is the Front-Mu point of the Liver, removes Liver Qi stagnation, stimulates blood or |
| **LV 6** (Zhongdu) | is the Xi point of the Liver channel, removes the Liver Qi stagnation, stimulates blood circulation |

- for psychological disorders (e.g. insomnia, irritability):

| **PC 6** (Neiguan) | is the Luo point of the Pericardium channel, nourishes the Heart and sedates the mind |
| **H 7** (Shenmen) | is the Yuan-Source point of the Heart channel, calms the Heart and mind |

E.P. Anmian for treating insomnia

- for blood stagnation

| **SP 8** (Diji) | is the Xi point of the Spleen channel, regulates the blood and removes stagnation |
| **LI 4** (Hegu) | is the Yuan-Source point of the Large Intestine channel, regulates Qi and blood |

ST 29 (Guilai)   cools Lower Jiao, removes blood stagnation, regulates the uterus

- The aggression of Cold

Therapeutic principle: warm the channels, support the circulation of blood

Prescription:

RM 5 (Shimen)   warms the Kidney, strengthens the Yang, regulates menstruation

RM 8 (Shenque)   warms the Kidney Yang, controls Cold and removes stagnation

ST 36 (Zusanli)   stimulates Qi and blood circulation, has a generally fortifying effect

LI 4 (Hegu)   regulates Qi and blood

SP 10 (Xuehai)   regulates menstruation in cases of blood stagnation due to Cold

Other points can be used in alternative prescription:

RM 4 (Guanyuan)   warms the Kidney, tones Qi and regulates the uterus

LV 8 (Ququan)   is the He point of the Liver channel, regulates Qi and blood and removes stagnation

Acupuncture is given with the reinforcing method and moxibustion is used for the points located on the Ren Mai Vessel. For RM 8, use moxa with salt.

- Damp-Heat in the Spleen and Stomach

Therapeutic principle: remove perverse Damp and Phlegm

Prescription:

RM 3 (Zhongji)   regulates menstruation, regulates Lower Jiao, removes pathogenic Heat and Damp

SP 9 (Yinlingquan)   is the He point of the Spleen channel, strengthens the Spleen and removes pathogenic Heat, stimulates circulation within Lower Jiao

BL 20 (Pishu)   is the Back-Shu point of the Spleen, tones the Spleen function for removing Damp

BL 28 (Pangguangshu) is the Back-Shu point of the Urinary Bladder, cools and drains Lower Jiao and regulates the fluids pathway

Other points can be used in alternative prescriptions:

RM 6 (Qihai)   tones Qi, regulates Qi and blood circulation

SP 6 (Sanyinjiao)   regulates Qi and blood, regulates the channels and collaterals, strengthens the Spleen and removes Damp

ST 40 (Fenglong)   is the Luo point of the Stomach channel, removes Damp and Heat.

Usually the treatment begins 3 to 4 days before the presumed date of menstruation and lasts for another 3 to 4 days after that date; one cure monthly, for 2 to 3 months. Each daily session is approximately 15 to 30 minutes in duration, using the reducing or reinforcing method to stimulate the selected acupoints, relative to the needs of each individual, every 5 to 15 minutes.

Auricular Therapy: points Uterus, Ovary, Hormones, Kidney, Adrenals. The stimulation is moderate, the needles are left in place for 20 minutes. One session is conducted daily, a week before and after menstruation.

THE MENOPAUSE

Menopause is the central element of the climacteric and corresponds to ceasing of the menstrual function due to the exhaustion of ovarian follicles. The definitive disappearance of menstruation is a physiologic phenomenon.

Clinically the exhaustion of ovarian follicles causes the disappearance of ovulation and definitive infertility. The cessation of the ovarian activity causes the disappearance of the feedback mechanisms, leading to a significant increase in the gonadotrophin level .

Initially, the symptoms are caused by a relative estrogen excess during perimenopause that progresses toward the estrogenous privation of menopause:

- disorders of menstrual cycle: abnormal uterine bleeding or amenorrhea
- psychological symptoms: irritability, insomnia, vertigo, anxiety,

fluctuations of mood, depression, lack of memory
- vasomotor symptoms: hot flushes
- genitourinary atrophy: causing dyspareunia, atrophic vaginitis, urethritis, urinary incontinence

The major risk of complications concerns the bones (osteoporosis) and the cardiovascular system. The treatment consists of hormonal replacement therapy and symptom-relieving drugs.

In Chinese traditional medicine, certain manifestations are recognized:
- menstrual cycle disorders
- vertigo, vision disturbances
- palpitations etc.

Su Wen (Chap.1) states the conditions of the menopause onset: the progressive decrease of the Kidney Qi, the deficiency of the Ren Mai and Chong Mai vessels and the exhaustion of sexual energy.

The lack of balance between the Yin and Yang has repercussions for the body resistance and the emotional factors.

The main deficiency is that of the Kidney Qi:
- the deficiency of Kidney Yang can cause an excess of Yin affecting the Spleen
- the deficiency of the Kidney Yin can cause an excess of Yang of the Liver or Heart

Etiopathogenesis

a) The Yin Deficiency of the Liver and Kidney

The Yin blood can be affected by severe emotional disorders, overstrain or stress and chronic diseases that consume the Yin of the Liver and Kidney. The head and eyes are not nourished and the deficiency of Yin can produce internal Heat. This conditions may result in damage to the Chong Mai and Ren Mai Vessels.

b) Disharmony Between the Heart and Kidney

This lack of balance is caused by chronic diseases, overstrain, stress, and excessive sexual activity that can affect the Yin of the Heart and Kidney. It can also be caused by severe emotional disorders that obstruct

Qi, which can turn into Fire. The Fire of the Heart can become hyperactive in the upper part of the body because Fire, as a Yang pathogenic factor, is characterized by ascending movement. The result is a lack of balance between the Heart and Kidney, disturbing the regulation of Water and Fire, and consuming the Kidney Essence causing a deficiency of the "Sea of Marrow".

c) The Yang Deficiency of the Spleen and Kidney

Yang deficiency results from chronic diseases that consume the Qi and damage the Spleen Yang and the Kidney. This may also be caused by the deficiency of the Kidney Yang and subsequent damage of the Spleen. The body is not warmed and the digestion, transporting and transforming functions will be damaged, including the transporting and transforming of the body fluids.

d) The Deficiency of the Kidney

The Kidney deficiency can be global or can affect only the Yin or the Yang of the Kidney. Long Shu (Chap. 65) mentions that the deficiency of the Kidney Yin is much more important than the deficiency of the Kidney Yang.

The causal factors can include: constitutional deficiency, chronic diseases, excessive sexual activity, or weakness of the Kidney at old ages.

In cases with deficiency of the Kidney Yang, the warming function of Yang is damaged and the nourishment of the bones, brain, ears and marrow is deficient. The reproductive function is damaged and infertility appears.

The deficiency of the Kidney Yang causes the deficiency of the Yang Spleen with the loss of Heat from the vessels and production of internal Cold with specific symptoms.

The deficiency of the Kidney Yin affects the Kidney functions of forming the marrow, dominating the bones and nourishing the brain.

The deficient Yin will cause an excess of Yang with the production of internal Heat and symptoms of excess type. The Yin of the Liver can no longer control the Yang of the Liver which ascends and the Yang of the Heart will be excessive.

Clinical Manifestations

a) The Yin Deficiency of the Liver and Kidney

Main symptoms include a flushed face, a wave-like depression, anxiety, irritability, nervousness, insomnia, memory disorders, headache, tinnitus, dizziness, vision disturbances, and a sensation of weakness in the knees and lumbar area. When there is an excess of Yang the following symptoms may also be present: a sensation of heat in the palms, feet and precardiac region; scanty menstrual blood loss, light or dark colored blood; a red tongue with a thin coating; and a rapid, thready pulse.

b) Disharmony Between Heart and Kidney

Main symptoms include insomnia, palpitations, memory disorders, depression, easy crying, dizziness, tinnitus, dry mouth, and sudden sweating. Lumbar pain, scanty menstrual flow, a red tongue with a thin coating, and a deep, rapid and thready pulse may also be noted.

c) The Yang Deficiency of the Spleen and Kidney

Main symptoms include apathy; lack of appetite; pallor; cold extremities; aversion to cold; edema of the face and lower limbs; a sensation of weakness in the knees and lumbar area; possible excessive menstrual flow, with light colored blood; loose stools and pollakiuria. A pale, swollen tongue with a thin coating and a deep, weak pulse may be recorded.

d) The Deficiency of the Kidney

Main symptoms include dizziness, headache, lumbar weakness sensation, pollakiuria, clear and white leukorrhea, a pale tongue with a thin coating and a weak, thready pulse.

With deficiency of the Kidney Yin, signs of Yang excess are: nervousness, hot flushes, dry mouth, dizziness, palpitations, hypertension, tinnitus, menstrual flow with dark colored blood, a red tongue with a thin coating and a rapid and thready pulse.

With deficiency of the Kidney Yang, signs of internal Cold can be observed: pallor, cold extremities, abdominal pain and cold sensation, apathy, aversion to cold, edema, pollakiuria, possible menstrual flow with light colored blood, a pale tongue with a white coating and a deep, weak pulse.

Treatment

a) The Yin Deficiency of the Liver and Kidney

Therapeutic principle: nourish the blood and Yin of the Liver and Kidney

Prescription:

BL 23 (Shenshu)	is the Back-Shu point of the Kidney, tones the Kidney, nourishes the Yin, strengthens the brain and marrow
BL 18 (Ganshu)	is the Back-Shu point of the Liver, regulates the Liver and Gall Bladder, removes pathogenic Heat, stimulates the brain and improves visual activity
SP 6 (Sanyinjiao)	is the Crossing point of the three Yin channels of the foot, the Liver, Kidney and Spleen, nourishes the Yin of the Liver and Kidney, regulates Qi and blood
LV 3 (Taichong)	is the Yuan-Source point of the Liver channel, strengthens the Liver, regulates Qi and blood circulation
K 3 (Taixi)	is the Yuan-Source point of the Kidney channel, nourishes the Kidney and Liver, regulates the Chong Mai and Ren Mai vessels
H 7 (Shenmen)	is the Yuan-Source point of the Heart channel, calms the Heart and mind

Acupuncture is given with the reducing or reinforcing method according to the symptoms and selected points.

b) Disharmony Between Heart and Kidney

Therapeutic principle: favor the balance between the Heart and Kidney to strengthen the Yin and blood, calm the mind

Prescription:

BL 15 (Xinshu)	is the Back-Shu point of the Heart channel, nourishes the blood and calms the mind
BL 23 (Shenshu)	is the Back-Shu point of the Kidney channel, tones the Kidney, nourishes the Yin

PC 6 (Neiguan)   is the Luo point of the Pericardium channel, nourishes the Heart and calms the mind

BL 17 (Geshu)   is the Influential point of the blood, nourishes the blood, regulates the Spleen-Stomach couple

K 2 (Rangu)   is the Ying point of the Kidney channel, nourishes the Kidney Yin, cools the Heat

BL 43 (Gaohuangshu)stimulates Qi functions, tones the Kidney, strengthens the Spleen and regulates the Stomach, calms the Heart and mind

Other points can also be used:

H 7 (Shenmen)   is the Yuan-Source point of the Heart channel, calms the Heart and mind

DM 20 (Baihui)   is the Crossing point of the Yang channels with the Du Mai Vessel, cools the brain and calms the mind

Acupuncture is given with the even movement method.

c) The Yang Deficiency of the Spleen and Kidney

Therapeutic principle: warm and tone Kidney Yang, tone the Spleen to remove Damp

Prescription:

SP 6 (Sanyinjiao)   tones the Spleen

BL 20 (Pishu)   is the Back-Shu point of the Spleen, tones the Spleen and removes pathogenic Damp

BL 23 (Shenshu)   is the Back-Shu point of the Kidney, strengthens the Yang, tones the Kidney Yang

DM 4 (Mingmen)   strengthens the Yang, regulates Qi

RM 4 (Guanyuan)   restores the Yang, stimulates Qi and blood circulation, regulates the Chong Mai and Ren Mai Vessels

The stimulation with the reinforcing method uses acupuncture and moxibustion.

d) The Deficiency of the Kidney

Therapeutic principle: tone the Kidney, regulate the Chong Mai and Ren Mai Vessels

Prescription:

BL 23 (Shenshu)	is the Back-Shu point of the Kidney, tones the Kidney
K 3 (Taixi)	is the Yuan-Source point of the Kidney channel, tones the Kidney Qi, regulates Chong Mai and Ren Mai Vessels
RM 4 (Guanyuan)	is the Crossing point of the Ren Mai Vessel with the Kidney channel, strengthens the Kidney, regulates the Ren Mai and Chong Mai Vessels, regulates Qi and blood
K 7 (Fuliu)	is the Jing-River point of the Kidney channel, nourishes the Kidney, strengthens the lumbar regions

Depending upon the type of deficiency, other points can be added:
- The deficiency of the Kidney Yin

Therapeutic principle: tone Kidney Yin, control the Yang of the Liver, soothe the Heart

Prescription:

K 1 (Yongquan)	is the Jing-Well point of the Kidney channel, nourishes the Yin
K 2 (Rangu)	is the Ying point of the Kidney channel, nourishes the Yin and removes pathogenic Heat
SP 6 (Sanyinjiao)	is the Crossing point of the three Yin channels of the foot, strengthens the Kidney, regulates Qi and blood
H 7 (Shenmen)	is the Yuan-Source point of the Heart channel, soothes the Heart and mind
BL 5 (Wushu)	calms the Yang of the Liver, removes internal Heat, calms the mind

- The deficiency of the Kidney Yang

Therapeutic principle: tone the Yang, warm the Kidney, tone the Spleen

Prescription:

RM 3 (Zhongji)	strengthens the original Yang, can spread the Cold from the uterus, regulates menstruation
RM 8 (Shenque)	tones the Yang, regulates the circulation of the Yang of the Kidney
BL 29 (Zhonglushu)	warms the Yang and removes Cold, strengthens the lumbar region
RM 2 (Qugu)	strengthens the Yang of the Kidney, warms the Yang

Acupuncture is given with the reinforcing method. Moxibustion can be used—moxa with salt for RM 8.

Symptomatic Treatment

In cases with clinical manifestations that are hard to systematize and, depending upon the etiopathogenic type, one can begin with a symptomatic treatment.

Hot Flushes

a) **LV 8** (Ququan) + **SP 9** (Yinlingquan) + **PC 3** (Quze) + **SJ 10** (Tianjing)

b) **K 7** (Fuliu) + **BL 23** (Shenshu) + **PC 9** (Zhongchong) + **ST 34** (Liangqiu) + **BL 67** (Kunlun)

c) **SP 4** (Gongsun) + **RM 22** (Tiantu) + **LV 5** (Ligou) + **DM 3** (Yaoyangquan) + **DM 4** (Mingmen)

d) **LV 14** (Qimen) + **SP 6** (Sanyinjiao) + **BL 20** (Pishu)

e) **LV 1** (Dadun) + **RM 6** (Qihai) + **H 7** (Shenmen) + **K 2** (Rangu) + **SI 3** (Houxi) + **K 7** (Fuliu)

The acupuncture sessions are weekly, each lasting for approximately 15 minutes and strong stimulation of the selected points is given.

Psychical Disorders

- anxiety

a) **BL 20** (Pishu) + **LV 13** (Zhangmen) + **RM 17** (Shanzhong)

b) **PC 7** (Daling) + **PC 6** (Neiguan) + **SI 3** (Houxi) + **RM 12** (Zhongwan)

- irritability

a) **LV 2** (Xingjian) + **LV 3** (Taichong) + **LV 14** (Qimen) + **BL 20** (Pishu)

b) **GB 38** (Yangfu) + **L 1** (Zhongfu) + **H 9** (Shaochong) + **SI 4** (Wangu) + **L 7** (Lieque)

- insomnia

a) **K 6** (Zhaohai) + **BL 62** (Shenmai) + **SP 9** (Yinlingquan) + **SP 6** (Sanyinjiao) + **RM 15** (Jiuwei)

b) **PC 6** (Neiguan) + **L 7** (Lieque) + **SP 4** (Gongsun) + **SP 6** (Sanyinjiao)

Constipation

a) **GB 34** (Yanglingquan) + **SI 3** (Houxi) + **SI 2** (Qiangu) + **LV 3** (Taichong) + **LV 2** (Xingjian)

b) **BL 25** (Dachangshu) + **ST 25** (Tianshu) + **SJ 6** (Zhigou) + **K 6** (Zhaohai) + **RM 12** (Zhongwan) + **LV 3** (Taichong)

Palpitations

BL 15 (Xinshu) + **RM 14** (Juque) + **H 7** (Shenmen) + **PC 6** (Neiguan)

Other points can be added:

- in the deficiency of the Spleen and Heart

BL 20 (Pishu), **BL 21** (Weishu), **ST 36** (Zusanli)

- in the deficiency of Yin with excessive Fire

BL 14 (Jueyinshu), **BL 23** (Shenshu), **K 3** (Taixi)

Vertigo

BL 65 (Shugu) + **BL 2** (Zanzhu) + **LI 4** (Hegu)

Sweating

a) **LI 4** (Hegu) + **K 2** (Rangu) + **K 7** (Fuliu)

b) **K 2** (Rangu) + **SJ 5** (Waiguan) + **BL 17** (Geshu)

Memory Disorders

BL 15 (Xinshu) + **BL 20** (Pishu) + **ST 36** (Zusanli) + **BL 23** (Shenshu) + **K 6** (Zhaohai) + **E.P.** Sishecong

LEUKORRHEA

The term leukorrhea refers to persistent vaginal discharge caused by pathological transforming of the vaginal contents.

Leukorrhea is a frequent clinical manifestation in the inflammatory diseases of the genital tract: vaginitis, cervicitis, endometritis, salpingitis etc.

From the perspective of Chinese traditional medicine, the notion of "Dai Xia" refers, in particular, to "a mucous, filamentous vaginal discharge" and was mentioned for the first time in Su Wen (Chap.60): "If Ren Mai is deficient there is leukorrhea (Dai Xia) and masses (Jia Fu) ... in women."

Seven types of leukorrhea are described, differentiated by color:
- Bai Dai is an excessive, white, fluid, glue-like discharge
- Chi Dai is a red, filamentous discharge
- Chi Bai Dai, is white with a red hue and filamentous
- Qing Dai is a greenish-blue, malodorous discharge
- Huang Dai is a yellowish, mucous, filamentous discharge
- Hei Dai is a "dark," clammy discharge, with an odor of tainted fish
- Wu Se Dai is a malodorous discharge, varied in color.

Etiopathogenesis

It is believed that "Dai Xia" is caused by damage to the Extraordinary Vessels Ren Mai and Du Mai, and weakness of the Dai Mai Vessel, involving the Spleen, Liver and Kidney.

Usually five etiopathogenic conditions are described:

a) The Deficiency of the Spleen Qi

This condition derives from inadequate food intake, with excessive consumption of raw, cold, sweet food or cold drinks that may weaken the Qi of the Middle Jiao. Overstrain and stress can be associated. All of these factors affect the Spleen function of transforming and transporting. The Spleen cannot control fluid distribution and endogenous Damp forms. Damp is heavy and has a tendency to descend, accumulating in the Lower Jiao and injuring the Ren Mai Vessel, resulting in leukorrhea.

b) The Stagnation of the Liver Qi

Emotional factors disorders are the prevalent element causing stagnation of the Liver Qi. The Qi congestion is maximum in the week that precedes menstruation, characterized by an increase of Yang and, consequently, an excess of internal Heat. The stagnant Liver Qi can also turn into Heat during this period.

The Liver and Spleen are closely related according to the dominating and counter-dominating cycles: the excess of the Liver will cause Spleen deficiency and the deficient Spleen favors the excess of the Liver. The association of Heat with endogenous Damp forms Damp-Heat that accumulates in the Lower Jiao causing leukorrhea.

These two pathogenic circumstances, the Spleen deficiency and the Liver stagnation are frequently associated.

c) Phlegm-Damp Accumulation

The excess of Phlegm-Damp can be constitutional in obese women. It becomes a pathogenic factor, as Phlegm accumulates in the Lower Jiao and forms abundant leukorrhea. Usually a congenital deficiency of the Spleen Qi is involved or it is compounded by the stagnation of the Liver Qi and/or the deficiency of the Spleen.

d) The Excess of Damp-Heat

Exogenous pathogenic Damp and Heat can enter into the body in conditions such as pregnancy, delivery, abortion, or uterine curettage, when the Ren Mai and Chong Mai vessels are weakened. Their excess can block the Dai Mai Vessel and affect the Spleen function with sinking of the Spleen Qi. Transforming and distribution within the body are deficient, the descending of Damp-Heat injures the Ren Mai and Dai Mai Vessels, and leukorrhea appears.

The exogenous excess of Damp-Heat can be favored by a diet rich in shellfish, shrimp, lobster or chicken.

e) The Deficiency of the Kidney Yang

The Kidney deficiency can be congenital or may be caused by chronic disease, sexual abuses, premature marriage, multiparity, or overstrain.

If the Kidney Yang is deficient, the control function of the Dai Mai Vessel is damaged. The Ren Mai Vessel loses its ability to consolidate and becomes incapable of transforming fluids, which are then eliminated as leukorrhea.

Clinical Manifestations

a) The Deficiency of the Spleen Qi

Main symptoms include a white, watery, odorless, saliva-like leukorrhea. Associated symptoms include pallor, asthenia, cold limbs, lack of appetite, loose stools, clear and abundant urine, a pale tongue with a white coating and a weak, slow pulse.

b) The Stagnation of the Liver Qi

Main symptoms include a white, thick, persistent leukorrhea accompanied by an irregular menstrual cycle and dysmenorrhea. Associated symptoms are depression, a sensation of fullness in the thorax, painful distension in the hypochondriac region, a yellowish complexion, constipation, a white tongue coating and a wiry pulse.

The thick consistency of this type of leukorrhea usually identifies it as Candidiasis leukorrhea.

The association of Heat gives a red hue to leukorrhea. It is sanguinolent and malodorous. Additional symptoms include a dry mouth, bitter taste, irritability, dizziness, palpitations, a red tongue with a yellow coating and a wiry pulse.

c) Phlegm-Damp Accumulation

Main symptoms include abundant, mucous, dense, persistent leukorrhea, usually in obese women. Asthenia, a sensation of heaviness in the head, thoracic oppression, tachypnea, abdominal distension or the appearance of tumoral masses, a moist, thick tongue coating and a sliding pulse are associated symptoms.

d) The Excess of Damp-Heat

Main symptoms include abundant, thick, yellow or reddish, extremely malodorous leukorrhea. Also characteristic of this condition are asthenia, anxiety and restlessness, insomnia, a sensation of heaviness in the head, thirst without desire to drink, hematuria, a moist, yellow tongue coating and a superficial, small and rapid pulse.

e) The Deficiency of the Kidney Yang

Main symptoms include a clear, white, watery, abundant, persistent, glue-like leukorrhea. Associated symptoms are pallor, a cold body, a sensation of cold and compression in the lower abdomen, lumbar pain, weakness of the knees, polyuria with diluted urine, loose stools, a pale tongue with a white coating, and a thready pulse. This type of leukorrhea is similar to that described as Bai Ying.

Treatment

In acute cases, and those of excess type, the treatment consists of frequent sessions, 1 to 2 daily with long duration and a short course of treatment. For chronic cases, and those of deficiency type, 1 to 2 sessions are conducted weekly and the course of treatment is typically long.

Regardless of the etiopathogenic type, each prescription involves certain major points:

GB 26 (Daimai)	is the Crossing point of the Dai Mai Vessel with the Gall Bladder channel, regulates the Dai Mai Vessel and is particularly effective in the treatment of leukorrhea
RM 6 (Qihai)	regulates Qi circulation, balances the Ren Mai Vessel and stimulates the Qi to transport and transform fluids
SP 6 (Sanyinjiao)	is the Crossing point of the three Yin channels of the foot, the Kidney, Liver and Spleen; tones the Spleen and Kidney; removes Damp

Secondary points are added, based upon the etiopathogenic type:

a) The Deficiency of the Spleen Qi

Therapeutic principle: tone the Spleen to remove Damp, regulate Ren Mai and Dai Mai Vessels

Prescription:

BL 20 (Pishu)	is the Back-Shu point of the Spleen, tones the Spleen Qi, favors the removal of Damp
SP 9 (Yinlingquan)	strengthens the Spleen and removes Damp, favors the circulation in Lower Jiao
ST 36 (Zusanli)	is the He point of the Stomach channel, regu-

lates the Stomach and tones the Spleen, regulates Qi and blood

Other points can also be used to strengthen the Spleen and remove Damp:

SP 8 (Diji)	is the Xi point of the Spleen channel, tones the Spleen
ST 25 (Tianshu)	regulates the Stomach, strengthens the Spleen to remove Damp
RM 12 (Zhongwan)	is the Front-Mu point of the Stomach and the Influential point of the Fu organs, regulates the Stomach, strengthens the Spleen and removes Damp

Acupuncture is given with the reinforcing method. For a strong stimulation, moxibustion can also be used.

b) The Stagnation of the Liver Qi

Therapeutic principle: disperse the stagnation of the Liver Qi, cool the Heat and remove Damp

Prescription:

LV 3 (Taichong)	is the Yuan-Source point of the Liver channel, removes Liver Qi stagnation, regulates Qi circulation and removes Damp
LV 6 (Zhongdu)	is the Xi point of the Liver channel, reduces Liver Fire
LV 2 (Xingjian)	is the reducing point of the Liver channel, reduces Liver Fire
SJ 6 (Zhigou)	is the Jing-River point of the San Jiao channel, regulates Qi in the San Jiao channel, regulates the Zang-Fu organs
BL 18 (Ganshu)	is the Back-Shu point of the Liver, removes Liver Qi stagnation

When the stagnation of the Liver Qi is accompanied by internal Damp-Heat formation, other points can be added:

LV 5 (Ligou)	is the Luo point of the Liver channel, spreads pathogenic Heat and Damp, removes Fire

from Lower Jiao or

LV 8 (Ququan)   is Reinforcing point of the Liver channel and blood and cools Damp-Heat

RM 3 (Zhongji)   regulates Lower Jiao to eliminate Damp-Heat

The reducing method is used to stimulate the selected acupoints.

c) *Phlegm-Damp Accumulation*

Therapeutic principle: tone the Spleen, disperse Damp and remove Phlegm

Prescription:

ST 40 (Fenglong)   is the Luo point of the Stomach channel, regulates the Stomach and removes Phlegm

ST 25 (Tianshu)   regulates the Stomach, regulates Qi, strengthens the Spleen for transforming Damp

RM 12 (Zhongwan)   is the Front-Mu point of the Stomach, strengthens the Spleen and removes Damp

d) *The Excess of Damp-Heat*

Therapeutic principle: disperse Heat, remove Damp and relieve Lower Jiao

Prescription:

RM 3 (Zhongji)   is the Crossing point of the Ren Mai Vessel with the Spleen, Liver and Kidney channels; removes pathogenic Damp and Heat from Lower Jiao

LV 3 (Taichong)   is the Yuan-Source point of the Liver channel, regulates Qi circulation, resolves Damp and Heat

SP 9 (Yinlingquan)   is the He point of the Spleen channel, tones the Spleen to remove Damp, favors the circulation within the San Jiao

ST 29 (Guilai)   cools Lower Jiao

In cases of leukorrhea caused by Damp-Heat, acupuncture is given with the reducing method, with strong stimulation, and the needles are left in place for approximately an hour. One to two sessions are conducted daily until acute symptoms alleviate.

e) The Deficiency of the Kidney Yang

Therapeutic principle: stimulate the Yang, tone the Kidney, regulate the Chong Mai and Ren Mai vessels

Prescription:

BL 23 (Shenshu)	is the Back-Shu point of the Kidney, strengthens the Yang of the Kidney, tones the lumbar region
K 7 (Fuliu)	nourishes the Kidney, favors the draining of the Lower Jiao
RM 4 (Guanyuan)	is the Crossing point of the Ren Mai Vessel with the three Yin channels of the foot, tones Qi, warms the Kidney, favors the Yang, regulates the Ren Mai and Dai Mai vessels
DM 4 (Mingmen)	restores the original Qi and tones the Yang of the Kidney

Strong stimulation is given and moxibustion is used for BL 23, RM 4 and DM 4.

VULVAR PRURITUS

A frequent symptom, vulvar pruritus or vaginitis may or may not be accompanied by leukorrhea.

Chinese traditional medicine addresses vulvar pruritus and three etiopathogenic types are differentiated:

Etiopathogenesis

a) Excessive Damp-Heat

Damp-Heat formation is closely related to Spleen deficiency and Liver stagnation. Being a pathogenic factor characterized by heaviness and descending movement, Damp-Heat will accumulate in the Lower Jiao producing leukorrhea and vulvar pruritus.

b) The Deficiency of the Kidney Yin

Chronic diseases, excessive sexual activity, feverish conditions in late stages, and the aging process can all consume the Kidney Yin. Typically, pruritus appears or is aggravated after menstruation, when the blood from the Chong Mai Vessel is weakened and causes a Yin deficiency of the whole body. The deficiency of Yin will produce internal Heat and symptoms of excess will appear.

c) Heat in the Blood

The Heat may be a consequence of the aggression of exogenous Heat, intake of piquant food, hot drinks, or alcohol. It may also be endogenous, caused by a constitutional excess of Yang, by Liver Qi stagnation that turns into Fire, or by the deficiency of the Yin body fluids in old age.

Because the insufficient Yin cannot lubricate and nourish the skin, mucous membranes, and orifices (vaginal and vulvar), Heat will produce dryness and pruritus.

Clinical Manifestations

a) Excessive Damp-Heat

Main symptoms include abundant, thick, clammy, yellowish, malodorous leukorrhea, and genital pruritus. Associated symptoms include nervousness, bitter taste, dry mouth, thirst, sometimes pollakiuria and urgent urination with a urethral burning sensation, and constipation. The patient may have a red tongue with yellow, thick coating and a rapid, wiry pulse.

b) The Deficiency of the Kidney Yin

Main symptoms include vaginal pruritus without leukorrhea, asthenia, anxiety or restlessness, nocturnal sweating, insomnia, palpitations, and dizziness. A sensation of weakness in the knees and lumbar area; a sensation of heat in the chest, palms and feet; dry skin; nocturia; scanty menstrual flow; bleeding gums; a red tongue with a scanty yellow coating, or a cracked tongue; and a rapid, thready pulse are associated symptoms.

This type of vaginitis can be observed in women after total hysterectomy, in menopause, or in cases without hormonal replacement therapy.

c) Heat in the Blood

Main symptoms include pruritus and a vaginal burning sensation, congestion of the vaginal mucous, and rough and dry skin, with lesions. Irritability, insomnia, a sensation of thoracic fullness, dry mouth, thirst with no desire to drink, a dark red tongue, and a rapid pulse are also characteristic.

Treatment

a) Excessive Damp-Heat

Therapeutic principle: remove Damp, cool the Heat

Prescription:

RM 3 (Zhongji)	is the Front-Mu point of the Urinary Bladder, stimulates blood circulation, regulates Lower Jiao and removes Damp
LV 5 (Ligou)	is the Luo point of the Liver channel, removes Liver Qi stagnation, removes Damp-Heat from the channel
LV 8 (Ququan)	is the He point of the Liver channel, regulates Qi and blood, disperses Heat and Damp
SP 6 (Sanyinjiao)	is the Crossing point of the three Yin channels of the foot, strengthens the Spleen, removes Damp and disperses Liver Fire
BL 54 (Zhibian)	regulates Lower Jiao, cools Damp Heat
LI 11 (Quchi)	is the He point of the Large Intestine channel, regulates Qi and blood, removes Damp and cools the Heat

Acupuncture is given with the reducing method, stimulating 2 to 3 acupoints together with one of the main points, either LV 5 or LV 8. Depending upon the severity of the symptoms, 1-2 sessions may be conducted daily.

b) The Deficiency of the Kidney Yin

Therapeutic principle: nourish the Yin, tone the Kidney

Prescription:

SP 6 (Sanyinjiao)	is the Crossing point of the Yin channels of the foot—the Kidney, Spleen and Liver; tones the Kidney and Spleen; regulates Qi and blood
K 3 (Taixi)	is the Yuan-Source point of the Kidney channel, tones the Kidney, nourishes the Liver, regulates the Chong Mai and Ren Mai vessels
LV 3 (Taichong)	is the Yuan-Source point of the Liver channel, regulates the Liver that stores the blood

| **K 2** (Rangu) | nourishes the Yin of the Kidney, regulates Lower Jiao, cools the Heat |

Other points located on the Kidney channel can also be used as follows:

| **K 10** (Yingu) | is the He point of the Kidney channel, nourishes the Kidney and disperses pathogenic Heat |
| **K 11** (Henggu) | is the Crossing point of the Kidney channel with the Chong Mai Vessel and is the local point for the treatment of external genital pain |

Acupuncture is given with the reinforcing method.

c) *Heat in the Blood*

Therapeutic principle: cool the blood and remove Heat

Prescription:

RM 1 (Huiyin)	is the Crossing point of the Ren Mai, the Du Mai and the Chong Mai vessels, regulates Chong Mai and Ren Mai, removes Heat, is an efficient point for genital pruritus
LV 11 (Yinlian)	stimulates blood circulation, regulates the Chong Mai and Ren Mai vessels, regulates blood and nourishes the uterus, is indicated for the treatment of genital pruritus
LV 8 (Ququan)	is the He point of the Liver channel, disperses and cools the Heat from the Liver channel

The acupoints located on the Liver channel are effective in the treatment of vulvar pruritus because the course of the channel is in the area of the external genitalia.

| **SP 10** (Xuehai) | cools the Heat from blood and stops the pruritus |

Acupuncture is given with the reducing method, one session daily. Treatments of 10 sessions each can be done, repeated at 3 day intervals, if necessary.

Auricular Therapy: points Ovary, Endocrine, Shenmen, External genitalia. Usually two auricular points are selected and moderate stimulation is given. The needles are left in place for approximately 15 to 20 minutes.

ACUTE ENDOMETRITIS

An acute and rare chronic uterine infection, endometritis is caused by bacterial aggression against the endometrium. Circumstances favoring development of the infection include pregnancy and postpartum, abortion or obstetrical maneuvers, local trauma, malnutrition, metabolic or consumptive diseases, and endocrine deficiencies etc. The clinical manifestations include fever; excessive, pus-filled and frequently malodorous uterine discharge, with uterine pain. The therapy consists of antibiotics and symptom-relieving medications.

From the perspective of Chinese traditional medicine, the onset of endometritis is determined by the aggression of exogenous pathogenic factors and the deficiency of certain Zang-Fu organs.

Etiopathogenesis

a) The Aggression of Damp-Heat

Exogenous pathogenic Damp is characterized by viscosity and stagnation. Damp can produce Heat which, being stagnant, attacks the uterus.

b) The Deficiency of Blood

The postpartum and postabortum periods are favorable conditions for development of the infection because of the deficiency of Qi and blood. The deficiency of blood that disturbs the menstrual cycle can also favor the aggression of the exogenous pathogenic factors, with damage to the Chong Mai and Ren Mai vessels and the uterus.

c) The Deficiency of the Kidney Qi

This deficiency can be constitutional or may be caused, as is often the case, by sexual abuses (e.g., early onset of sexual life, sexual excess, multiparity). The deficiency of Qi causes an insufficient nourishment of the uterus which is closely related to the Kidney.

Clinical Manifestations

a) The Aggression of Damp-Heat

Main symptoms include fever, lower abdominal pain with abundant, yellowish, malodorous leukorrhea, and pruritus of the external genitalia. Associated symptoms are asthenia, frequently with a sensation of heaviness in the body; a sensation of fullness in the thorax; anxiety; insomnia; thirst; a red tongue with a thick, yellow coating; and a string-taut, sliding pulse.

b) The Deficiency of Blood

Main symptoms include lower abdominal pain, low fever, and leukorrhea. Associated symptoms are a dark complexion; dizziness; vertigo; headache; insomnia; palpitations; dyspnea; a pale tongue, with a white coating; and a deep, fine, forceless pulse.

c) The Deficiency of the Kidney Qi

Main symptoms include pelvic and lumbar pain, clear, watery leukorrhea, a sensation of weakness in the lumbar region and lower limbs, and fever. Associated symptoms include a dark complexion, vertigo, aversion to cold, a pale tongue with thin coating, and a deep, low pulse.

Treatment

a) The Aggression of Damp-Heat

Therapeutic principle: cool the Heat, remove Damp

Prescription:

RM 3 (Zhongji)	regulates Lower Jiao and removes Damp
SP 6 (Sanyinjiao)	is the Crossing point of the three Yin channels of the foot, strengthens the Spleen, removes Damp
SP 9 (Yinglingquan)	is the He point of the Spleen channel, tones the Spleen to remove Damp and stimulates circulation within the Lower Jiao
LV 5 (Ligou)	is the Luo point of the Liver channel, cools Heat and removes Damp, removes Fire from the Lower Jiao
BL 34 (Yanglingquan)	is the He point of the Gall Bladder channel, disperses the Heat and removes Damp

Acupuncture is given with the reducing method.

b) The Deficiency of Blood

Therapeutic principle: tone Qi, nourish blood

Prescription:

RM 6 (Qihai)	tones the Qi
RM 4 (Guanyuan)	tones the Qi, regulates circulation within the Chong Mai and Ren Mai vessels

SP 6 (SanyinJiao)	strengthens the Spleen and Stomach, regulates Qi and blood
ST 36 (Zusanli)	tones the Stomach, regulates Qi and blood, has a generally fortifying effect
BL 17 (Geshu)	is the Influential point of blood, nourishes the blood

Acupuncture is given with the reinforcing method.

c) The Deficiency of the Kidney Qi

Therapeutic principle: tone the Qi

Prescription:

RM 4 (Guanyuan)	warms the Kidney, tones the Essence, regulates the Qi and the circulation in the Chong Mai and Ren Mai vessels
BL 23 (Shenshu)	is the Back-Shu point of the Kidney, nourishes the Yin and strengthens the Yang, tones the Kidney
K 12 (Dahe)	tones the Kidney Qi and regulates the uterus
E.P. Weibao	regulates Chong Mai and Ren Mai
SP 6 (Sanyinjiao)	is the Crossing point of the three Yin channels of the foot, the Spleen, Kidney and Liver; strengthens Kidney Qi

Other points can also be used in alternative prescriptions:

DM 4 (Mingmen)	strengthens the Kidney Yang, tones the Essence, stops leukorrhea
K 3 (Taixi)	is the Yuan-Source point of the Kidney channel, nourishes the Kidney and Liver, regulates the Chong Mai and Ren Mai vessels
RM 2 (Qugu)	warms and tones the Kidney Yang, regulates menstruation and stops leukorrhea

Acupuncture is given with the reducing method, except for E.P. Weibao which is stimulated with even movement.

Auricular Therapy: points Uterus, Endocrine, Ovary, Shenmen. The stimulation is moderate, one session daily and the needles are left in place for approximately 15 to 20 minutes.

PELVIC INFLAMMATORY DISEASE

In western medicine, this term refers to salpingitis, parametritis, and peritonitis with acute or chronic evolution. In cases of acute pelvic infections approximately two thirds are polymicrobial and their signs and symptoms are generally nonspecific. The treatment primarily relies upon antibiotic therapy.

From the perspective of Chinese traditional medicine, several clinical entities are described:

- dysmenorrhea: Tong Jing
- leukorrhea: Dai Xia
- menstrual cycle disorders: Yue Jing Bu Jiao
- pelvic tumoral masses: Zheng Jia

These conditions are caused by the stagnation of Qi and blood or the aggression of pathogenic factors with damage to the Chong Mai and Ren Mai vessels.

Etiopathogenesis

a) Prosperous Damp-Heat

This is a frequent etiopathogenic condition in acute and chronic cases. It can appear after the attack of exogenous or endogenous constitutional Damp or after birth, abortion or menstruation when the vessels of the uterus are deficient. If exogenous Damp enters inward, it will block the Dai Mai Vessel and it will accumulate in the Lower Jiao. The circulation of Qi and blood will be obstructed, causing abdominal pain and leukorrhea. Pelvic tumoral masses may appear as a result of persistent stagnation.

b) The Stagnation of Qi and Blood

Qi and blood stagnation is seen only in chronic stages. It appears after an abortion or birth, when blood is not entirely removed and is stagnant within the uterus. The circulation of Qi and blood is not free within the channels and the Ren Mai and Chong Mai vessels can no longer nourish the uterus.

Clinical Manifestations

The symptoms and signs belong to the acute or chronic type of pelvic inflammatory disease:

1) Acute pelvic inflammatory disease has the following manifestations: fever; sweating; lower abdominal distension with abdominal
tenderness; menstrual cycle disorders, usually with excessive flow; and
an excessive white-yellowish, malodorous discharge.

2) Chronic pelvic inflammatory disease has the following manifestations: abdominal, lumbar and sacral pain; menstrual cycle disorders;
dysmenorrhea; abundant leukorrhea; and, occasionally, a sensation of
heaviness in the anal region.

According to the etiopathogenic type, other symptoms and signs can
be observed and reported:

a) Prosperous Damp-Heat

Main symptoms include fever; chills with aversion to cold; thirst
without desire to drink; lower abdominal pain with muscular contracture,
aggravated on pressure; abdominal distension; and a sensation of fullness
in the thorax. Associated symptoms include oliguria; constipation; a
yellow, abundant, malodorous leukorrhea; a yellow, thick tongue coating; and a sliding, rapid or string-taut pulse.

b) The Stagnation of Qi and Blood

Main symptoms include abdominal and lumbosacral pains,
unaggravated by palpation and palpable, fixed or mobile tumoral masses.
Associated symptoms include abundant leukorrhea and menstrual cycle
disorders, menstrual flow with clots, dysmenorrhea, constipation, a pale,
dry complexion, a red tongue or one with purplish spots, and a deep, wiry,
string-taut pulse.

Treatment

a) Prosperous Damp-Heat

Therapeutic principle: tone the Spleen to remove Damp, cool the
Heat and transform Phlegm

Prescription:

SP 9 (Yinlingquan)	is the He point of the Spleen channel, tones the Spleen and removes Damp, stimulates circulation within San Jiao
SP 6 (Sanyinjiao)	is the Crossing point of the three Yin channels of the foot, the Spleen, Kidney and Liver,

	tones the Spleen and regulates the Stomach, favors the transporting and transforming of Phlegm, regulates Qi and blood
RM 3 (Zhongji)	regulates the Chong Mai and Ren Mai vessels, regulates menstruation, removes Damp-Heat
ST 29 (Guilai)	regulates Lower Jiao, regulates the Qi of the Chong Mai and Ren Mai vessels, regulates the uterus
GB 26 (Daimai)	removes pathogenic Damp and Heat, drains the channels, regulates menstruation, stops leukorrhea

Other points can be used in alternative prescriptions as follows:

K 13 (Qixue)	regulates the Chong Mai and Ren Mai vessels, favors the draining of the Lower Jiao
BL 24 (Qihaishu)	regulates Qi and blood
BL 26 (Guanyuanshu)	regulates Lower Jiao, tones the Kidney and lumbar pain
BL 28 (Pangguangshu)	is the Back-Shu point of the Urinary Bladder, tones Qi, removes pathogenic Qi from Lower Jiao
BL 31 (Shangliao)	is the Crossing point of the Gall Bladder and Urinary Bladder channels, tones blood and has an analgesic effect

Acupuncture is given with the dispersion method.

b) The Stagnation of Qi and Blood

Therapeutic principle: stimulate Qi and blood circulation to transform stagnation

Prescription:

RM 3 (Zhongji)	regulates Qi and blood, regulates Lower Jiao and the Chong Mai and Ren Mai Vessels, regulates menstruation
SP 6 (Sanyinjiao)	tones the Qi, strengthens the Spleen and Stomach, regulates Qi and blood circulation
LV 2 (Xingjian)	is the Ying point of the Liver channel, re-

moves pathogenic Heat of the Liver and cools the blood, regulates Liver Qi

RM 6 (Qihai)   regulates Qi and blood circulation, regulates the Chong Mai and Ren Mai Vessels

E.P. Weidao   regulates the circulation of Qi within Chong Mai and Ren Mai

Other points can be used in alternative prescriptions:

ST 25 (Tianshu)   regulates the Stomach and strengthens the Spleen, regulates the Qi and menstruation

BL 32 (Ciliao)   stimulates Qi and blood circulation, calms pain

BL 27 (Xiaochangshu) is the Back-Shu point of the Small Intestine, spreads pathogenic Heat and Damp from the Lower Jiao

BL 25 (Dachangshu) is the Back-Shu point of the Large Intestine, regulates the Qi of Fu organs, removes stagnation and pathogenic Damp

ST 36 (Zusanli)   regulates Qi and blood, has a generally fortifying effect

Different prescriptions can also be used:

a) RM 4 + RM 3 + ST 29 + ST 28

RM 4 (Guanyuan)   regulates Qi and blood, regulates circulation within the Chong Mai and Ren Mai vessels

RM 3 (Zhongji)   tones the Qi, regulates Qi and blood circulation within the Chong Mai and Ren Mai Vessels

SP 6 (Sanyinjiao)   tones the Spleen, regulates Qi and blood circulation

ST 29 (Guilai)   regulates the Lower Jiao, regulates the uterus

ST 28 (Shuidao)   regulates Lower Jiao, removes pathogenic Damp

LV 5 (Ligou)   is the Luo point of the Liver channel, removes Liver Qi stagnation, removes pathogenic Heat and Damp

LV 6 (Zhongdu)	is the Xi point of the Liver channel, removes Liver Qi stagnation, drains the channels, sedates the pain

b) RM 4 + ST 28 + ST 36 + SP 6

RM 4 (Guanyuan)	regulates and tones the Qi, regulates the Chong Mai and Ren Mai vessels
ST 28 (Shuidao)	removes pathogenic Damp
ST 36 (Zusanli)	and
SP 6 (Sanyinjiao)	tones the Qi, stimulates Qi and blood circulation

If necessary, several symptomatic points can be added to each prescription as follows:

- fever

LI 11 (Quchi)	regulates Qi and blood, regulates the channels, cools the Heat
LI 4 (Hegu)	cools the Heat, removes inflammation and sedates pain, regulates Qi and blood

- painful abdominal distension

RM 6 (Qihai)	regulates Qi and blood, regulates circulation within the Chong Mai and Ren Mai vessels
LV 14 (Qimen)	is the Front-Mu point of the Liver, removes Liver Qi stagnation, removes other stagnation, stimulates blood
ST 25 (Tianshu)	stimulates Qi circulation, drains the channels, removes pathogenic Damp

- excessive leukorrhea

SP 8 (Diji)	is the Xi point of the Spleen channel, stimulates the Spleen-Stomach couple, regulates menstruation, stops leukorrhea

- adhesions

RM 12 (Zhongwan)

- hypermenorrhea

ST 44 (Neiting)	is the Ying point of the Stomach channel, disperses pathogenic Heat and Damp

LV 1 (Dadun)	is the Jing-Well point of the Liver channel, regulates Lower Jiao, regulates menstruation, calms the spirit
SP 1 (Yinbai)	is the Jing-Well point of the Spleen channel, strengthens the Spleen, increases Qi and maintains blood
- abdominal masses	
SP 13 (Fushe)	is the Crossing point of the Spleen and Liver channels with the Yin Wei Mai Vessel, regulates the circulation of Qi
SP 9 (Yinlingquan)	strengthens the Spleen, stimulates circulation within San Jiao
- nervousness	
SJ 5 (Waiguan)	is the Luo point of the San Jiao channel, calms the spirit
H 7 (Shenmen)	is the Yuan-Source point of the Heart channel, calms the mind
- constipation	
BL 25 (Dachangshu)	is the Front-Mu point of the Large Intestine, promotes the circulation of Qi in the large intestine
K 6 (Zhaohai)	regulates blood, cools and drains the Lower Jiao
SJ 6 (Zhigou)	is the Jing-River point of the San Jiao channel, stimulates Qi circulation in San Jiao

Stimulation of the points is performed daily or every two days for acute cases. Deep insertion of the needles is necessary and needles are left in place for 20 minutes or more. Insertion in inflamed areas or where abdominal masses can be felt on palpation should be avoided. Moxibustion should be used in tender areas. One should avoid acupuncture sessions during menstruation.

Another prescription uses the following points:

E.P. Weidao

K 13 (Qixue)

BL 20 (Pishu)

The acupoints sensitive on pressure are selected. A 0,5 ml intradermic injection, consisting of 25 mg vitamin B1 diluted with 5 ml saline solution is injected.

Treatment duration is from 5 to 7 days, with one session being conducted daily. If necessary, another treatment series can be repeated.

Auricular Therapy: points Uterus, Ovary, Hormones, Adrenals. A session is performed daily and stimulation is moderate. The needles are left in place for approximately 20 minutes (or longer, for chronic cases).

PELVIC TUMORAL MASSES

The existence of abdominal tumoral masses has been recognized from ancient times. In Chinese traditional medicine this pathology is called Zheng Jia:

- Zheng refers to fixed masses of hard consistency, with a fixed location
- Jia refers to mobile masses with no specific location and no fixed pain

On palpation, these masses seem to be movable and they can disappear spontaneously. "That is why it is said the Zheng ones are manifest, they have a shape that one can feel; the Jia ones are apparent, they take the shape."

Observed in both males and females, the Zheng Jia diseases are more frequent in females.

Three circumstances contribute to this pathology:

- the stagnation of Qi
- the stagnation of blood
- Phlegm accumulation

On abdominal palpation, the hard, fixed, painful masses indicate a stagnation of blood. Soft masses that are not delimited and which have variable painful areas indicate the stagnation of Qi. The mass with soft consistency, usually with fixed location and pain, indicates the accumulation of Phlegm.

The ovarian cyst and uterine leiomyomata are both classified as Zheng Jia. Pharmacotherapy is employed as the first step in treating these masses.

OVARIAN CYST

Ovarian masses can be benign or malignant. Proper clinical assessment is necessary and ultrasonography or other imaging modalities can help to establish a precise diagnosis. Benign ovarian cysts are usually inflammatory in nature. Oral contraceptive therapy can resolve many of them. Surgery may be required in certain circumstances (e.g., masses 8 cm in diameter; an ovarian mass before menarche or in menopause; a persistent mass after 8 weeks of contraceptive therapy etc.), and cystectomy usually is preferred.

From the perspective of Chinese traditional medicine, an ovarian cyst is caused by the stagnation of Qi.

Etiopathogenesis

The stagnation of Qi appears when the Qi of one part of the body or of a Zang-Fu organ is obstructed. Frequently this is the consequence of emotional factors disorders or of the invasion of exogenous pathogenic factors such as Cold and Damp. The retardation in the circulation of Qi is followed by Qi obstruction that causes distension and pain.

a) The Stagnation of the Liver Qi

Frequently the stagnation of Qi affects the Liver, disturbing the Liver's function of maintaining the free circulation of Qi, resulting in retardation of Qi circulation. Liver Qi can injure the Spleen and Stomach, and the retardation of Qi favors Damp accumulation and transformation into Phlegm. Prolonged Liver Qi obstruction causes Qi and blood stagnation and the formation of palpable, painful tumoral masses.

b) The Stagnation of the Liver Qi Accompanied by Cold

Because Cold causes stagnation and constriction, it will cause Qi obstruction and retardation. As a Yin pathogenic factor, Cold consumes the Yang and affects the body's warming function.

Clinical Manifestations

a) The Stagnation of Qi

Main symptoms include the presence of a palpable, mobile mass of increased consistency and indefinite size and shape. Associated symptoms include abdominal distension and pain with no fixed location and with possible exacerbation during menstruation. Distension is more severe than pain; it can be temporarily alleviated by belching or flatulence. Depression may be present. A dark-colored complexion; leukor-rhea; a pink tongue with a thin, sometimes yellow, coating; and a string-taut, sliding pulse are also characteristic.

b) The Stagnation of the Liver Qi

Main symptoms include pain in the costal region, aggravated by pressure, and painful distension in the hypochondriac and hypogastric regions. Lack of appetite; belching; an irregular menstrual cycle with dark-colored blood; a dark red tongue or one with purplish spots; and a string-taut pulse are associated symptoms.

c) The Stagnation of Qi Accompanied by Cold

Main symptoms include a sensation of thoracic and epigastric fullness with pain, nausea, belching, cold limbs, aversion to Cold, menstrual cycle disorders (long menstrual cycle and menstrual flow with clots), and pollakiuria. A thin, white tongue coating and a string-taut, retarded pulse.

Treatment

a) The Stagnation of Qi

Therapeutic principle: regulate Qi, remove stagnation

Prescription:

RM 4 (Guanyuan)	is the Crossing point of the Ren Mai Vessel with the three Yin channels of the foot, strengthens the original Qi, regulates Qi and blood circulation, regulates the Chong Mai and Ren Mai vessels
SP 6 (Sanyinjiao)	is the Crossing point of the Spleen Kidney and Liver channels, stimulates Qi and blood circulation, regulates the channels
ST 29 (Guilai)	regulates the Lower Jiao, regulates the uterus, removes Qi and blood stagnation
ST 30 (Qichong)	removes Qi and blood stagnation, is an important energetic point

E.P. Zigong

Stimulation is given with the reducing method. The needles can also be inserted intradermally, surrounding the area in which the tumoral masses are located.

b) The Stagnation of the Liver Qi

Therapeutic principle: remove stagnation, regulate the Liver Qi

Prescription:

LV 2 (Xingjian)	is the Ying point of the Liver channel and the reducing point, removes the stagnation of the Liver Qi
LV 5 (Ligou)	is the Luo point of the Liver channel, drains the Liver, regulates Liver Qi
LV 6 (Zhongdu)	is the Xi point of the Liver channel, removes stagnation from the Liver, regulates the channels, sedates pain
LV 9 (Yinbao)	removes stagnation, regulates the Chong Mai and Ren Mai vessels
LV 14 (Qimen)	is the Front-Mu point of the Liver, regulates the Liver, stimulates free circulation of Qi, smooths the hypochondriac region

Any of the acupoints mentioned above can be added to the main point selected for the stagnation of Qi. Acupuncture is given with the reducing method.

c) The Stagnation of Qi Accompanied by Cold

Therapeutic principle: warm the blood, stimulate Qi and blood circulation

Prescription:

BL 29 (Zhonglushu)	warms the Yang and removes pathogenic Cold, strengthens the Kidney
BL 33 (Zhongliao)	is the Crossing point of the Urinary Bladder and Gall Bladder channels, regulates the channels, stimulates blood circulation, removes pathogenic Cold, sedates pain
K 3 (Taixi)	is the Yuan-Source point of the Kidney channel, nourishes and tones Lower Jiao, regulates Chong Mai and Ren Mai
RM 5 (Shimen)	is the Front-Mu point of the San Jiao, warms the Kidney, strengthens the Yang, regulates the menstrual cycle

RM 7 (YinJiao)   warms Kidney Yang, regulates menstruation

SP 14 (Fujie)   warms the Middle Jiao and stimulates Qi circulation, favors the descending of perverse Qi

DM 3 (Yaoyangguan) tones the Kidney, removes Cold and Damp, regulates the Chong Mai and Ren Mai vessels, regulates the uterus

One or more acupoints are selected and added to those points used to remove the stagnation of Qi.

Acupuncture treatment can be used only in cases with benign, functional tumors and precise diagnosis based upon pelvic examinations and diagnostic techniques (e.g. ultrasound) is mandatory.

UTERINE LEIOMYOMATA

Uterine leiomyomata is a benign disease that appears only during the period of ovarian activity. The etiology is multifactorial, and the hormonal state, even if important, is not the only factor involved in the formation of leiomyomas.

One or more tumoral masses can be palpated allowing assessment of the location, volume and form, consistency, and mobility. Uterine polyfibromatosis refers to multiple nodes.

Different complications can aggravate the evolution of the uterine leiomyomas: hemorrhagic, infectious, mechanical—related to location, vascular and degenerative changes.

From the perspective of Chinese traditional medicine, abdominal tumoral masses—uterine leiomyomata are believed to be caused by stagnation of blood or Phlegm.

Etiopathogenesis

a) The Stagnation of Blood

The stagnation of blood results from disturbance of blood circulation. The entering of Wind and Cold in the uterus during the postpartum period will cause the constriction of vessels and Qi and blood "coagulation." With the circulation of Qi affected, and with Qi as the commander of blood, disturbance of the emotional factors and Liver Qi stagnation negatively influence blood circulation. Traumatic injuries at menstruation or after birth can cause bleeding and accumulation of blood that stagnates. The deficiency of Qi, constitutional or by consumption of Qi as a result of overstrain, can affect Qi circulation and cause stagnation.

b) The Accumulation of Phlegm

The excess of Phlegm can be constitutional, especially in obese patients. Phlegm accumulation can lead to obstruction of the channels and to Qi, blood and Phlegm stagnation. Clinical manifestations are different depending upon the involved area.

Clinical Manifestations

a) The Stagnation of Blood

Main symptoms include a palpably hard, fixed, and sometimes painful, mass in the lower abdomen. The pain is aggravated on pressure. Menstrual cycles are irregular with excessive flow and long duration. Associated symptoms include abundant leukorrhea; fever; dysuria; constipation; a dark complexion; a dark, bluish tongue or one with purplish spots and a thin coating; and a string-taut, wiry, sliding pulse.

The deficiency of blood will worsen in cases with prolonged stagnation of blood. In these instances, a hardening of the abdominal mass will occur and may be accompanied by extreme pallor with yellowish tone; dry skin; increased loss of weight; vertigo; vision disturbances; insomnia; tinnitus; a dark red tongue, possibly with no coating; and a thready pulse.

If blood stagnation is accompanied by Cold, the following symptoms can appear: irregular menstruation, a menstrual cycle with dark blood and clots, dysmenorrhea and sometimes amenorrhea. Painful abdominal distension that alleviates with application of warmth; cold extremities; a pale tongue with a bluish cast and a white, thin coating; and a deep, wiry and strong pulse may also be present.

If blood stagnation coexists with Qi deficiency clinical manifestations include apathy, vertigo, vision disturbances, sweating, pollakiuria, loose stools, a pale, bluish tongue with a thin coating and a wiry or hollow, weak pulse.

b) The Accumulation of Phlegm

Main symptoms include a soft abdominal mass, fixed and accompanied by pain. The patients are usually obese with a constitutional predisposition to Phlegm accumulation. Associated symptoms are an irregular menstrual cycle; possible amenorrhea; abundant, white, clammy leukorrhea; vertigo; insomnia; a sensation of heaviness in the head; a white, thick tongue coating; and a string-taut, sliding pulse.

Treatment

a) The Stagnation of Blood

Therapeutic principle: stimulate blood to remove stagnation

Prescription:

RM 3 (Zhongji)	is the Crossing point of the Ren Mai with the Yin channels of the foot, the Kidney, Spleen and Liver; regulates Qi and blood; regulates the Lower Jiao and menstruation
SP 6 (Sanyinjiao)	is the Crossing point of the Yin channels of the foot, the Kidney, Spleen and Liver; regulates Qi and blood circulation; drains the channels; tones Spleen and Stomach; a source of blood
LV 3 (Taichong)	is the Yuan-Source point of the Liver channel, regulates Qi and blood circulation
LV 6 (Zhongdu)	is the Xi point of the Liver channel, regulates Qi and blood circulation
ST 29 (Guilai)	is a point of the Stomach channel, rich in Qi and blood; regulates Qi and stimulates blood circulation

The selected points can be used in alternative prescriptions. The acupuncture sensation should spread towards the external genitalia.

- If blood deficiency is associated:

Therapeutic principle: tone and stimulate blood circulation

Prescription:

BL 17 (Geshu)	is the Influential point of blood, tones the Spleen and regulates the Stomach, regulates blood and removes stasis, regulates Qi circulation
ST 36 (Zusanli)	regulates Spleen and Stomach, a source of blood, regulates Qi and blood

SP 8 (Diji)   is the Xi point of the Spleen channel, stimulates Spleen and Stomach, regulates blood and menstruation

LV 14 (Qimen)   is the Front-Mu point of the Liver and the Crossing point of the Liver and Spleen channels with Yin Wei Mai Vessel, strengthens the Spleen and Stomach, stimulates blood circulation and removes stasis

Acupuncture is given with the reducing and even movement method, according to the selected points.

- If blood stagnation is accompanied by Cold

Therapeutic principle: remove Cold and transform clots

Prescription:

BL 23 (Shenshu)   is the Back-Shu point of the Kidney, tones Kidney Yang

RM 4 (Guanyuan)   is the Crossing point of the Ren Mai Vessel with the Kidney, Spleen and Liver channels; tones the Yang; regulates the Chong Mai and Ren Mai vessels; stimulates Qi circulation

RM 5 (Shimen)   warms the Kidney, strengthens Yang, regulates menstruation

DM 3 (Yaoyangguan) strengthens the Kidney, removes pathogenic Cold, regulates the Chong Mai and Ren Mai vessels

Strong stimulation of the selected points is necessary and moxibustion can be used, except for BL 23.

Other points can be included in alternative prescriptions as follows:

RM 7 (Yinjiao)   is the Crossing point of the Ren Mai and Chong Mai vessels with the Kidney channel, tones the Kidney Yang, regulates blood and menstruation

BL 29 (Zhonglushu)   warms the Yang and removes pathogenic Cold

ST 29 (Guilai)   warms the Lower Jiao, regulates the uterus

DM 2 (Yaoshu)   warms the Lower Jiao, stimulates circulation within the channels

- If there is also a deficiency of Qi:

Therapeutic principle: tone the correct Qi and remove the pathogenic Qi (care must be taken to avoid injuring the correct Qi).

Prescription:

ST 36 (Zusanli)   is the He point of the Stomach channel and one of the four Dominant points, regulates the Stomach and tones the Spleen, regulates Qi and blood, supports the correct Qi

RM 4 (Guanyuan)   tones the Qi, regulates Qi and blood, regulates the Chong Mai and Ren Mai vessels

BL 23 (Shenshu)   is the Back-Shu point of the Kidney, tones Kidney Qi, strengthens the Kidney Yang

K 13 (Qixue)   is the Crossing point of the Kidney channel with the Chong Mai Vessel, tones Kidney Qi, regulates the Chong Mai and Ren Mai vessels, drains the Lower Jiao

K 8 (Jiaoxin)   is the Confluent point of the Yin Qiao Mai Vessel, tones the Kidney, regulates the Chong Mai and Ren Mai vessels, regulates Qi and blood, stimulates the uterus

K 15 (Zhongzhu)   nourishes Kidney Qi, drains the Lower Jiao, regulates the uterus

From the above mentioned points, two or three are selected in alternative prescriptions. Acupuncture is given with the reinforcing method.

b) The Accumulation of Phlegm

Therapeutic principle: stimulate blood circulation and drain the channels, transform Phlegm, remove stasis

Prescription:

SP 6 (SanyinJiao)   tones the Spleen to transform Phlegm, stimulates Qi and blood circulation, drains the channels

RM 17 (Shanzhong) is the Influential point of Qi, regulates Qi functions and stimulates blood, transforms Phlegm

ST 29 (Guilai)   drains Lower Jiao, regulates Qi, regulates menstruation

ST 40 (Fenglong)   is the Luo point of the Stomach channel, regulates the Stomach and transforms Phlegm

SP 9 (Yinlingquan) is the He point of the Spleen channel, strengthens the Spleen, removes Damp, stimulates circulation within the Lower Jiao

LV 5 (Ligou)   is the Luo point of the Liver channel, supports Qi and drains the channels, removes Damp-Heat from the genital area

The selected acupoints are stimulated with the even movement method.

UTERINE RETROVERSION

Uterine retroposition is one of the most frequently seen disorders of the uterus. It can be congenital or acquired, mobile or fixed and irreductible. The congenital form usually occurs in women with low tissular tonus. The acquired forms are typically a consequence of obstetrical traumas. Frequently retroflexion appears within the context of pelvic inflammatory pathology.

If there are any symptoms these are usually lumbar and lower back pains, dysmenorrhea and dyspareunia. Treatment consists of manual replacement and relief of symptoms.

Etiopathogenesis

From the perspective of Chinese traditional medicine, uterine retroversion is caused by a deficiency of Kidney Yang. This type of deficiency can be constitutional or acquired through Kidney damage. The deficiency of Kidney Yang manifests as an inability of Yang to sustain the functions of the organs and tissues. This has implications for the Chong Mai, Ren Mai and Dai Mai Vessels with the likelihood of uterine deviation onset.

Clinical Manifestations

The mobile forms of uterine retroversion are usually asymptomatic, but can coexist with dysmenorrhea, lumbar and lower back pain, menstrual cycle disorders and dyspareunia.

Irreducible retroposition can cause compression pollakiuria and constipation. This condition may be associated with pallor, cold limbs, white leukorrhea, infertility, a pale tongue with a thin coating, and a deep, weak pulse.

Treatment

Acupuncture treatment affords an alternative therapy for redressing the uterine position, in mobile forms, and alleviating the symptoms in cases with posterior adherences.

Prescription:

a) RM 12 + RM 3 + SJ 4 + E.P. Baomen + E.P. Zihu

RM 12 (Zhongwan)	is the Front-Mu point of the Stomach, the Influential point of the Fu organs and the Crossing point of Ren Mai Vessel with the Small Intestine, San Jiao and Stomach channels; stimulates the ascent of Qi; strengthens the Spleen and regulates the Stomach
RM 3 (Zhongji)	is the Front-Mu point of the Urinary Bladder and the Crossing point of Ren Mai and the Spleen, Kidney and Liver channels; tones Kidney Yang, regulates menstruation
SJ 4 (Yangchi)	is the Yuan-Source point of the San Jiao channel, regulates San Jiao, regulates the Qi
E.P. Baomen	located 2 cun to the left of RM 4
E.P. Zihu	located 2 cun to the right of RM 4

b) SP 6 + LV 1 + K 6 + ST 36

SP 6 (Sanyinjiao)	is the Crossing point of the three Yin channels of the foot, the Kidney, Liver and Spleen; tones the Spleen and Kidney, regulates Qi and blood
LV 1 (Dadun)	is the Jing-Well point of the Liver channel, regulates the Chong Mai and Ren Mai vessels
K 6 (Zhaohai)	is the Confluent point of the Yin Qiao Mai vessel, regulates the Lower Jiao, regulates menstruation

ST 36 (Zusanli)   is the He point of the Stomach channel, tones Qi and blood, has a generally fortifying effect

Stimulation of the acupoints is given with the reinforcing method, mostly using moxibustion. The number of sessions needed—usually between 10 and 20— is determined by noting the progressive alleviation of signs and symptoms.

UTERINE PROLAPSE

Uterine prolapse refers to herniation through the urogenital diaphragm and the descent of the uterus and vaginal walls. This movement of the uterus can result in prolapse of the adjacent organs.

The main initiating factor is obstetrical trauma, especially multiple deliveries for which a constitutional factor can associate. A constitutional predisposition can exist separately, causing prolapse in nulliparas and even in sexually inactive women. The pelvic relaxation is progressive, usually becoming manifest during menopause, when an endocrine factor is associated. Treatment usually involves the local or systemic administration of estrogen and surgical repair in postmenopausal women, while exercises and pessary support can help in younger patients.

Chinese traditional medicine recognizes three degrees of uterine prolapse, called "Yin Ting" or "Yin Tuo."

- first degree: ptosis without symptoms, the cervix remains inside the vaginal canal
- second degree: the cervix reaches the level of the vaginal introitus and may protrude with straining
- third degree: the cervix and uterus are beyond the hymeneal ring and ulcerations are possible

Etiopathogenesis

a) The Sinking of Qi

The following factors can be involved in the uterine prolapse:

- weak constitution
- early physical effort in postpartum period, before Qi and blood are restored
- exhausting labor, with excessive efforts that can injure the Chong Mai and Ren Mai vessels
- overstrain due to chronic efforts that increase intra-abdominal

pressure: constipation, coughing, etc.

All of these circumstances can cause the sinking of Qi, that is no longer able to keep the uterus in its physiologic position. Spleen and Stomach weakness, lack of Heart nourishment, and the descent of the pathogenic Damp appear as consequences of Qi deficiency.

b) The Deficiency of the Kidney Qi

This type of deficiency can be caused by:

- sexual abuses (e.g., early marriage, excessive sexual activity)

- frequent pregnancies and deliveries

- advanced age

The Kidney Qi can be consumed in these circumstances resulting in the weakness of the Chong Mai and Ren Mai vessels and causing the Du Mai Vessel to lose its function of restriction, leading to uterine prolapse.

Rare cases of neglected uterine prolapse with ulceration and infection are related to lower accumulation of Damp-Heat and the appearance of symptoms of excess.

Clinical Manifestations

a) The Sinking of Qi

Main symptoms include uterine prolapse aggravated by a prolonged upright position, with a bearing down sensation in the lower abdomen. Associated symptoms include asthenia, palpitations, pollakiuria, leukorrhea, a pale tongue with a thin coating and a weak pulse.

b) The Deficiency of the Kidney Qi

Main symptoms include uterine prolapse, tumefaction and weakness of the back and feet, and a sensation of pressure in the lower abdomen. Lumbar weakness, vaginal dryness, pollakiuria, tinnitus, dizziness, a pink tongue, and a weak pulse are associated symptoms.

In cases with accumulation of Damp-Heat:

Main symptoms include uterine prolapse with a swollen and painful uterus. Fever, spontaneous sweating, a dry mouth, nervousness, a sensation of thoracic fullness, oliguria, constipation, abundant, malodorous leukorrhea with sanguinolent fluid secretions, a red tongue with a yellow, thick coating, and a sliding, rapid pulse are also characteristic.

Treatment

a) The Sinking of Qi

Therapeutic principle: strengthen the Qi and restore the uterine position

Prescription:

DM 20 (Baihui)   is the Crossing point of the Yang channels, facilitates the ascent of Yang Qi

Use of this point is based upon the principle of treating lower body diseases with acupoints located in the upper body.

RM 6 (Qihai)   tones the Qi, favors the ascending of Yang

ST 29 (Guilai)   warms the Lower Jiao, is a local point located in the area of the broad ligament

RM 12 (Zhongwan)   and

ST 36 (Zusanli)   rebuilds the Qi of the Middle Jiao, has a generally fortifying effect

GB 28 (Weidao)   is the Crossing point of the Gall Bladder channel with the Dai Mai Vessel, is located on the fallopian ligament

Stimulation is given using the reinforcing method with acupuncture and, possibly, moxibustion afterward.

b) The Deficiency of the Kidney Qi

Therapeutic principle: tone the Kidney

Prescription:

RM 4 (Guanyuan)   tones Qi, strengthens the Kidney, regulates Qi and blood, regulates circulation within the Chong Mai and Ren Mai vessels

BL 23 (Shenshu)   is the Back-Shu point of the Kidney, strengthens the Kidney

SP 6 (Sanyinjiao)   is the Crossing point of the three Yin channels of the foot, the Kidney, Liver and Spleen, tones the Kidney, regulates Qi and blood circulation

K 6 (Zhaohai)   strengthens the Kidney; together with LV 8, nourishes the tendons supporting the uterus

LV 8 (Ququan)	is the He point of the Liver channel, regulates Qi and blood
E.P. Weibao	and
E.P. Zigong	are both indicated in uterine prolapse

The reinforcing method of stimulating the selected acupoints is used and acupuncture or moxibustion is given. Every two days a session is conducted and the needles are left in place for approximately 15 minutes.

In cases of accumulation of Damp-Heat:

Therapeutic principle: cool the Heat and remove Damp

Prescription:

LV 3 (Taichong)	is the Yuan-Source point of the Liver channel, resolves Damp-Heat, stimulates Qi and blood circulation
LV 8 (Ququan)	is the He point of the Liver channel, cools Damp-Heat, regulates Qi and blood, strengthens the tendons
SP 9 (Yinlingquan)	strengthens the Spleen to remove Damp, restores circulation within San Jiao
RM 3 (Zhongji)	regulates the Lower Jiao and removes Damp-Heat, regulates the uterus

Acupuncture is given with the reducing method in this case, with daily stimulation of the acupoints.

Auricular Therapy: points Uterus, Endocrine, Subcortical. A session is conducted every day. The needles are left in place for approximately 20 minutes, with strong stimulation or may be implanted for long-term stimulation in neglected cases.

INFERTILITY

Infertility is the failure to conceive in a couple with a normal sexual life and no use of contraceptive methods. There are two types: primary and secondary infertility. Primary infertility refers to absence of conception after one year in a couple's normal sexual life. Secondary infertility describes an inability to conceive again after one or more pregnancies have occurred.

The assessment of an infertile couple includes multiple factors: cervical, uterine, tubal, peritoneal, ovulatory. Infectious and mechanical problems represent the main etiologic factors. The management of infertility aims to address an etiology, if one can be identified.

Since ancient times, Chinese traditional medicine, when approaching an infertile couple, differentiated primary infertility from secondary infertility and male infertility. Male infertility is believed to be caused by the deficiency of the Kidney Qi and the weakness of the Essence.

From the perspective of Chinese traditional medicine there are two etiologic categories:

- congenital deficiencies
- acquired pathological disturbances

Congenital Deficiencies

There are five congenital deficiencies, known as Wu Bu Mu (the five unfeminities):

Luo "Spiral": a spiral shaped fold of the vaginal orifice

Wen "Bent": narrow vagina

Gu "Strain": the constriction of the vaginal orifice as if there is no orifice

Jiao " Horn": clitoridean hypertrophy

Mai "Flux": primary amenorrhea

The first four deficiencies are untreatable by pharmacotherapy or acupuncture and require surgical procedures to be corrected. The fifth deficiency ties infertility to the menstrual cycle and thus suggests certain therapeutic possibilities.

Acquired Disturbances

The main structures involved in the etiopathogenesis of infertility are the Kidney, Spleen and Liver in permanent relationship with the Extraordinary Vessels.

A parallel with the etiologic perspective of western medicine is drawn because the pattern of injury to these structures, especially of the Extraordinary Vessels, has repercussions for female infertility, causing:

- primary amenorrhea - involves the Ren Mai and Chong Mai vessels and, in the adrenogenital syndrome, includes damage to the

Spleen function

- secondary amenorrhea

a) anovulation - involves the Ren Mai, Chong Mai, and Du Mai vessels, and the Spleen and Lung

b) psychical disorders - involves the seven emotional factors, the Liver and Shen Qi

c) consumptive diseases - due to organ pathology

- menstrual cycle disorders, especially spaniomenorrhea, involve the deficiency of Qi and blood and injury of the Chong Mai, Ren Mai, Du Mai, and Yin Qiao Mai vessels and the Regular channels
- infectious factors (vaginitis, cervicitis, endometritis, pelvic inflammatory disease) - involve the Liver (channel and organ), due to aggression of Damp-Heat and Wind, and the Chong Mai and Ren Mai vessels
- functional changes of cervical mucus - involve Qi/blood balance, the Spleen and Liver, the Chong Mai Vessel, Shen Qi
- tubal spasm - involves the attack of Cold upon the Liver, the damage of the Yin Wei Mai Vessel circulation and distribution
- endometriosis - involves the Qi/blood lack of balance with Qi and blood stagnation, the Extraordinary Vessels, the Spleen and Liver
- uterine malpositions - involves the Dai Mai, Ren Mai, and Chong Mai vessels, the Spleen and Liver
- infertility due to nidation disturbances - involves a lack of Qi/ blood balance, as well as the Yin Wei Mai and Ren Mai vessels, the Kidney, Spleen, and Shen Qi
- miscarriage, premature labor - involves the Chong Mai, Ren Mai, and Yin Qiao Mai vessels, and the lack of Qi/blood balance
- infertility of no apparent cause - involves Shen Qi, the Extraordinary Vessels, the Liver, Heart, Lung, San Jiao

Etiopathogenesis

Infertility may be caused either by deficiency or by excess; these types are often seen together in practice.

a) The Deficiency of the Kidney Qi

The Kidney deficiency can be congenital or acquired. Chronic diseases, physical and psychological overstrain can weaken the Kidney Qi. Excessive sexual activity can affect the Kidney, causing the deficiency of Kidney Yang with repercussions for the reproductive function. The lack of balance between Yin and Yang will affect the Chong Mai and Ren Mai vessels.

In *Sheng Ji Zhong Lu* (a medical encyclopedia from the 12th century) it is mentioned: "Women's infertility is due to a deficiency of the Chong Mai and Ren Mai Vessels. Then the Qi of the Kidney is collapsed and cold."

b) The Deficiency of Blood

The deficiency of blood can be caused by insufficient production (in cases where the Spleen and Stomach, as blood producers, are damaged), by excessive blood loss, or by severe emotional changes that consume the body Yin.

The encyclopedia cited above refers to this circumstance of infertility: "Women's infertility is usually due to a lack of blood that is insufficient to retain Essence."

c) The Deficiency of the Spleen Qi

The affecting of the Spleen Qi is caused by overstrain, stress, inadequate food intake, or chronic diseases. The persistence of these factors or failure to rectify the lack of energetic balance will cause the Yang deficiency of the Spleen. The deficient Spleen and Stomach can no longer nourish the Chong Mai and Ren Mai vessels, which has repercussions for Qi/blood balance and contributes to menstrual cycle disorders and infertility.

d) The Excess of Phlegm-Damp

Phlegm-Damp excess is frequent in obese women, in whom it may be constitutional. Exposure to Damp, an excess of greasy food, alimentary and alcoholic abuses can cause the accumulation of Damp. Damp is characterized by viscosity and stagnation, with obstruction of Qi circulation. The accumulation of Phlegm-Damp in the Lower Jiao will obstruct the uterus, affecting reproduction.

Classical literature (Ge Zhi Yu Lun in the14th century) states that: "Obese women concerned about food and drinks have irregular menstruation and cannot conceive because their body is abundant in fat and Phlegm-Damp obstructs the uterus."

e) Heat in the Blood

One cause of infertility is the internal excess of Heat in the blood. Yin fluids will be consumed and will drain and dry the blood, affecting the uterus.

The Chinese classics mention this pathology as an infertility factor: "In thin, weakened women who are infertile, internal Heat turns into Fire, the uterus blood is dry, and it can no longer condense the Essence."

f) The Stagnation of the Liver Qi

Emotional factors disorders can affect the Liver's function of maintaining free circulation of Qi, causing Liver Qi stagnation. It will cause Spleen aggression. The delay in Qi circulation will allow the accumulation of Damp and Phlegm. As Qi dysfunction also damages the blood circulation, the Chong Mai and Ren Mai vessels will be affected, causing menstrual cycle disorders.

Clinical Manifestations

a) The Deficiency of the Kidney Qi

Main symptoms include infertility; long menstrual cycles with scanty menstrual flow and light colored blood; and white, watery, glue-like leukorrhea. A pale complexion and lumbar pain with nocturia can be associated as can a pale tongue with a thin coating and a weak, thready pulse.

If there is a Yang deficiency of the Kidney, symptoms may include a sensation of cold in the abdomen, lumbar weakness, eventual urinary incontinence, dizziness, and tinnitus. The effect of the deficiency on the reproductive function is expressed as infertility in females and impotence in males. A pale tongue and a deep, weak pulse may also be present.

b) The Deficiency of Blood

Main symptoms include infertility and oligomenorrhea with scanty menstrual flow and light colored blood. A pale, withered complexion with dry skin, asthenia, vertigo, vision disturbances, palpitations, dyspnea, a pale tongue with a thin coating, and a fine, weak pulse are also characteristic.

If a Yin deficiency is associated, clinical symptoms mimic those of Yang excess: short menstrual cycles with scanty flow and red blood, red lips, a dry mouth, afternoon fever, nervousness, irritability, a red tongue with a very thin coating and a string-taut pulse, that is weak on deep palpation.

c) The Deficiency of the Spleen Qi

Main symptoms include infertility; long menstrual cycles with scanty flow and abundant, saliva-like leukorrhea. Associated symptoms include asthenia, lack of appetite, a sensation of heaviness in the body, abdominal distension, loose stools, a white tongue, and a weak, slow, deep and delayed pulse.

d) The Excess of Phlegm-Damp

Main symptoms include infertility; irregular menstrual cycles with excessive flow and light-colored blood, abundant, white leukorrhea, and a dark complexion. Obesity, dizziness, palpitations, a thick tongue with a white, thick, moist coating and a sliding pulse may also be present.

e) Heat in the Blood

Main symptoms include infertility and, possibly, delayed menstruation with dark-colored blood. Associated symptoms are palpitations, insomnia, nervousness, a flushed face, a dry mouth, a red tongue with a yellow coating, and a rapid, wide, superficial pulse.

f) The Stagnation of the Liver Qi

Main symptoms include infertility; long, irregular menstrual cycles, alternating excessive with scanty menstruation, dysmenorrhea, and white, sometimes pink leukorrhea. A sensation of painful distension in the hypochondriac area, thoracic fullness, and depression may be reported. A normal tongue with a thin, white coating and a string-taut pulse may also be observed.

Treatment

The treatment seeks mainly to regulate the Chong Mai and Ren Mai vessels.

The following acupoints can also regulate the two Extraordinary Vessels, Chong Mai and Ren Mai:

RM 4 (Guanyuan)

RM 6 (Qihai)

K 3 (Taixi)

K 5 (Shuiquan)

K 13 (Qixue)

K 14 (Siman)

Usually in cases with pathology of the Extraordinary Vessels, the specific treatment involves less use of the Confluent point, which is reserved for a major lack of energetic balance (up-down, right-left, anterior-posterior).

Prescription:

- for Chong Mai Vessels

RM 4 (Guanyuan)

SP 4 (Gongsun)   when the Spleen branch is damaged

ST 30 (Qichong)

- for Ren Mai Vessel

RM 3 (Zhongji)

RM 2 (Qugu)

RM 4 (Guanyuan)

RM 5 (Shimen)

- for Du Mai Vessel

DM 1 (Changqiang)

RM 2 (Qugu)

SI 3 (Houxi)

- for Dai Mai Vessel

GB 26 (Daimai)

GB 41 (Zulinqi)

- for Yin Wei Mai Vessel

K 9 (Zhubin)

PC 6 (Neiguan)

- for Yin Qiao Mai Vessel

K 6 (Zhaohai)

K 8 (Jiaoxin)

Special attention should be paid to the following factors: psychological status, life style, physical activity, sexual life and hygiene.

The treatment proceeds according to the etiopathogenic type:

a) The Deficiency of the Kidney Qi

Therapeutic principle: warm the Kidney, support blood and regulate the Chong Mai and Ren Mai Vessels

Prescription:

RM 4 (Guanyuan)	is the Crossing point of the Ren Mai Vessel with the Kidney, Spleen and Liver channels; tones Kidney Qi
BL 23 (Shenshu)	is the Back-Shu point of the Kidney, nourishes the Yin and warms the Yang, tones the Kidney and the lumbar region
SP 6 (Sanyinjiao)	is the Crossing point of the three Yin channels of the foot, tones the Kidney, stimulates Qi and blood circulation
K 3 (Taixi)	is the Yuan-Source point of the Kidney channel, nourishes the Kidney and Liver, regulates the Chong Mai and Ren Mai vessels
ST 36 (Zusanli)	is the He point of the Stomach channel, tones the Spleen and regulates the Stomach (sources of blood), has a generally fortifying effect

In cases with deficiency of the Kidney Yang, the following points can be used in alternative prescriptions:

DM 14 (Mingmen)	strengthens the Kidney, tones the Yang, regulates menstruation, stops leukorrhea
RM 5 (Shimen)	is the Front-Mu point of the San Jiao warms the Kidney and tones the Yang, regulates menstruation
BL 33 (Zhongliao)	is the Crossing point of the Urinary Bladder and Gall Bladder channels, stimulates blood

circulation, disperses Cold, is indicated in infertility

b) The Deficiency of Blood

Therapeutic principle: nourish blood, nourish Yin

Prescription:

BL 17 (Geshu)	is the Influential point of blood, regulates blood, tones and regulates the Stomach
BL 20 (Pishu)	is the Back-Shu point of the Spleen, tones the Spleen, supports blood
SP 6 (Sanyinjiao)	stimulates the function of the Spleen and Stomach, supports blood, stimulates Qi and blood circulation
LV 13 (Zhangmen)	is the Front-Mu point of the Spleen, strengthens the Spleen and enhances the therapeutic effect
BL 21 (Weishu)	is the Back-Shu point of the Stomach, strengthens the Stomach and supports blood formation
SP 3 (Taibai)	is the Yuan-Source point of the Spleen channel, tones the Spleen

- If a deficiency of Yin is associated:

Therapeutic principle: nourish the Yin, nourish blood

Prescription:

RM 6 (Qihai)	reduces weakness, regulates Qi circulation, regulates the Chong Mai and Ren Mai Vessels
SP 6 (Sanyinjiao)	is the Crossing point of the three Yin channels of the foot, strengthens the Spleen, tones the Yin
K 2 (Rangu)	is the Ying point of the Kidney channel, nourishes the Yin, regulates the Chong Mai and Ren Mai vessels
BL 17 (Geshu)	is the Influential point of blood, nourishes the blood

K 14 (Siman)   strengthens the Kidney, regulates the Chong
                          Mai and Ren Mai vessels

c) The Deficiency of the Spleen Qi

Therapeutic principle: tone the Spleen

Prescription:

ST 36 (Zusanli)   strengthens the Spleen and Stomach, increases
                          body resistance

SP 3 (Taibai)   is the Yuan-Source point of the Spleen chan-
                          nel, tones the Spleen, regulates the Spleen and
                          Stomach

LV 13 (Zhangmen)   is the Front-Mu point of the Spleen regulates
                          the organs, tones the Spleen and Stomach

BL 21 (Weishu)   is the Back-Shu point of the Stomach, tones
                          the Spleen and regulates the Stomach

BL 20 (Pishu)   is the Back-Shu point of the Spleen, promotes
                          Spleen functions, regulates Spleen Qi

d) The Excess of Phlegm-Damp

Therapeutic principle: resolve the Phlegm, remove Damp

Prescription:

BL 20 (Pishu)   is the Back-Shu point of the Spleen, strength-
                          ens the Spleen and removes Damp

BL 21 (Weishu)   is the Back-Shu point of the Stomach, regu-
                          lates the Stomach and tones the Spleen, re-
                          moves pathogenic Damp

RM 12 (Zhongwan)   is the Front-Mu point of the Stomach and the
                          Influential point of the Fu organs, regulates
                          the Stomach, tones the Spleen and stimulates
                          the dispersion of Damp

ST 40 (Fenglong)   is the Luo point of the Stomach channel,
                          related to the Spleen channel, regulates the
                          Stomach, reduces Phlegm, calms the mind

ST 25 (Tianshu)   regulates the Stomach, tones the Spleen to
                          transform Damp, regulates Qi and menstrua-
                          tion

| **SP 6** (Sanyinjiao) | tones the Spleen and Stomach, stimulates the Spleen function of transforming Damp, regulates Qi and blood |

e) The Stagnation of the Liver Qi

Therapeutic principle: drain the Liver, stimulate blood circulation, nourish blood

Prescription:

RM 6 (Qihai)	regulates free circulation of Qi, regulates the Chong Mai and Ren Mai vessels
LV 2 (Xingjian)	is the Ying point of the Liver channel, removes Liver stagnation, removes pathogenic Heat from the Liver
LV 8 (Ququan)	is the He point of the Liver channel, regulates Qi and blood circulation, removes pathogenic Heat
LV 14 (Qimen)	is the Front-Mu point of the Liver and the Crossing point of the Liver and Spleen channels with the Yin Wei Mai Vessel, removes Liver Qi stagnation, stimulates blood circulation and remove stasis, tones the Spleen
SP 8 (Diji)	is the Xi point of the Spleen channel, stimulates the Spleen and Stomach, regulates menstruation, stops leukorrhea
K 21 (Youmen)	is the Crossing point of the Kidney channel and the Chong Mai Vessel, regulates the Liver and stimulates Qi circulation, strengthens the Spleen, removes pathogenic Heat from the abdomen, soothes spasms
PC 7 (Daling)	is the Yuan-Source of the Pericardium channel, sedates the mind
BL 32 (Ciliao)	regulates Qi, regulates menstruation, reduces pain, promotes blood

The following can be added:

E.P. Zigong

E.P. Weibao

ST 29 (Guilai)   regulates menstruation

The stimulation of the selected acupoints is done with the reducing or reinforcing method, according to the etiopathogenic type, of excess or deficiency. Moxibustion can be effective when strong stimulation is needed.

Usually a treatment series is repeated several times.

Infertility Caused by Tubal Factors

The causes that transform the fallopian tubes and interfere with their reproductive function vary: inflammation, mechanical factors, tubal endometriosis, uterine malpositions or tumoral masses which can cause an external compression and change the normal position of the fallopian tubes. In more than 40% of cases, the etiology is infection.

Etiopathogenesis

From the perspective of Chinese traditional medicine, infertility due to tubal obstruction results from stagnation of the Liver Qi. The Liver dysfunction can damage the Spleen function of transporting and transforming. This condition is known as "stagnation of the Liver Qi leading to the deficiency of the Spleen." Thus the Spleen can no longer transform Damp, which becomes Phlegm. The accumulation of Phlegm in the Lower Jiao will obstruct the uterus and injure the Chong Mai and Ren Mai Vessels.

Clinical Manifestations

Main symptoms include infertility; irregular menstrual cycles, accompanied by abdominal distension and a pressing sensation and yellowish, thick, adherent, malodorous, and irritating leukorrhea. Associated symptoms include oliguria, constipation, a sensation of heaviness in the body, and apathy. A yellow tongue coating and a rapid, sliding, strained pulse may also be present.

Treatment

Therapeutic principle: remove Damp, transform Phlegm, maintain the free circulation within the channels

Prescription:

RM 3 (Zhongji)	regulates the uterus, regulates the Lower Jiao, disperses Damp
SP 6 (Sanyinjiao)	tones the Spleen to remove Damp, stimulates Qi and blood circulation
ST 36 (Zusanli)	strengthens Spleen and Stomach, regulates Qi and blood circulation, removes Damp
ST 30 (Qichong)	is the Crossing point of the Stomach channel with the Chong Mai Vessel, removes Qi and blood obstruction
SP 9 (Yinlingquan)	is the He point of the Spleen channel, removes Damp from the Lower Jiao, disperses stasis
BL 18 (Ganshu)	is the Back-Shu point of the Liver, removes Qi stagnation, removes Damp
LV 5 (Ligou)	is the Luo point of the Liver channel, removes Liver Qi stagnation
E.P. Zigong	is located at 3 cun from RM 3, regulates the uterus, is indicated in cases of distal tubal obstruction

Acupuncture is given with the reinforcing method. For RM 3, a sensation of abdominal distension should be obtained, which allows the opening of the Chong Mai and Ren Mai vessels. A session is conducted daily.

ORAL CONTRACEPTIVE EFFECTS AND ACUPUNCTURE

The action of oral contraceptives is based upon the interference with the hypothalamic-pituitary-ovarian function. Among the contraceptive effects, structural and functional changes at different levels of the genital system occur and systemic effects can be associated. Their incidence and severity is related to the hormonal composition and the dose of each pill's component. Using low-dose pills has reduced many possible complications. There are cases of persistent symptoms and discomfort that may require discontinuation of oral contraceptives.

Acupuncture can help to restore the damaged energetic balance evidenced by some of the clinical manifestations. It may increase tolerance to the pills, allowing their continued use.

Breast Tenderness

Prescription:

a) **K 23** (Shengfu) + **RM 17** (Shanzhong) + **SP 21** (Dabao) + **ST 13** (Qihu)

b) **K 7** (Fuliu) + **K 10** (Yingu) + **K 27** (Shufu) + **ST 36** (Zusanli) + **ST 40** (Fenglong)

c) **BL 16** (Dushu) + **BL 17** (Geshu) + **BL 18** (Ganshu) + **RM 17** (Shanzhong) + **LI 6** (Pianli)

d) **LV 3** (Taichong) + **GB 41** (Zulinqi) + **ST 18** (Rugen) + **SI 1** (Shaoze)

Acupuncture treatment is given during the second phase of the menstrual cycle, every three or four days. Needles are retained for 15 minutes and stimulation is given with the even movement method.

Breakthrough Bleeding and Spotting

These symptoms usually disappear spontaneously after 3 to 4 months of oral contraceptive administration. Their persistence may require treatment and acupuncture offers an easy alternative.

Prescription:

a) **SP 5** (Shangqiu) + **SP 9** (Yinlingquan) + **SP 10** (Xuehai) + **ST 30** (Qichong)

b) **BL 31** (Shangliao) + **BL 32** (Ciliao) + **BL 33** (Zhongliao) + **BL 34** (Xialiao) + **L 7** (Lieque) + **SP 6** (Sanyinjiao)

Acupuncture is given in every two days and stimulation uses the even movement method. Needles are retained for approximately 15 to 20 minutes.

Postpill Amenorrhea

Postpill amenorrhea can affect up to 5% of the users of oral contraceptives. Amenorrhea can persist up to six months or more after birth control pills are discontinued.

The onset of amenorrhea with the use of oral contraceptives first requires that pregnancy—intrauterine or ectopic— and/or a pituitary adenoma be ruled out.

Acupuncture treatment as an alternative therapy can avoid side effects of hormonal therapy.

Prescription:

a) **RM 3** (Zhongji) + **RM 4** (Guanyuan) + **SP 13** (Fushe) + **ST 25** (Tianshu)

b) **LI 4** (Hegu) + **LI 7** (Lieque) + **K 10** (Yingu) + **SP 4** (Gongsun)

c) **SP 6** (Sanyinjiao) + **BL 18** (Ganshu) + **SP 10** (Xuehai) + **RM 6** (Qihai) + **RM 4** (Guanyuan)

d) **RM 4** (Guanyuan) + **ST 29** (Guilai) + **SP 6** (Sanyinjiao) + **SP 10** (Xuehai) + **LV 3** (Taichong) + **LI 4** (Hegu)

e) **RM 4** (Guanyuan) + **BL 20** (Pishu) + **BL 23** (Shenshu) + **ST 36** (Zusanli) + **SP 6** (Sanyinjiao)

Auricular Therapy: points Uterus, Ovary, Shenmen can also be used alone or in different prescriptions.

Oligomenorrhea

Prescription:

a)**ST 25** (Tianshu) + **K 13** (Qixue) + **SP 8** (Diji) + **LV 3** (Taichong)

b) **RM 4** (Guanyuan) + **RM 6** (Qihai) + **SP 6** (Sanyinjiao) + **H 7** (Shenmen)

Acupuncture treatment starts three or four days before the date when menstruation should begin and is continued for three or four days after that date. A daily session is given and needles are retained for approximately 15-20 minutes.

Auricular Therapy can also be used.

In a study of women who have used oral contraceptives in the last five years, it was observed that patients who had used birth control pills for more than 2 to 3 years required more treatment. The same observation was true for patients with a history of menstrual disorders before use of oral contraceptives was instituted.

Circulatory Disorders

Circulatory disorders are related to the pathology of the Spleen channel, following the course of the internal saphenous vein.

Prescription:

a) **SP 6** (Sanyinjiao) + **SP 9** (Yinlingquan) + **SP 11** (Jimen) + **RM 2** (Qugu)

b) **SP 6** (Sanyinjiao) + **LV 3** (Taichong) + **LV 8** (Ququan)

c) **SP 9** (Yinlingquan) + **SP 13** (Fushe) + **PC 6** (Neiguan) + **ST 25** (Tianshu)

d) **SP 2** (Dadu) + **SP 3** (Taibai) + **ST 34** (Liangqiu) + **ST 36** (Zusanli) + **GB 34** (Yanglingquan)

e) **GB 26** (Daimai) + **GB 27** (Wushu) + **GB 41** (Zulinqi) + **SJ 8** (Sanyangluo)

One to two sessions are given weekly; with 8 to 10 sessions forming one treatment. Needles are retained for approximately 15 to 20 minutes.

Asthenia

Acupuncture treatment can be used after possible organic causes have been excluded.

Prescription:

a) **BL 23** (Shenshu) + **DM 3** (Yaoyangquan) + **K 7** (Fuliu)

b) **L 7** (Lieque) + **LI 4** (Hegu) + **ST 36** (Zusanli) + **BL 67** (Zhiyin)

c) **ST 36** (Zusanli) + **BL 8** (Luoque) + **SJ 3** (Zhongzhu) + **RM 6** (Qihai) + **GB 34** (Yanglingqaun)

d) **SI 3** (Houxi) + **BL 62** (Shenmai) + **LV 8** (Ququan) + **SJ 5** (Waiguan) + **H 9** (Shaochong)

e) **RM 12** (Zhongwan) + **DM 20** (Baihui) + **L 1** (Zhongfu) + **LV 14** (Qimen)

Auricular Therapy: points Heart, San Jiao, Sympathetic nervous system can be used.

ACUTE MASTITIS

The inflammatory breast pathology consists of several entities: lymphangitis, acute mastitis and acute suppurative infections. They occur most frequently in postpartum during lactation and more rarely during pregnancy. The most common etiologic agent is *Staphylococcus aureus* which spreads through nipple fissures and erosions in primiparas and as a result of inadequate breast hygiene. The treatment consists of applying heat and continuing nursing from the affected breast; artificial drainage; anti-inflammatory drugs and antibiotics; and surgical treatment (incision and drainage in the suppurative forms).

Acupuncture treatment can be effective in early stages but not in cases of abscess formation.

In Chinese traditional medicine, acute mastitis is called "Ru Yong," while "Waichui Ru Yong" defines external mastitis that begins with the start of breast-feeding. It was believed that as the newborn fell asleep at the breast, the air from its nostrils entered into the milk and mixed with the Heat of the milk.

Etiopathogenesis

The nipple is located on the course of the Liver channel and the breast is in the distribution area of the Stomach channel.

Mastitis is due to milk retention in the breast as a result of several factors:

- the stagnation of the Liver Qi due to emotional factors disturbance (cares, anxiety, depression, irritability) that is favored during the postpartum period
- the stagnation of Heat in the Stomach channel due to excessive intake of sweet and greasy food
- constitutional excess of Yang, with excessive Heat in the Liver and Stomach
- the invasion of pathogenic exogenous factors such as Wind and Fire, favored by the existence of nipple lesions

All these circumstances can cause the obstruction of the channels, blocking the circulation of Qi and leading to the development of stasis.

Clinical Manifestations

Main symptoms include redness, swelling, heat and pain of the involved breast, this phenomenon is rarely seen bilaterally. A tumoral mass may be palpated, the consistency of which will depend upon its degree of formation and the stage of pus accumulation. Associated symptoms may include high fever, a generally disturbed condition, headache, nausea, thirst, nervousness, and constipation. The expression of milk is difficult. In severe cases, axillary lumps can be felt on palpation. A red tongue with a yellow, thick coating and a string-taut, sliding, rapid pulse may also be noted.

Treatment

Therapeutic principle: regulate Liver Qi and the Qi of the Stomach channel, remove stagnation and disperse the Heat

Prescription:

GB 21 (Jianjing)   is the Crossing point of the Gall Bladder, Stomach, San Jiao channels and the Yang Wei Mai Vessel, whose courses cross the thoracic and/or breast area; regulates the channels Qi; removes Heat and disperses stasis; is an efficient point for mastitis

ST 18 (Rugen)   regulates Qi and blood circulation, removes Heat from the Stomach channel

ST 36 (Zusanli)   is the He point of the Stomach channel, regulates the Stomach, removes Heat from the channel and increases the body resistance

RM 17 (Shanzhong)   is the Influential point of the Qi, regulates Qi functions and removes the obstruction of lactation

SI 1 (Shaoze)   is the Jing-Well point of the Small Intestine channel, removes the channels obstruction, regulates Qi, allows the expression of milk, is an empirical point in treatment of mastitis

LV 3 (Taichong)   is the Yuan-Source point of the Liver channel, removes Qi stagnation, stimulates Qi and blood circulation, removes pathogenic Heat

The selected acupoints are stimulated with the reducing method and the needles are left in place for approximately 15 to 20 minutes. For GB 21 the insertion is oblique, avoiding deep insertion to prevent pneumothorax and strong stimulation to prevent the syncope. For RM 17 the needle insertion is also oblique, waiting for the acupuncture sensation to spread towards the involved breast. SI 1 is pricked for bleeding. A session is conducted daily. In the early stages of mastitis, acupuncture is effective after 3 to 6 sessions.

Other points can also be used in alternative prescription as follows:

LV 14 (Qimen)   is the Front-Mu point of the Liver, removes

	Liver Qi stagnation, stimulates blood circulation and removes stasis
LI 11 (Quchi)	is the He point of the Large Intestine channel, removes pathogenic Heat, removes channels obstruction, regulates Qi and blood
DM 14 (Dazhui)	is the Crossing point of the Yang channels of the hand and foot with Dai Mai Vessel, stimulates the circulation of Yang and removes Heat, stimulates circulation and calms the mind
GB 41 (Zulinqi)	is the Shu-Stream point of the Gall Bladder channel and the Confluent point of the Dai Mai vessel, removes Liver Qi stagnation, removes pathogenic Heat

Another therapeutic method involves selecting the site for needle insertion in the following way: bilaterally, between T4 and T 7 vertebrae, the pores form depressions that approximate the size of a millet bean. Seven to ten such depressions can exist. The needles are inserted in the selected points and stimulation is given with the reducing method, after the needles are withdrawn. Usually the points on the opposite side are also stimulated; 2 to 3 sessions are required.

Bleeding is another method that should be considered for the treatment of mastitis. On inspection, between the T7 and T12 vertebrae, small red points of about 0,5 mm in diameter can be observed. These points maintain their red color on pressure. They are usually located on the same side with the affected breast, though they also exist, more rarely, on the opposite side. After the skin is disinfected, the needle is inserted in the red points, and these are pricked for bleeding, pressing the area with one finger. A single session is usually enough as the red points and the breast pain disappear after 9 hours on the average.

FIBROCYSTIC BREAST DISEASE

Fibrocystic breast disease is a benign pathology caused by ovarian dysfunction. Neuropsychologic imbalance favors the development of this condition. Fibrocystic breast disease occurs most frequently in women younger than 30 years of age and during perimenopause, when it can affect as many as 60% of women.

The mammary lesions can be:

- diffuse, affecting the mammary gland globally, with cyclic variations in consistency
- circumscribed, in the form of multiple nodules, of different size and increased consistency, well-delimited and usually located in the upper external quadrant. The associated pains are bilateral, with cyclic evolution according to menstruation. The treatment is local or systemic, using progestins.

From the perspective of Chinese traditional medicine, the existence of benign tumoral masses in the breast shows disorders in the circulation of Qi and blood or Qi and blood deficiency with delayed circulation.

Etiopathogenesis

a) The Stagnation of the Liver Qi

Frequently Liver Qi stagnation is caused by depression that affects the Liver function of maintaining free circulation of Qi, causing Qi stagnation. The delay of Qi and blood circulation affects the Chong Mai and Ren Mai vessels causing menstrual cycle disorders. Prolonged obstruction of Liver Qi, resulting in Qi and blood stagnation, can cause palpable breast tumoral masses, as the nipple is located on the course of the Liver channel.

b) The Ascending of the Yang Liver

Liver Qi obstruction, caused by depression, anxiety, or anger can turn into Fire. As a Yang pathogenic factor, the Fire consumes the internal Yin and is characterized by ascending movement, causing symptoms of excess to appear in the upper part of the body. The formation of the tumoral masses shows prolonged Qi obstruction.

c) The Yin Deficiency of the Kidney and Liver

This type of deficiency can be attributed to emotional factors disturbance, overstrain and stress, consumption of Yin in chronic disease, or the process of aging. The Yin deficiency produces internal Heat and affects the Chong Mai and Ren Mai vessels with menstrual cycle disorders as a consequence. The circulation of Qi is delayed, causing tumoral masses to appear.

d) The Deficiency of Qi and Blood

The deficiency of Qi and blood can be constitutional or may be caused by chronic disease, inadequate food intake, or physical and psychological overstrain. Qi deficiency prevents the ascent of Yang, with insufficient nourishment of the upper part of the body. The delay of Qi and blood circulation causes tumoral masses to form.

Clinical Manifestations

Upon palpation of the breast, tumoral masses can be detected. Typically these are well-delimited, with a smooth contour and moderate consistency, mobile or seeming to be locally distended, without alterations of the supradjacent skin.

Based on the etiopathogenic type, additional symptoms may be present:

a) The Stagnation of the Liver Qi

Main symptoms include painful breast distension, exacerbated during menstruation, and an irregular menstrual cycle with scanty flow and dark-colored blood, with dysmenorrhea. Associated symptoms include distension in the hypochondriac region, depression, and a sensation of thoracic fullness and constriction alleviated by deep and frequent sighing. A bluish tongue (or one with purplish spots on the borders) and a wiry, string-taut pulse may be observed.

b) The Ascending of Yang Liver

Main symptoms include local tumefaction and a sensation of internal heat, dry mouth, bitter taste, ocular congestion and pruritus, headache, vertigo, tinnitus, irritability, insomnia, palpitations, and oliguria. A red tongue with a yellow coating and a wiry, rapid pulse may also be noted.

c) The Yin Deficiency of the Kidney and Liver

Main symptoms include menstrual cycle disorders with scanty menstrual flow, dizziness, vision disturbances, and a sensation of heat in the chest, palms and feet. Associated symptoms include a sensation of weakness in the knees and lumbar area. The patient may evidence a pale tongue with a white, thin coating and a thready and rapid pulse.

d) The Deficiency of Qi and Blood

Main symptoms include a long menstrual cycle with scanty flow and light red blood, accompanied by dysmenorrhea which is alleviated by warmth and pressure. Pallor, persistent asthenia, lack of appetite, cold limbs, palpitations, dizziness, a pale tongue with a thin coating and a weak, thready pulse may also be observed.

Treatment

Therapeutic principle: remove Qi stagnation, remove stasis and obstruction of the channels, tone the deficiencies

Prescription:

RM 17 (Shanzhong) is the Crossing point of the Kidney, Spleen, Small Intestine and Pericardium channels and the Influential point of Qi; regulates the movement of Qi; stimulates Qi circulation and removes stagnation

SI 1 (Shaoze) is the Jing-Well point of the Small Intestine channel, removes obstruction of the channels and removes breast tumoral masses

GB 21 (Jianjing) regulates the Qi of the channels and disperses stasis

Associating the acupoints SI 1 and GB 21 is effective in the treatment of breast tumoral masses.

LV 3 (Taichong) is the Yuan-Source point of the Liver channel, removes Liver Qi stagnation and restores the normal functions of the Liver

LV 8 (Ququan) is the He point of the Liver channel, nourishes the Yin Liver, regulates Qi and blood

ST 36 (Zusanli) is the He point of the Stomach channel on which the breast is located, regulates Qi and blood

LI 4 (Hegu) is the Yuan-Source point of the Large Intestine channel, regulates Qi and blood, removes stagnation

Acupuncture is given with the reducing method and the needles are left in place for approximately 30 minutes, except for SI 1 which is pricked for bleeding.

ST 18 (Rugen)   is located in the mammary area and has the local effect of removing the obstruction of the channel

For stimulating this last point moxibustion is used, with moxa cones and continuous movement around the point for approximately 20 minutes per session. There should be no crust formation.

Adding this point, after a series of 10 sessions during which the above prescription is used, can reduce the size of the tumoral mass. A session is conducted daily, for many weeks, until the complete disappearance of the tumoral masses.

FIBROADENOMA OF THE BREAST

Fibroadenoma of the breast is a benign tumor that appears in young women who experience excessive estrogenic stimulation. The evolution is very slow, with visible changes appearing after years. Usually this condition is asymptomatic.

In Chinese traditional medicine, the fibroadenoma belongs to the categories named Ru Li, Ru He or Ru Ya, and has a progressive onset and a long evolution.

Etiopathogenesis

Several conditions are involved in the etiopathogenesis of the breast fibroadenoma: Liver Qi stagnation, Phlegm accumulation and the obstruction of the channels.

a) The Stagnation of the Liver Qi

The disturbance of emotional factors affects the Liver function and causes Liver Qi stagnation. The circulation of Qi is damaged and as "Qi is the commander of blood," this will also cause the stagnation of blood. Affecting Qi and blood circulation causes obstruction of the channels. This phenomenon will manifest clinically by the appearance of breast tumoral masses, as the breast is located on the course of the Liver channel.

b) The Accumulation of Phlegm

A constitutional tendency to Phlegm accumulation is particularly likely to exist in obese women. This will damage the circulation of Qi, causing the stagnation of Phlegm, Qi and blood.

Clinical Manifestations

The main symptom is the tumoral mass, usually located in the upper external quadrant of the breast. It is well-delimited, round or oval in shape, has a hard or elastic consistency, and is normal in aspect. The volume is 1 to 10 cm in diameter and is not cyclically influenced. Other clinical manifestations can be present, according to the etiopathogenic type:

a) The Stagnation of the Liver Qi

Main symptoms include menstrual cycle disorders and dysmenorrhea, painful distension in the hypochondriac region and lower abdomen, breast distension, depression, irritability, and lack of appetite. A dark, red tongue (or one with purplish spots on the borders) and a string-taut pulse may be noted.

b) The Accumulation of Phlegm

Main symptoms include menstrual cycle disorders, occasional amenorrhea, abundant leukorrhea, a sensation of thoracic fullness, vision disturbances, vertigo, tinnitus, insomnia, a sensation of heaviness in the head, lack of appetite, and pallor. The patient may also have a white, thick tongue coating and a string-taut, sliding pulse.

Treatment

Several prescriptions can be used:

a) Association of Ashi points with secondary points

GB 21 (Jianjing)	regulates the Qi of the channels that pass on the area of breast location, removes stasis
ST 36 (Zusanli)	is the He point of the Stomach, regulates Qi, removes obstruction
RM 17 (Shanzhong)	is the Influential point of Qi, regulates Qi and removes obstruction
SP 6 (SanyinJiao)	regulates the Stomach and tones the Spleen to remove Damp, regulates Qi and blood circulation, removes the obstruction of channels

b) The needles are inserted in the tumoral mass, 3 to 5 needles according to the size of tumor, with a depth of insertion of 0,3-0,5 cun. Acupuncture is given with the reducing method, twisting and scratching the needle for 3 to 5 minutes.

Other points can be added:

GB 21 (Jianjing)

RM 17 (Shanzhong)

ST 36 (Zusanli)

SP 6 (Sanyinjiao)

The stimulation of these acupoints is of very short duration during a daily session. The treatment consists of more series, of 10 sessions each, repeated after 2 to 3 days.

CHAPTER 4

ASPECTS OF SEXUAL DYSFUNCTION

From ancient times, Chinese civilizations considered sexual activity an integral part of the natural order of the Universe. The union between male and female is the union of the Yang and Yin, Sky and Earth. Sexual dysfunction has repercussions for the individual, for the couple and family life and, indirectly, for the entire community.

Chinese texts, dating from as early as the 11th century B.C., such as the "Guide to the Art of the Bedroom" and the most famous work, "Su Nu King" (Classic of the innocent girl), reveal the cultural value for sexual harmony. This kind of literature was never vulgar or pornographic and periodically has been revised and reissued.

Ideas about sexual health and sexual functioning have been long established and well formulated. Sexual harmony of a couple and sexual satisfaction are essential to maintain balance for the indidividual, family and community. Sexual dysfunction can lead to a variety of disease states. Normal sexual activity is an integral part of overall health and is fundamental to longevity. From the Chinese perspective, the woman has the right to satisfy her sexual needs and her partner is obliged to meet those needs. Unfounded sexual abstinence is out of conformity with this concept of harmonious integration.

Sexual pathology is varied in type and intensity. Conditions ranging from frigidity (deficiency) to nymphomania (excess), as well as abnormal sexual behavior, can be encountered in practice. Although prevalent, sexual problems are seldom the sole reason for medical examination. A careful, delicate, but thorough, history can uncover poor sexual health, helping to confirm its all too frequent implication as a cause of other illnesses.

Because sexuality is one of the major functions of the Ego, restoring normal sexual activity should always be an objective of treatment. Some of the most frequent aspects of practice are presented below.

DECREASE OR ABSENCE OF LIBIDO

When the reason for the medical examination is the decrease or absence of libido, establishing the etiologic circumstances is very important. The onset of sexual dysfunction may be very rapid or slow and progressive. Many events may precede its onset: family concerns, medical, surgical, or psychoaffective concerns.

Sudden Onset of Decreased Libido

Previous to the onset of sexual dysfunction, women who report decreased libido typically have experienced sexual satisfaction. The decrease of libido is rapid and often can be attributed to the following etiologic factors.

a) Emotional Causes

Sexual dysfunction frequently is caused by emotional trauma, e.g., the death of a family member or familial discord. In time, as the unpleasant event passes, sexual dysfunction can spontaneously regress. Conjugal conflicts, whether actual or perceived, can have lingering consequences. A negative pattern involving rejection of the sexual partner and refusal of sexual activity may be established and maintained, even when the woman desires to resume a sexual relationship.

Prescription:

ST 14 (Kufang) is used in cases of physical or psychological disorders caused by shock; psychic or moral hypersensitivity, or unwillingness to be touched or seen

SP 5 (Shangqiu) is indicated in cases characterized by excessive worry, pessimism, or anxiety

Psychotherapy may play an important role as a means of uncovering the cause of the dysfunctional behavior and of divesting the cause of its power to result in symptoms.

b) Medical and Surgical Causes

Medical and surgical concerns are often the basis of disorders of the libido and are also the most easily treated. A typical etiologic factor is a surgical procedure of the lower abdomen, e.g., uterine curettage, hysterosalpingography, or cesarean section. Such procedures represent circumstances during which the body's resistance can be lowered and made susceptible to the invasion of exogenous pathogenic Cold which will accumulate in the Lower Jiao.

Prescription:

RM 4 (Guanyuan) warms the Kidney and Lower Jiao, supports the return of the Yang, preserves the Essence

RM 5 (Shimen)   is the Front-Mu point of San Jiao, warms the
                          Kidney and tones the Yang

The acupoint RM 5, called the "Gate of Stone" is also indicated in cases which have a psychological etiology. If stimulated, this acupoint generates and increases sexual desire.

RM 6 (Qihai)   tones the Yang and Kidney Essence, stimu-
                          lates Yang to ascend and tones Qi, is indicated
                          in conditions of Cold in the genital system

ST 28 (Shuidao)   regulates the Lower Jiao

ST 29 (Guilai)   regulates the Lower Jiao and warms the uterus

ST 30 (Qichong)   regulates the Chong Mai and Ren Mai vessels
                          and the uterus

The notion of "Cold in the genital system" refers to the invasion of exogenous pathogenic Cold in the Lower Jiao, but it also signifies listlessness, insensibility, and lack of desire.

Progressive Onset of Libido Disturbances

A thorough history can disclose the causes of progressive loss of libido. From the perspective of traditional Chinese medicine, this pathology is of the deficiency type.

Etiopathogenesis

a) The Deficiency of Heart Qi

This deficiency is caused by chronic disease, by damage to the Yang from severe, acute illness, or as a consequence of the aging process. The deficiency of Qi will result in hypofunctioning of the Zang-Fu organs and blood circulation disorders. Because the Heart houses mentality, deficiency of Heart Qi will cause psychological disorders that affect sexual functioning.

b) The Deficiency of the Kidney

Deficiency of the Kidney Yang can be caused by chronic disease, excessive sexual activity, or consumption of Yang with aging. The warming function of Yang is damaged as is the nourishing support of the marrow, brain and bones. The reproductive function is diminished, possibly as a result of sexual dysfunction. A deficiency of the Yang of the Spleen may be associated with this condition.

Kidney Yin may become deficient in relation to chronic disease, aging (especially during menopause), and convalescence from febrile disease. The deficient Yin causes an excess of internal Heat that ascends and is manifested as psychic disorders.

Clinical Manifestations

a) The Deficiency of Heart Qi

The main symptoms include physical, psychological, and sexual asthenia, palpitations, cold limbs, and spontaneous sweating. A pale tongue may be noted as may a weak and thready pulse.

b) The Deficieny of the Kidney

The deficiency of the Kidney Yang is characterized by asthenia, depression, aversion to cold, cold limbs, a sensation of lumbar weakness, and edema of the lower limbs. A pale tongue with a white coating may be observed accompanied by a deep, weak pulse.

The main symptoms of deficiency of the Kidney Yin include asthenia, depression, insomnia, memory disorders, behavioral disturbances, hot flushes, and noctural sweating. Oliguria, constipation, and dryness of the vaginal mucosa may be associated with this condition. A red tongue with a thin coating may be noted; a thready, rapid pulse may be palpated.

Treatment

a) The Deficiency of the Heart Qi

Therapeutic principle: strengthen the Qi, calm the Heart

Prescription:

RM 4 (Guanyuan)	stimulates the return of Yang and preserves the Essence
DM 1 (Changqiang)	is the Luo point of the Du Mai Vessel, removes sexual asthenia
BL 15 (Xinshu)	is the Back-Shu point of the Heart, regulates the Heart
H 1 (Jiquan)	stimulates Qi circulation
H 3 (Shaohai)	is the He point of the Heart channel, sooths the mind, regulates Qi and blood circulation
H 9 (Shaochong)	is the Jing-Well point of the Heart channel,

calms the Heart and sedates the mind, restores the Yang

b) The Deficiency of the Kidney

- The Deficiency of the Kidney Yang

Therapeutic principle: tone the Yang, warm the Kidney and strengthen the Spleen

Prescription:

BL 23 (Shenshu)	is the Back-Shu point of the Kidney, nourishes the Yin and strengthens the Yang, supports the brain and marrow
BL 20 (Pishu)	is the Back-Shu point of the Spleen, strengthens the Spleen
RM 4 (Guanyuan)	warms the Kidney, tones Jing, tones the Qi, stimulates the return of Yang, regulates Qi and blood
RM 7 (Yinliao)	warms the Kidney Yang
K 12 (Dahe)	tones the Kidney Qi and regulates the uterus
BL 43 (Gaohuang)	strengthens the functions of Qi and tones the Kidney, calms the Heart and mind

- The Deficiency of the Kidney Yin

Therapeutic principle: tone the Kidney Yin, calm the Heart

Prescription:

RM 4 (Guanyuan)	warms the Kidney, regulates Qi and blood, regulates the uterus
BL 23 (Shenshu)	nourishes the Kidney Yin
K 2 (Rangu)	is the Ying point of the Kidney channel, nourishes the Kidney Yin, cools the Heat, regulates the Lower Jiao.
K 3 (Taixi)	is the Yuan-Source point of the Kidney channel, nourishes and tones the Lower Jiao and regulates the Chong Mai and Ren Mai vessels.
H 6 (Yinxi)	is the Xi point of the Heart channel, regulates the Heart and mind, cools the blood, and

| | reduces sweating. |
| **SP 8** (Diji) | is the Xi point of the Spleen channel, tones the sexual energy and increases the vaginal secretions. |

Acupuncture is given with the reinforcing method.

The involvement of the Liver, which governs sexual desire, should also be mentioned. Damage to the Liver, caused by disturbance of emotional factors, can affect the libido.

In such cases other points can be associated:

LV 1 (Dadun)	is the Jing-Well point of the Liver channel, regulates the Lower Jiao, calms the mind and feelings.
LV 2 (Xingjian)	is the Ying point of the Liver channel, disperses the Liver Fire, cools the Heat and the Lower Jiao.
LV 14 (Qimen)	is the Front-Mu point of the Liver; removes Liver Qi stagnation; stimulates blood circulation.
BL 18 (Ganshu)	is the Back-Shu point of the Liver; removes Liver Qi stagnation; removes pathogenic Fire; stimulates the mind.

Other prescriptions can also be used:

a) **DM 4** (Mingmen) + **DM 2** (Yaoshu) + **LV 8** (Ququan) + **SI 5** (Yanggu)

b) **RM 5** (Shimen) + **RM 6** (Qihai) + **ST 28** (Shuidao) + **ST 45** (Lidui)

c) **SP 9** (Yinlingquan) + **K 12** (Dahe) + **ST 36** (Zusanli) + **LV 13** (Zhangmen) + **PC 6** (Neiguan)

ANORGASMIA

Anorgasmia has feminine and masculine causes. The attitude and behavior of the partner during sexual intercourse are extremely important. The absence of the prelude, short duration of sexual intercourse, premature ejaculation, and disorders of sexual behavior are circumstances that can lead to anorgasmia in women.

From ancient times, the weight of opinion, from the Chinese perspective, has held that the male should develop the ability to delay ejaculation until the woman has reached orgasm. Because the woman is Yin, the achievement of sexual satisfaction is slower than for the man, who is Yang.

The feminine causes can be somatic diseases (e.g., dyspareunia, vaginismus) or psychological issues, such as the absence of the libido or inability to relax and enjoy the experience. In the latter case, repeated failures establish a vicious cycle.

K 4 (Dazhong)	is the Luo point of the Kidney channel; helps to diminish a sense of inferiority, as well as the effects of repeated failure; helps to lessen fear and anxiety.
SP 5 (Shangqiu)	is indicated in cases of pessimism, anxiety about the future, obsession, or lack of self control.
ST 15 (Wuyi)	is indicated for difficult orgasm.

After the organic pathologies (e.g., genital infections, prolapse, endometriosis, cervical lesions etc.) are excluded, acupuncture can prove helpful in the treatment of other causes of anorgasmia.

DYSPAREUNIA

Dyspareunia is defined as painful sexual intercourse. It can cause an abnormal sexual life and multiple psychosomatic difficulties. The pain may be felt as a burning sensation during sexual intercourse, pelvic pain especially in the iliac fossa, or lower abdominal pain after intercourse.

a) Superficial pain that appears at the beginning of sexual intercourse impedes pleasure and orgasm.

From the perspective of Chinese traditional medicine, this condition is caused by Yin stagnation and an excess in the Lower Jiao. Pain is the primary manifestation of that stagnation.

Therapeutic principle: drain and regulate Lower Jiao, remove stagnation.

Prescription:

SP 1 (Yinbai)	is the Jing-Well point of the Spleen channel, promotes blood circulation and supports Qi, is indicated in cases of genital stagnation.

SP 8 (Diji)	is the Xi point of the Spleen channel, regulates blood, is indicated in pelvic stagnation.
SP 9 (Yinlingquan)	is the He point of the Spleen channel, tones the Spleen, stimulates the circulation within San Jiao.
BL 53 (Baohuang)	regulates the Qi of Fu organs, regulates the Lower Jiao, is indicated in pelvic congestion and all diseases of the uterus.
RM 3 (Zhongji)	regulates the Lower Jiao.
RM 4 (Guanyuan)	tones Qi, regulates Qi and blood.
LV 1 (Dadun)	is the Jing point of the Liver channel, regulates the Lower Jiao and sedates the mind.
K 13 (Qixue)	drains the Lower Jiao, regulates the Chong Mai and Ren Mai Vessels.

Acupuncture is given with the reinforcing or reducing method according to the selected points, moxa to RM 3, RM 4.

b) Profound pain that appears during sexual intercourse allows sexual pleasure to develop but interferes with the ability to achieve orgasm.

From the perspective of Chinese traditional medicine, this condition is believed to be the consequence of stagnation in the Lower Jiao and is often attributed to blood deficiency and/or Qi deficiency. Blood deficiency may be caused by consumption of the Yin in cases where severe emotional trauma or excessive sexual activity has occurred. Because of the blood deficiency, the Zang-Fu organs and the channels cannot be properly nourished. Qi deficiency may appear as a result of stress, strain, or the aging process.

Prescription:

RM 4 (Guanyuan)	strengthens the original Qi, regulates Qi and blood circulation.
RM 5 (Shimen)	increases the libido.
K 2 (Rangu)	is the Ying point of the Kidney channel, regulates the Lower Jiao, is useful in cases of delay or absence of orgasm.

K 3 (Taixi)   is the Yuan-Source point of the Kidney channel, nourishes the Yin and strengthens the Yang; tones Kidney Qi

In order to regulate and drain the Lower Jiao, other points located on the Kidney channel can also be selected: **K 5** (Shuiquan), **K 6** (Zhaohai), **K 7** (Fuliu), **K 13** (Qixue) or **K 15** (Zhongzhu).

SP 9 (Yinlingquan)   promotes circulation in San Jiao.

LV 3 (Taichong)   is the Yuan-Source point of the Liver channel, promotes Qi and blood circulation, transforms stagnation, is indicated in painful sexual intercourse.

In all cases the association of points that can calm the Heart and mind is useful:

H 7 (Shenmen)   is the Yuan-Source point of the Heart channel, soothes the mind.

PC 6 (Neiguan)   is the Luo point of the Pericardium channel, nourishes the Heart and sedates the mind.

Acupuncture is given with the reducing method.

VAGINISMUS

Vaginismus is the reflexive, violent and lasting contracture of the lower vaginal muscles. The spasm of the vaginal entrance makes penetration impossible. Vaginismus can be primary, usually related to one's first experience of sexual intercourse. A secondary vaginismus is also described. Vaginismus is frequently associated with and related to dyspareunia. A variety of organic and anatomic factors, as well as psychosocial and educational issues, can be involved.

From the perspective of Chinese traditional medicine, vaginismus can be the consequence of any of the three etiologic circumstances which follow:

a) The Deficiency of the Kidney Yin

This may be caused by excessive sexual activity or chronic diseases. If there is a Yin deficiency, the Yang, without control, becomes hyperactive and symptoms of the excess type appear.

b)The Deficiency of the Liver Yin

In chronic diseases or in cases where blood production is insufficient, this type of deficiency can occur. The insufficient Yin of the Liver is not able to adequately nourish the muscles; thus, spasms and muscular contractions develop. The "Sea of blood" is empty; consequently, disorders of the menstrual cycle relative to deficiency (e.g. amenorrhea) appear.

c) The Deficiency of the Kidney and Liver Yin

This type of deficiency may result from injury to the Yin blood in cases of severe emotional trauma, stress, strain, or consumption of the Yin of the Kidney and Liver in older subjects (e.g. in menopause). The Yin deficiency causes endogenous Heat and symptoms of false excess. The Chong Mai and Ren Mai vessels are injured.

Cases of incidental vaginismus are considered to be the consequence of excessive sexual activity that causes the deficiency of Yin in the Lower Jiao.

Treatment

Therapeutic principle: strengthen the deficient Yin.

Prescription:

RM 7 (Yinjiao)   is indicated for constrictive vaginal pains.

SP 6 (Sanyinjiao)   is the crossing point of the three Yin channels of the foot, the Kidney, Liver and Spleen, strengthens Yin.

LV 3 (Taichong)   is the Yuan-Source point of the Liver channel, promotes Qi and blood circulation and is selected for its antispastic effect.

LV 9 (Yinbao)   can smooth the perineal area.

GB 26 (Daimai)   is indicated in muscular spasm.

GB 34 (Yanglingquan) is the reunion point of the muscles.

According to the etiopathogenesis, other points can be added:

a) The Deficiency of the Kidney Yin

K 2 (Rangu)   is the Ying point of the Kidney channel, regulates the lower Jiao.

K 3 (Taixi)	is the Yuan-Source point of the Kidney channel, nourishes the Kidney Yin, supports the Lower Jiao.
K6 (Zhaohai)	strengthens the Kidney and regulates the Lower Jiao, sedates pain.
BL 23 (Shenshu)	is the Back-Shu point of the Kidney, nourishes the Yin, tones the Kidney.

Acupuncture is given with the reinforcing method.

b) The Deficiency of the Liver Yin

LV 2 (Xingjian)	is the Ying point of the Liver channel, drains and cools the Lower Jiao.
LV 4 (Zhongfeng)	is the Jing-River point of the Liver channel.
BL 18 (Ganshu)	is the Back-Shu point of the Liver, strengthens the Liver Qi, regulates blood.

These points are indicated in vaginal spasm and painful vaginal contractions. Acupuncture is given with the reinforcing method.

c) The Deficiency of the Kidney and Liver Yin

| RM 4 (Guanyuan) | is the crossing point of the Ren Mai Vessel with the three Yin channels of the foot, tones the Yin, strengthens the Kidney and Liver. |
| K 3 (Taixi) | is the Yuan-Source point of the Kidney channel, nourishes the Kidney and Liver, regulates the Chong Mai and Ren Mai Vessels. |

Acupuncture is given with the reinforcing method and moxibustion can be used to stimulate acupoint RM 4.

In cases of incidental vaginismus, the following may be associated:

| ST 33 (Yinshi) | restores the Yin/Yang balance within the pelvis. |

Other prescriptions include:

a) LV 1 (Dadun) + SP 6 (Sanyinjiao)

b) LV 1 (Dadun) + RM 4 (Guanyuan)

c) LV 1 (Dadun) + LV 3 (Taichong)

d) LV 2 (Xingjian) + LV 3 (Taichong) + LV 10 (Zuwuli) + RM 2 (Qugu) + DM 3 (Yaoyangquan)

e) **ST 25** (Tianshu) + **K 6** (Zhaohai) + **PC 6** (Neiguan) + **H 3** (Shaohai)

Psychotherapy is a major component of the treatment. It is known that the psychological effect is dependent upon Shen Qi and that acupuncture stimulation can promote this energy.

FRIGIDITY

Frigidity is the sexual dysfunction that involves the loss of libido and inability to achieve orgasm. In complete frigidity both libido and orgasm are absent; disassociated frigidity refers only to the inability to reach orgasm. Frigidity may be primary or secondary, caused by anxiety or depression, or it may be one aspect of sexual aversion. It is believed that about 10% of women do not attain orgasm and more than 50% of women may experience situational absence of orgasm.

Prescription:

a) **SP 2** (Dadu) + **SP 3** (Taibai) + **SP 9** (Yinlingquan) + **SP 13** (Fushe) + **PC 6** (Neiguan)

b) **BL 23** (Shenshu) + **DM 3** (Yaoyangquan) + **BL 10** (Tianzhu) + **GB 20** (Fengchi)

c) **SJ 5** (Waiguan) + **LI 4** (Hegu) + **DM 13** (Taodao) + **DM 19** (Houding) + **BL 26** (Guanyuanshu) + **ST 30** (Qichong)

d) **SJ 5** (Waiguan) + **ST 30** (Qichong) + **RM 3** (Zhongji) + **RM 4** (Guanyuan) + **K 11** (Henggu)

e) **ST 25** (Tianshu) + **PC 3** (Quze) + **H 9** (Shongji) + **K 27** (Shufu)

In cases of dissociated frigidity the following prescriptions can be used:

a) **LV 3** (Taichong) + **LV 10** (Zuwuli) + **ST 34** (Liangqiu) + **BL 67** (Zhiyin)

b) **BL 31** (Shangliao) + **BL 32** (Ciliao) + **BL 33** (Zhongliao) + **BL 34** (Xialiao) + **L 7** (Lieque) + **SP 4** (Gongsun) + **DM 3** (Yaoyangquan)

c) **SP 4** (Gongsun) + **PC 6** (Nciguan) + **ST 36** (Zusanli) + **GB 34** (Yanglingquan)

Acupuncture is given in 8 to 10 weekly sessions and needles are retained for 15 to 20 minutes. The even movement technique is used for stimulation of the selected points.

NYMPHOMANIA

Sexual hyperexcitability can manifest as either erotomania or nymphomania. These dysfunctions usually start during childhood or at puberty and are temporary. When they are associated with psychological disorders, they may become persistent and require therapy.

Acupuncture therapy is an easy alternative treatment that affords decrease and control of sexual excitation.

Prescription:

a) LV 14 (Qimen) + K 1 (Yongquan) + BL 23 (Shenshu) + RM 17 Shanzhong)

b) ST 14 (Kufang) + L 1 (Zhongfu) + K 22 (Tiantu) + SJ 3 (Quze)

c) SP 21 (Dabao) + PC 6 (Neiguan) + SP 6 (Sanyinjiao) + RM 6 (Qihai)

d) ST 12 (Quepen) + K 2 (Rangu) + SP 5 (Shangqiu) + SJ 10 (Tianjing)

The number of sessions required depends upon the level of sexual dysfunction.

In order to improve the therapeutic effects of acupunture upon a couple's sexual life, consideration should be given to the partner's possible contribution to the dysfunctional condition. Masculine pathologies such as oligospermia, premature ejaculation, impotence or behavioral disturbances can also be treated with the use of acupuncture.

CHAPTER 5

DISEASES OF THE URINARY TRACT

Often a causal relationship exists between gynecologic and urinary diseases. Inflammatory diseases such as cystitis, urethritis, or pyelonephritis can support or aggravate an inflammatory adnexal process. Urinary tract infections, renal colic or urinary retention may have repercussions upon the genital system. Infection can spread directly, in acute cases, from the genital to the urinary system or it may develop secondary to chronic pelvic inflammatory disease, causing urinary symptoms that alleviate or disappear after the genital disease is treated.

LIN SYNDROME

Chinese traditional medicine refers to the "Lin syndrome," which includes urinary disorders such as frequent urination, dysuria, and urinary incontinence. Based upon clinical manifestations, five entities can be differentiated:

- **Re** (Heat) **Lin:** corresponds to acute urinary tract infections (cystitis, pyelonephritis, etc.)
- **Xue** (Blood) **Lin:** corresponds to the presence of bloody urine from urinary tract infections, but also refers to tuberculosis or a neoplastic process in this location
- **Shi** (Calculi) **Lin:** corresponds to renal, ureteral or vesical calculi
- **Gao** (Milky) **Lin:** corresponds to diseases with milky, turbid urine
- **Lao** (Consumptive) **Lin:** corresponds to chronic diseases

The Lin syndrome is usually caused by two etiopathogenic circumstances: deficiency of the Kidney Qi and accumulation of Damp-Heat in the Lower Jiao, favored by the deficiency of the Kidney and Urinary Bladder.

Etiopathogenesis

a) The Deficiency of Kidney Qi

The consumption of Kidney Qi may be caused by: physical and psychological overstrain, excessive sexual activity (e.g., sexual abuses, early marriage, multiparity), advancing age or congenital deficiency. These conditions lead to a deficiency of Kidney Qi and the dysfunction of the Urinary Bladder in controlling urination. The deficiency of the Kidney Qi can also generate a deficiency of the Spleen Qi, with sinking of Qi of the Lower Jiao.

b) The Accumulation of Damp-Heat in Lower Jiao

Damp-Heat can have an endogenous origin caused by an excessive intake of sweet, piquant and greasy food and alcohol intake. The stagnation of the Liver Qi can turn into Fire, with the accumulation of Qi and Fire in the Lower Jiao.

Accumulation of Damp-Heat in the Lower Jiao causes the dysfunction of the Urinary Bladder. The different aspects of the Lin syndrome can be described as follows:

Re (Heat) Lin

Accumulation of Heat in the Lower Jiao impedes the activity of the Urinary Bladder. Urination is difficult and can be accompanied by a burning sensation; dysuria may develop.

Xue (Blood) Lin

If Damp-Heat accumulates in the Urinary Bladder, or Fire damages the Urinary Bladder, the blood vessels can be injured leading to blood extravasation and painful urination, with bloody urine.

Shi (Calculi) Lin

Prolonged accumulation of Damp-Heat in the Lower Jiao causes the evaporation of fluids. Urine condenses, forming stones of different sizes and in different locations, from the Kidney to the urethra and urinary bladder. Urination is difficult, dysuria may develop and, occasionally, secondary anuria may occur as a result of calculi obstruction.

Gao (Milky) Lin

Damp-Heat can also affect the Kidney function of filtering impurities. As the Urinary Bladder is also damaged, it can no longer control the excretion of impurities, and turbid, milky or creamy urine may appear.

Clinical Manifestations

The clinical manifestations are dominated by pollakiuria and dysuria, sometimes even with false incontinence, in relation to which a sensation of lumbar weakness may develop.

Other signs and symptoms specific to the five types of Lin syndrome may be associated.

Re (Heat) Lin

Main symptoms include oliguria with concentrated urine, a burning sensation during urination, fever, aversion to cold, dry lips, and bitter taste. A red tongue with a yellow, sticky coating and a rapid, wiry pulse may be present.

Xue (Blood) Lin

Main symptoms include urgency of urination with bloody urine and dysuria, a burning sensation during urination, and lower abdominal pain with a fixed location. A yellow, thin tongue coating and a forceful and rapid pulse may also be noted.

Shi (Calculi) Lin

Main symptoms include the presence of calculi or sand in the urine, dysuria, possibly acute urinary retention consequent to urinary tract obstruction caused by calculi, colic pain with lumbar and abdominal involvement spreading toward the external genitalia, and bloody urine. The patient may have a normal or yellow, sticky tongue coating and a rapid, thready, tense pulse.

Gao (Milky) Lin

Main symptoms include turbid urine, with a milky or creamy aspect, a urethral burning sensation during urination, and a dry mouth. A red tongue with a sticky coating and a rapid, thready pulse may be detected.

Lao (Consumptive) Lin

Main symptoms include difficult urination with incontinence exacerbated by overstrain, lumbar weakness, and lower abdominal pain. Associated symptoms include asthenia, restlessness, a pale tongue with a thin coating and a weak pulse.

Treatment

When selecting a certain prescription, the etiopathogenic type to which the symptoms belong should be taken into account:
- excess type: Re Lin, Shi Lin

Therapeutic principle: remove Heat and Damp, promote urination
- deficiency type: Xue Lin, Gao Lin and Lao Lin (which may, in fact, also be seen among the conditions caused by excess, but may be complicated with deficiency)

Therapeutic principle: tone the Kidney and Spleen

Prescription:

BL 23 (Shenshu)	is the Back-Shu point of the Kidney, nourishes the Kidney Yin and strengthens the Yang, tones the Kidney
RM 3 (Zhongji)	is the Front-Mu point of the Urinary Bladder, stimulates the functions of the Urinary Bladder
SP 6 (Sanyinjiao)	is the Crossing point of the three Yin channels of the foot, the Kidney, Spleen and Liver; strengthens the Yin, tones the Kidney and Spleen, regulates Qi and blood
SP 9 (Yinlingquan)	is the He point of the Spleen channel, tones the Spleen and removes Damp, promotes urination

Acupuncture is given with the reinforcing method.

According to the etiopathogenic type, other points can be added:

a) Re (Heat) Lin

Prescription:

BL 28 (Pangguangshu)	is the Back-Shu point of the Urinary Bladder, removes pathogenic Heat from the Lower Jiao, tones the original Qi, regulates fluid transport
LI 11 (Quchi)	is the He point of the Large Intestine channel, removes pathogenic Heat, regulates Qi and blood
K 10 (Yingu)	is the He point of the Kidney channel, nourishes the Kidney and removes pathogenic Heat

Acupuncture is given with the reducing method.

b) Xue (Blood) Lin

Prescription:

SP 10 (Xuehai)	removes Heat from the Lower Jiao and stops blood extravasation

c) Shi (Calculi) Lin

The treatment is presented in the discussion about Urinary Calculi.

d) Gao (Milky) Lin

Prescription:

K 3 (Taixi)	is the Yuan-Source point of the Kidney channel, nourishes the Kidney and Liver, tones the Lower Jiao
K 6 (Zhaohai)	is the Confluent point of the Yin Qiao Mai Vessel with the Kidney channel, tones the Kidney, regulates the Lower Jiao
RM 4 (Guanyuan)	is the Crossing point of Ren Mai with the three Yin channels of the foot, the Kidney, Spleen and Liver; tones Qi and strengthens the Kidney Yang, stimulates and regulates Qi and blood circulation

e) Lao (Consumptive) Lin

Prescription:

DM 20 (Baihui)	is the Crossing point of all Yang channels, strengthens Qi
RM 4 (Guanyuan)	tones the Kidney Qi
RM 6 (Qihai)	strengthens the Essence and Yang, tones the Qi
BL 20 (Pishu)	is the Back-Shu point of the Spleen, tones the Spleen and regulates the Stomach, supports blood
ST 36 (Zusanli)	is the He point of the Stomach channel, tones Qi and blood, has a generally reinforcing effect

Acupuncture is given with the reducing method in cases of Re (Heat) Lin and Shi (Calculi) Lin and with the reinforcing method in other cases. When strong stimulation is necessary, moxibustion is used to stimulate the points located on the abdomen and back.

URINARY CALCULI

There are multiple causes that determine the formation of calculi at the level of the urinary tract. These range from disorders of the calcium metabolism to urinary tract infections.

The major symptom of urinary calculi is renal colic. Pain is severe with a sudden onset and lumbar location. It spreads along the ureteral course toward the flanks and external genitalia through the thighs. It is accompanied by dysuria, urgency of urination and, possibly, acute urinary retention. Sympathetic phenomena are frequently associated.

Etiopathogenesis

From the perspective of Chinese traditional medicine, there are three etiologic circumstances involved:

a) Accumulation of Damp-Heat in the Lower Jiao

Exogenous pathogenic Damp-Heat, resulting from excessive intake of hot, greasy and sweet food, can accumulate in the Lower Jiao and affect the functions of the Urinary Bladder. When Damp-Heat is excessive, it leads to evaporation of the fluids and transformation of impurities into calculi with the onset of urinary disturbances as a result.

b) The Deficiency of Yin

The deficiency of Yin can be congenital or caused by the following circumstances: consumption of Yin fluids as a function of chronic disease and chronic hemorrhages which occur during the postpartum period or as a consequence of pathogenic Fire. The deficiency of Yin causes an excess of Yang that stimulates the consumption of fluids. The urine is thus "burned" and forms calculi through condensation.

c) The Deficiency of Kidney Yang

The deficiency of the Kidney Yang can be due to congenital Yang deficiency, chronic disease, or excessive sexual activity that affects the Kidney. The Yang function of warming and nourishing the brain, marrow, bones and ears is damaged. The Kidney and Urinary Bladder dysfunction of controlling the urine is evidenced by the formation of the calculi and the appearance of urinary disturbances.

Clinical Manifestations

Renal colic is an extremely strong pain of Yang type with a sudden onset and accompanying restlessness. Urinary disturbances and other symptoms and signs characteristic of urinary calculi may also be present.

a) Accumulation of Damp-Heat in Lower Jiao

Main symptoms include recurrent renal colic with abdominal spreading, oliguria with turbid urine or bloody urine accompanied by dysuria and a urethral burning sensation and, possibly, false urinary incontinence. Thirst with lack of desire to drink, constipation, and sensations of heaviness and fullness in the lower abdomen are associated symptoms. A red tongue with a yellow, sticky or (rarely) a white coating and a rapid, sliding pulse may also be noted.

b) The Deficiency of Yin

Main symptoms include recurrent, lasting renal colic, oliguria with concentrated urine and a mild urethral burning sensation, and abdominal pain. Associated symptoms include asthenia, palpitations, insomnia, vision disturbances, tinnitus, dry mouth, a pale and dry complexion, a red tongue with a thin, dry coating and a weak, thready pulse.

c) The Deficiency of Kidney Yang

Main symptoms include recurrent renal colic and chronic renal disease (hydronephrosis). A sensation of lumbar weakness, pallor, cold limbs, aversion to cold, dizziness, tinnitus and infertility are associated symptoms. A pale tongue with a thin coating and a deep, weak pulse may also be present.

Depending upon the location of the calculi, the following symptoms may appear:

- renal and ureteral calculi: paroxysmal pain located in the lumbar area or flanks, possibly accompanied by bloody urine and symptoms of urinary tract infection
- vesical calculi: dysuria, difficult urination, bloody urine, possible acute urinary retention, pain spreading towards the perineal area
- urethral calculi: difficult urination with possible acute urinary retention, accompanied by dysuria and bloody urine

Treatment

When selecting the prescription, several factors should be considered:

- the moment of treatment, during the renal colic or between the crises
- the etiopathogenic circumstances
- the location of the urinary calculi on the urinary tract

1. Renal Colic Treatment

Therapeutic principle: promote urination and remove the calculi

Prescription:

K 3 (Taixi)	is the Yuan-Source point of the Kidney channel, nourishes the Kidney and Liver, tones the Lower Jiao
K 4 (Dazhong)	is the Luo point of the Kidney channel and regulates the Kidney
LV 3 (Taichong)	is the Yuan-Source point of the Liver channel, stimulates Qi and blood circulation, drains the channels, relieves dysuria
GB 39 (Xuanzhong)	is the Great Luo point of the three Yang channels of the foot and also the Lower-He point of San Jiao channel, strengthens the Urinary Bladder function, drains Damp-Heat from the Lower Jiao
BL 23 (Shenshu)	is the Back-Shu point of the Kidney, tones the Kidney
RM 2 (Qugu)	regulates and tones the Kidney
BL 60 (Kunlun)	is the He point of the Urinary Bladder, promotes urination

Strong stimulation is usually necessary, either manual or electrical, especially when the patient is experiencing little pain relief. For acupoints K 3 and LV 3, the acupuncture sensation should be perceived as spreading toward the knee joint.

No matter the location of the calculi, their expulsion is accompanied by pain, beginning 10 to 30 minutes after the start of stimulation and increasing during the course of treatment. The pain is considered a good sign that the calculi are moving and stimulation should be not discontinued. Expulsion is, of course, easier in cases with small, smooth calculi than for those in which the stones are irregular, though small.

Acupuncture can help calculi to change position and thus affords their expulsion by ureteral relaxation, especially when ureteral obstruction has occurred.

The following prescription can be useful:

K 7 (Fuliu)

RM 5 (Shimen)

Depending upon the location of the calculi, several prescriptions can be selected as follows:

- renal and upper ureteral calculi

BL 23 (Shenshu)	is the Back-Shu point of the Kidney, strengthens the Kidney, tones the Yang
BL 22 (Sanjiaoshu)	is the Back-Shu point of San Jiao, regulates San Jiao, strengthens the Spleen
ST 25 (Tianshu)	is the Front-Mu point of the Large Intestine, regulates the Stomach and Spleen, removes pathogenic Damp
RM 6 (Qihai)	strengthens the Yang, tones and regulates Qi

- middle and lower ureteral and vesical calculi

BL 23 (Shenshu)	tones the Kidney Qi
BL 32 (Ciliao)	stimulates Qi circulation and has an analgesic effect
BL 28 (Pangguangshu)	is the Back-Shu point of the Urinary Bladder, removes pathogenic Heat from the Lower Jiao, regulates the functions of the Urinary Bladder
RM 3 (Zhongji)	is the Front-Mu point of the Urinary Bladder, regulates its functions, promotes urination
ST 28 (Shuidao)	promotes urination and regulates fluid distribution, removes pathogenic Heat

Auricular Therapy: points Kidney, Urinary Bladder, Shenmen, Sympathetic nervous system can be used.

2. Long-Term Therapy

The goal is to remove, if possible, the etiopathogenic circumstances that favor the formation of calculi. Toward that end, therapy seeks to tone the Kidney and support the Urinary Bladder functions.

a) Accumulation of Damp-Heat in the Lower Jiao

Therapeutic principle: remove Damp-Heat and drain the Lower Jiao

Prescription:

SP 9 (Yinlingquan)	is the He point of the Spleen channel, tones the Spleen and removes pathogenic Damp, regulates fluid excretion
SP 6 (Sanyinjiao)	is the Crossing point of the Yin channels of the foot, tones the Kidney and strengthens the Spleen to remove Damp, regulates Qi and blood circulation
LV 2 (Xingjian)	is the Ying point of the Liver channel, removes Liver Qi stagnation, cools blood and the Lower Jiao
K 2 (Rangu)	is the Ying point of the Kidney channel, nourishes Kidney Yin, cools the Heat and regulates the Lower Jiao
RM 3 (Zhongji)	is the Front-Mu point of the Lower Jiao, removes Damp-Heat, regulates the Lower Jiao
BL 54 (Zhibian)	cools Damp-Heat, regulates the Lower Jiao

Acupuncture is given with the reducing method.

b) The Deficiency of Yin

Therapeutic principle: nourish the Yin

Prescription:

K 3 (Taixi)	is the Yuan-Source point of the Kidney channel, nourishes the Kidney
K 2 (Rangu)	is the Ying point of the Kidney channel, nourishes the Yin, regulates the Lower Jiao
SP 6 (SanyinJiao)	tones the Yin, nourishes the Kidney and Spleen, nourishes blood, regulates Qi and blood circulation

BL 17 (Geshu)	is the Influential point of blood, nourishes and supports blood
BL 23 (Shenshu)	is the Back-Shu point of the Kidney, nourishes the Yin, tones the Kidney
H 8 (Shaofu)	is the Ying point of the Heart channel, regulates Qi circulation, removes pathogenic Heat, calms the mind.

Acupuncture is given with the reinforcing method.

c) The Deficiency of Kidney Yang

Therapeutic principle: nourish the Yang, tone Kidney

Prescription:

DM 4 (Mingmen)	tones the Yang of the Kidney, strengthens the lumbar area
RM 4 (Guanyuan)	tones and regulates the Qi, stimulates Yang, regulates the Chong Mai and Ren Mai vessels
RM 6 (Qihai)	strengthens the Yang, tones and regulates the Qi
BL 23 (Shenshu)	is the Back-Shu point of the Kidney, tones the Kidney and strengthens the Yang

Stimulation is given with the reinforcing method and acupuncture or moxibustion is used.

Ashi points can also be used according to the location of the calculi.

A session is performed daily and needles are retained for 30 to 60 minutes, with needle stimulation every 10 minutes. Courses of 7 to 10 sessions can be repeated after a pause of a few days.

URINARY TRACT INFECTIONS

Urinary tract infections are the inflammatory diseases most frequently encountered in women's pathology. Different physiologic and pathologic circumstances of the genital system account for the frequency of their occurrence: functional changes during the menstrual cycle, vulvovaginal and metroadnexal inflammatory diseases, uterine malposition (uterine hyperanteversoflexion, uterine prolapse), trophic changes during menopause, and pregnancy.

The symptoms of the urinary tract infections vary according to their location (i.e., the upper or lower urinary tract), the clinical form, duration of evolution, and the absence or presence of complications.

Cystitis and acute pyelonephritis are more frequently encountered. Cystitis is located in the lower urinary tract and is evidenced by frequent urination, (which sometimes appears to be false incontinence of urine), dysuria and turbid urine. The major sign is the presence of pus in the urine. The absence of fever is a characteristic. Bloody urine may also be reported.

Acute pyelonephritis is the prototype of urinary infections located in the upper urinary tract. The clinical manifestations are the following: fever and chills, muscle pains, lumbar pain exacerbated on palpation (the Giordano sign is present on the affected side) and urinary disturbances due to vesico-urethral irritation: pollakiuria, dysuria, and a urethral burning sensation. The urine is turbid, sometimes bloody, and oliguria may be present in severe cases. The microscopic examination of the urine specimen shows pus, blood, bacteria and, sometimes, cylindrical casts in the urine. Diagnosis is based upon at least two positive urocultures.

From the perspective of Chinese traditional medicine, urinary tract infections occur as part of the Lin syndrome with the following etiopathogenic conditions:

- **Re** (Heat) **Lin**
- **Xue** (Blood) **Lin**
- **Gao** (Milky) **Lin**

Etiopathogenesis

a) Damp-Heat in the Urinary Bladder

The aggression of exogenous Damp-Heat manifests as inflammatory phenomena of the urinary tract. Endogenous Damp-Heat is a consequence of the excessive intake of hot, greasy, sweet food and alcoholic drinks. As a pathogenic factor characterized by heaviness and descending movement, Damp-Heat will accumulate in the Urinary Bladder, affecting its function by causing urinary disturbances. The injury of blood vessels leads to bloody urine. As the Urinary Bladder is related to the Kidney, the functions of the Kidney are also affected.

Accumulation of Damp-Heat in the Lower Jiao will affect the San Jiao function of filtering the impurities and turbid, milky urine appears.

b) The Hyperactivity of the Fire Heart

Retention of exogenous pathogenic factors within the body, prolonged depression or prolonged excess of piquant and hot food, alcoholic drinks and smoking can result in the formation of Fire. The Fire of the Heart, while ascending, affects the mind, consumes the Yin body fluids, and stimulates blood circulation. When Fire injures the blood vessels and causes blood extravasation, bloody urine will be seen.

c) The Deficiency of Yin

Excessive food intake, sexual abuses or severe emotional factors disorders can cause the consumption of the body Yin and the appearance of a false excess of Yang. This explains the presence of fever as one of the symptoms of this deficiency.

d) The Dysfunction of Qi

Damage of the Liver Qi caused by anger or depressive mood, conversion of the stagnant Qi to Fire, or the obstruction of Qi due to stagnation will cause the accumulation of Qi and Fire in the Lower Jiao, the stagnation of Qi of the Urinary Bladder, and resulting urinary disturbances.

Clinical Manifestations

a) Damp-Heat in the Urinary Bladder

Main symptoms include pollakiuria and dysuria, with possible false urinary incontinence, a urethral burning sensation, concentrated or turbid urine, and bloody urine. A sensation of lumbar weakness may also be present, as may a yellow, sticky tongue coating and a rapid, sliding pulse.

b) The Hyperactivity of the Fire Heart

Main symptoms include nervousness, restlessness, insomnia, a flushed face, thirst, concentrated urine, with dysuria and a sensation of urethral burning before urination, and, in severe cases, bloody urine. A red tongue with a yellow coating and a rapid pulse may also be noted.

c) The Deficiency of Yin

Main symptoms include dysuria, pollakiuria, oliguria with concentrated urine, afternoon fever, a flushed face, nervousness, anxiety, insomnia, vertigo, thirst, and a dry mouth. A red tongue with no coating or a yellowish, dry coating and a rapid, weak pulse may be observed.

d) The Dysfunction of Qi

Main symptoms include difficult urination and false urination and a sensation of fullness and pain in the lower abdomen. The patient may have a white, thin tongue coating and a deep, tense pulse.

Treatment

The etiologic treatment has been described with the Lin syndrome.

Cystitis

Prescription:

K 2 (Rangu)	is the Ying point of the Kidney channel, nourishes the Yin and removes pathogenic Heat, regulates the Urinary Bladder, regulates the Chong Mai and Ren Mai vessels and the Lower Jiao
K 3 (Taixi)	is the Yuan-Source point of the Kidney channel, nourishes the Kidney, tones the Lower Jiao
RM 3 (Zhongji)	is the Front-Mu point of the Urinary Bladder, tones the Kidney Yang, removes Damp-Heat, regulates the function of the Urinary Bladder and promotes urination
BL 28 (Pangguangshu)	is the Back-Shu point of the Urinary Bladder, regulates the Urinary Bladder, removes Heat from Lower Jiao, regulates urination
RM 6 (Qihai)	tones Qi, nourishes the Kidney, regulates the functions of Qi
PC 6 (Neiguan)	is the Luo point of the Pericardium channel, related to San Jiao channel, removes pathogenic Heat, stimulates Qi circulation, regulates San Jiao

Other points can also be selected in alternative prescriptions, when necessary:

LV 2 (Xingjian)	is the Ying point of the Liver channel, removes pathogenic Heat, cools the blood and the Lower Jiao

Acupoint LV 2 is considered extremely effective for difficult and painful urination.

K 6 (Zhaohai)	is the Confluent point of the Yin Qiao Mai Vessel, regulates the Lower Jiao, sedates pain
RM 2 (Qugu)	warms the Yang and tones the Kidney, is indicated in urinary disturbances
BL 27 (Xiaochangshu)	is the Back-Shu point of the Small Intestine, removes pathogenic Damp-Heat from the Lower Jiao, regulates the excretion

Acute Pyelonephritis

Prescription:

RM 3 (Zhongji)	tones the Kidney Yang, removes the pathogenic Damp-Heat, regulates urination
BL 23 (Shenshu)	is the Back-Shu point of the Kidney, strengthens the Kidney Qi, supports the Urinary Bladder functions
K 3 (Taixi)	is the Yuan-Source point of the Kidney channel, nourishes the Kidney
K 10 (Yingu)	is the He point of the Kidney channel, nourishes the Kidney and removes pathogenic Heat, regulates the Qi of the channels
LV 2 (Xingjian)	is Ying point of the Liver channel cools the blood, removes pathogenic Heat, is effective in painful urination
GB 34 (Yanglingquan)	is the He point of the Gall Bladder channel, stimulates the Liver and Gall Bladder, removes pathogenic Heat and Damp, is indicated in urinary disturbances caused by Cold and Heat
RM 4 (Guanyuan)	is the Front-Mu point of the Small Intestine and the Crossing point of Ren Mai with the Yin channels of the foot, tones the original Qi, strengthens the Yang, stimulates Qi and blood circulation, regulates the Chong Mai and Ren Mai vessels.

Other points can also be selected in alternative prescriptions, if needed:

SP 9 (Yinlingquan)   is the He point of the Spleen channel, restores Qi functions, promotes physiologic urination

BL 32 (Ciliao)   stimulates Qi circulation, strengthens blood circulation, alleviates pain

LV 8 (Ququan)   is the He point of the Liver channel, removes pathogenic Damp-Heat, drains the Urinary Bladder

- in cases with bloody urine, the following points can be used:

SP 10 (Xuehai)   removes Heat from the Lower Jiao, cools the blood, stops the extravasation of blood

SP 6 (Sanyinjiao)   tones the Spleen and Kidney, supports blood, regulates Qi and blood circulation

-in cases with fever, the following can be used:

LI 4 (Hegu)   is the Yuan-Source point of the Large Intestine channel, cools blood, regulates Qi and blood

DM 14 (Daznui)   is the Crossing point of the Du Mai Vessel with the Yang channels, removes pathogenic Cold, stimulates Qi circulation and calms the mind

SJ 5 (Waiguan)   is the Luo point of the San Jiao channel, promotes sweating, removes pathogenic Heat, drains the channels

Acupuncture is given with the reinforcing or reducing method, according to the selected acupoints.

ACUTE URINARY RETENTION

Urinary retention manifests as an inability to expel the urine that accumulates in the urinary bladder. The distension of the urinary bladder causes lower abdominal pain and, eventually, is accompanied by a constant sensation of urinary urgency with little or no actual excretion. Acute urinary retention is more frequent during the postpartum period and after surgery.

From the perspective of Chinese traditional medicine, acute urinary retention is caused by the dysfunction of Qi of the Urinary Bladder. The main function of the urinary bladder is to temporarily store the urine which later is excreted through the activity of Qi. This function of the urinary bladder is supported by the Kidney Qi. When Qi function is normal, urination is physiologic. The dysfunction of Qi generates urinary retention.

Etiopathogenesis

a) Accumulation of Damp-Heat in the Lower Jiao

Accumulation of Damp-Heat can be caused by the invasion of exogenous pathogenic Damp-Heat during feverish diseases and by excessive intake of hot, greasy, sweet food. The stagnation of Liver Qi, usually caused by emotional factors disturbance, if prolonged, can transform into Fire. The excess of the Liver lead to Spleen Deficiency. Damp-Heat accumulates in the Lower Jiao and affects the Qi function of controlling urination; urinary retention is the result.

b) The Deficiency of the Kidney Yang

This deficiency can arise from congenital deficiency of Yang or weakness of the Kidney as a function of aging. It also can be caused by other circumstances that injure the Kidney: chronic disease or excessive sexual activity (e.g., sexual abuses, multiparity). The excretory function of the urinary bladder depends upon the warming function of the Kidney Yang. When the Kidney Yang is deficient, the urinary bladder is too weak to excrete urine and urinary retention appears.

This condition is also observed in the postpartum period, because during labor and delivery loss of Qi and blood is frequent. The fluids, Yin and blood, have a tendency to be quickly restored, while Qi is restored much more slowly. The Kidney deficiency can become manifest and, among other signs and symptoms, urinary retention can appear.

c) Qi Dysfunction of the Urinary Bladder Channel

A traumatic injury or a surgical procedure on the lower abdomen can affect the Qi of the Urinary Bladder channel. The delay or obstruction of Qi circulation causes blood stagnation and dysfunction of the Urinary Bladder, with urinary retention.

Clinical Manifestations

Acute urinary retention is the main symptom, accompanied by a sensation of fullness in the urinary bladder and painful distension in the lower abdomen. Other signs and symptoms may appear, according to the etiopathogenic circumstances:

a) Accumulation of Damp-Heat in the Lower Jiao

Associated symptoms include thirst with lack of desire to drink, a sensation of heaviness and fullness in the lower abdomen, and constipation. The patient may have a sticky, yellow or white tongue coating and a rapid, sliding or wiry and forceful pulse.

b) The Deficiency of the Kidney Yang

Associated symptoms include a decrease of the excretory force of the urinary bladder and urinary retention, a pale complexion, asthenia, tinnitus, cold limbs, and a sensation of weakness in the knees and lumbar area. A pale tongue with a white, thin coating and a deep, weak and thready pulse may also be present.

c) Qi Dysfunction of the Urinary Bladder Channel

Painful abdominal distension, aggravated on pressure, is a symptom associated with this condition. Purplish tongue spots and a rapid, hesitant pulse may be detected.

Treatment

a) Accumulation of Damp-Heat in the Lower Jiao

Therapeutic principle: remove Damp-Heat, promote urination

Prescription:

RM 3 (Zhongji)	is the Front-Mu point of the Urinary Bladder, removes pathogenic Damp-Heat, regulates the Urinary Bladder function, promotes urination
RM 6 (Qihai)	tones the Qi, nourishes the Kidney, regulates Qi functions
BL 28 (Pangguangshu)	is the Back-Shu point of the Urinary Bladder, removes pathogenic Heat from the Lower Jiao, regulates the excretion of fluids

BL 39 (Weiyang)	is the Lower-He point of the San Jiao channel, regulates San Jiao, stimulates fluid circulation
SP 9 (Yinlingquan)	is the He point of the Spleen channel, removes pathogenic Heat, regulates fluid excretion
SP 6 (Sanyinjiao)	regulates Qi and blood circulation, removes Heat from the Lower Jiao

Acupuncture is given with the reducing method. A session lasts for approximately 20 to 30 minutes.

In cases with fever, the association of the points SP 6 and SP 9 is effective, with careful attention to the spread of the acupuncture sensation toward the knee joint. As for the point RM 3, a deep insertion of the needle is necessary, at 1.5-2 cun. The acupuncture sensation should be felt as local tumefaction and distension, spreading towards the external genitalia. Through RM 3, the point RM 2 (Qugu) can also be penetrated, with gentle stimulation; this measure may be repeated, if necessary.

b)The Deficiency of the Kidney Yang

Therapeutic principle: warm and tone the Kidney Yang

Prescription:

BL 23 (Shenshu)	is the Back-Shu point of the Kidney, nourishes the Yin and tones the Kidney Yang
DM 4 (Mingmen)	strengthens the Kidney Yang, regulates the Qi, tones the lumbar region
RM 4 (Guanyuan)	warms the Kidney, tones Qi and stimulates the return of Yang
DM 20 (Baihui)	is the Crossing point of the Yang channels, tones the Yang
SJ 4 (Yangchi)	is the Yuan-Source point of the San Jiao channel, tones the function of San Jiao and stimulates the water circulation
K 7 (Fuliu)	is the Jing-River point of the Kidney channel, tones the Kidney, regulates the water circulation.

Other points can also be selected:

SP 6 (Sanyinjiao)   strengthens the Kidney, regulates Qi and blood circulation

RM 6 (Qihai)   tones the Qi, nourishes the Kidney

Stimulation is given with the reinforcing method. Acupuncture or moxibustion in the points of the Ren Mai and Du Mai Vessels can be used.

c) Qi Dysfunction of the Urinary Bladder Channel

Therapeutic principle: stimulate Qi circulation and restore the function of the Urinary Bladder

Prescription:

RM 3 (Zhongji)   is the Front-Mu point of the Urinary Bladder, restores the Urinary Bladder function and promotes urination. Is selected as the main point

SP 6 (Sanyinjiao)   is the Crossing point of the three Yin channels of the foot, tones the Spleen and Kidney, regulates Qi and blood circulation in the damaged channels

K 5 (Shuiquan)   is the Xi point of the Kidney channel, regulates Qi and blood, drains and regulates the Urinary Bladder

ST 28 (Shuidao)   regulates fluid circulation, promotes urination and removes painful distension

BL 67 (Zhiyin)   is the Jing-Well point of the Urinary Bladder channel, promotes urination

For acute urinary retention (vesical globe) after surgical procedures, other prescriptions can also be selected:

K 10 (Yingu) + SP 9 (Yinlingquan) + RM 3 (Zhongji)

SP 6 (Sanyinjiao) + ST 28 (Shuidao)

The stimulation of the selected acupoints should be continuous and repeated several times a day. For the point ST 28, electrostimulation is very effective, the needle insertion is deep on both sides and toward the urinary bladder.

Stimulation of a point located at half distance between point RM 8

(Shenque) and the pubis symphysis is a simple method for treating urinary retention. With the patient in a recumbent position and the lower limbs flexed, the above mentioned point is pressed with the thumb of the right hand, slowly and gently, with an up and down movement, until spontaneous urination appears.

URINARY INCONTINENCE

Urinary incontinence is the involuntary loss of urine. Usually symptomatic, it is not painful but can sometimes be accompanied by a local straining sensation. Several causes can be involved: congenital factors, obstetrical trauma, surgical procedures in the genital area, uterine prolapse, and psychogenic causes.

From the perspective of Chinese traditional medicine, urinary incontinence is a clinical manifestation caused by the deficiency of the Qi of the Spleen and Kidney.

Etiopathogenesis

a) The Deficiency of Kidney Qi

The Kidney deficiency can be congenital or caused by the weakness of Kidney Qi in advanced age. The Kidney Qi can be consumed by physical and psychological overstrain and chronic disease. The deficient Qi can no longer nourish the affected area. The weakness of Kidney Qi causes the inability of the Urinary Bladder to control urination; this condition manifests as urinary disturbances and, in severe cases, urinary incontinence.

b) The Deficiency of Spleen Qi

Chronic diseases, physical overstrain, stress, and inadequate food intake can affect the Spleen Qi. The deficiency of the Spleen Qi may also be caused by the weakness of the Spleen associated with advanced age. The deficient Spleen is evidenced by dysfunction of transporting and transforming, with insufficient Qi and blood production. In severe cases the Spleen's inability to ascend the Qi causes the sinking of Qi; this phenomenon is called "the sinking of Qi of the Middle Jiao," as the Middle Jiao is most frequently involved. The sinking of Qi is made apparent by prolapse of the uterus, vesical or other organs. The prolapse can be accompanied by urinary incontinence.

Clinical Manifestations

a) The Deficiency of Kidney Qi

Main symptoms include urinary disturbances and, in severe cases, urinary incontinence . Associated symptoms include dizziness, tinnitus, a sensation of weakness in the lumbar area and the knee joint, clear leukorrhea, and vaginal dryness. The patient may have a red tongue with a white coating and a weak, thready pulse.

b) The Deficiency of Spleen Qi

Main symptoms include possible uterine prolapse accompanied by urinary incontinence and a bearing-down sensation in the abdominal region or prolapse/ptosis in other locations (anal, vesical prolapse, renal or gastric ptosis). A pale complexion, asthenia, weight loss, lack of appetite, lack of desire to speak, abdominal distension, a pale tongue with a white, thin coating and a slow, weak or soft, thready pulse are also characteristic.

Treatment

a) The Deficiency of Kidney Qi

Therapeutic principle: tone Kidney Qi, support the function of the Urinary Bladder

Prescription:

RM 3 (Zhongji)   is the Front-Mu point of the Urinary Bladder, regulates the Urinary Bladder function

RM 4 (Guanyuan)   is the Crossing point of the Ren Mai with the Kidney, Spleen and Liver channels, tones Qi, strengthens the Kidney, stimulates Qi circulation, regulates the Ren Mai Vessel

BL 23 (Shenshu)   is the Back-Shu point of the Kidney, nourishes the Yin and warms the Yang, tones the Kidney

BL 28 (Pangguangshu) is the Back-Shu point of the Urinary Bladder, tones Qi, regulates the Lower Jiao and Urinary Bladder, regulates urination

BL 33 (Zhongliao)   is the Crossing point of the Urinary Bladder and Gall Bladder channel, stimulates blood circulation and disperses Cold

K 3 (Taixi)   is the Yuan-Source point of the Kidney chan-
                         nel, nourishes the Kidney, regulates the Ren
                         Mai Vessel

K 7 (Fuliu)   is the Jing-River point of the Kidney channel,
                         tones the Kidney and regulates fluid circulation

b) The Deficiency of Spleen Qi

Therapeutic principle tone the Spleen, ascend Qi

Prescription:

BL 20 (Pishu)   is the Back-Shu point of the Spleen, strength-
                         ens the Spleen, supports and regulates blood

ST 36 (Zusanli)   is the He point of the Stomach channel and the
                         Dominant point, regulates the Stomach and
                         tones the Spleen, restores the Qi of Middle
                         Jiao

SP 6 (Sanyinjiao)   is the Crossing point of the three Yin channels
                         of the foot, tones the Spleen and Kidney,
                         regulates Qi and blood circulation

SP 9 (Yinlingquan)   is the He point of the Spleen channel, tones the
                         Spleen and warms the Middle Jiao, regulates
                         urination

RM 6 (Qihai)   restores Qi and tones the function of supporting

RM 12 (Zhongwan)   is the Front-Mu point of the Stomach and the
                         Influential point of the Fu organs, regulates
                         the Stomach and tones the Spleen, ascends the
                         Qi of the Middle Jiao

BL 39 (Weiyang)   is the Lower-He point of the Urinary Bladder
                         channel, regulates the Lower Jiao

RM 5 (Shimen)   is the Front-Mu point of San Jiao, regulates
                         San Jiao

Acupuncture is given with the reinforcing method in the above mentioned points, which may be selected in alternative prescriptions. A session is performed daily and needles are retained for approximately 15 to 20 minutes. Moxibustion can be used to stimulate SP 6 and ST 36 and the points located abdominally.

CHAPTER 6

ACUPUNCTURE ANALGESIA

Acupuncture analgesia refers to the analgesic effect and the regulation of the physiologic functions of the body, obtained after stimulation of certain acupoints on the patient about to undergo a surgical procedure. The method has developed in the 50's in China with the integration of traditional and western medicine.

The method consists of the insertion of acupuncture needles in different areas of the body (body, limbs, ears, face or nose and dorsal tongue), following which manual or electric stimulation of the selected points is performed. After a period of approximately 15 to 30 minutes, during which the analgesic effect is induced, the surgical procedure can begin and intraoperative stimulation of the acupoints is given.

THE ACTION MECHANISM
OF ACUPUNCTURE ANALGESIA

Several theories have been proposed to explain the action mechanism of acupuncture analgesia: the channels theory, the nervous system theory, and umoral factors involvement. None is able to explain completely the mechanism of acupuncture analgesia.

a) The Theory of Channels

The theory of channels has an important role in acupuncture analgesia. It is based upon the concept of free circulation of Qi within the channels in a certain sequence, governed by the Yin/Yang balance. The points for analgesia are thus selected from the points located on the channels that are in the area of the planned surgical field or from those related to the organ that is to be surgically treated.

Even though lacking the ability to provide a scientific explanation to acupuncture analgesia, the theory of channels allows us to understand the effects generated by needling the acupoints: analgesic, sedative, regulatory and anti-inflammatory. The acupuncture sensation spreads along the channels and, in this way, the channels establish internal-external connections, interactions among the Zang-Fu organs and, ultimately, the integration of the entire body.

b) The Theory of the Nervous System

For a better understanding of the way acupuncture can produce pain relief, the "gate control theory of pain" has an essential role (Melzack and Wall, 1965). According to this theory, the thick A beta fibers located in the substance of Rolando of the posterior spinal horn have an inhibiting effect upon A delta and C fibers that bring the nociceptive influx. It is believed that the analgesic effect obtained through acupuncture results from the action upon the A beta fibers.

Later, other "gates of control" have been emphasised. A "gate control" can be established by modulating the activity of Rolando's gelatinous substance, by the reticular formation through the reverberated circuits. A theory of a "second gate," located in the thalamus, has also been proposed. Professor Chang Hsiangtung has demonstrated the role of the thalamus and neurophysiological mechanisms involved in acupuncture analgesia.

The last "gate control" of pain, when conscience integration is accomplished, is the cerebral cortex. The projection of the different organs on the cortical areas helps explain the effect of certain acupuncture points upon the organs to which they are not anatomically related.

It has also been demonstrated that the acupuncture analgesic effects depend upon excitability of the cortical areas. This condition of cortical excitability is subject to the influence of emotional factors. This explains the role of emotional balance in obtaining therapeutic effects associated with acupuncture.

Another aspect of the relation between acupuncture and the nervous system is the involvement of the autonomic nervous system. In order to obtain acupuncture analgesia, an indispensable condition is the functional integrity of the nerves and nervous transmission. It has been observed that analgesia is efficient when the stimulated points are located near the nervous branch of the surgical field. The specificity of certain points in acupuncture analgesia is considered to be closely related to the plentiful distribution of nervous fibers in those points such as GB 30 (Huantiao) and DM 26 (Renzhong).

It is important to remember that there are some acupoints which correspond to a metameric distribution and their stimulation generates certain reactions in the organs afferent to those metamers. From this perspective, if limited to several acupoints, acupuncture analgesia can be considered a reflexotherapy.

c) The Umoral Theory

The discovery, beginning in 1975, of the endorphins have made possible a better understanding of the mechanism of acupuncture analgesia. Acupuncture has been shown to increase the pain threshold by means of naloxone blockage of beta endorphin.

Among endogenous opiates, other substances are also involved in the biochemic mediation of pain: P substance, cholecystokinines, and neurotensin etc. Acupuncture has been shown to increase the synthesis of serotonin, acetylcholine, catecholamines and to effect changes of the ionic concentrations (of K, Ca, Mg and change of the Mg/Ca rapport).

Mediating the analgesic response at the point of acupuncture by liberating different substances thus completes the complex mechanism of acupuncture analgesia.

ADVANTAGES AND DISADVANTAGES OF ACUPUNCTURE ANALGESIA

Advantages

Acupuncture analgesia is a method with no side effects (overdose, sensitivity to anesthetics etc.). As long as it is correctly used, acupuncture analgesia does not affect the physiological functions of the body and thus does not cause intraoperative incidents. The physiological functions— including blood pressure, pulse and breath— are maintained within normal parameters.

This method of analgesia is an important alternative for geriatric patients and for patients with hepatic, renal or pulmonary failure who may have a restricted tolerance to drugs.

Unlike the anesthesia used in western medical practice during which the central nervous system is inactivated, acupuncture activates the brain and the central nervous system, maintaining the vital functions. This explains why it is possible to use acupuncture analgesia without risk in emergencies, and in hypertensive or hypotensive patients, such as in shock, when acupuncture stimulation increases the blood pressure values and keeps them relative stable during surgery.

If acupuncture analgesia is used during surgery, the procedure is less hemorrhagic, much faster, with better healing of the incision and prompt reestablishment of internal organ function. The gastrointestinal function is minimally affected and the intestinal movements are quickly restored. Urinary retention and abdominal distension after surgery are very rare.

It has been observed that the frequency of postoperative infectious complications is much smaller after acupuncture analgesia. This phenomenon is explained by virtue of the fact that the action of acupuncture stimulates the immune mechanisms and phagocytosis.

Acupuncture analgesia allows a good collaboration between the physician and the patient during surgery. The patient is conscious and although insensitive to pain, is capable of all motor and sensitive functions. As the analgesic effect lasts a few hours after the surgical procedure is over, thus reducing postoperative pain, drugs usually needed to cover this period are less necessary

Acupuncture analgesia is a simple, easy and low-costing method. Applying this method of analgesia needs no special equipment and thus can be used in places where usual anesthetic equipment is not available.

Disadvantages

Acupuncture analgesia has three main disadvantages:

1.) The analgesia obtained is incomplete, even though the threshold of painful sensibility is high. When the patient feels pain, it is necessary to administer analgesic drugs.

2.) Using acupuncture analgesia, especially in abdominal surgery, does not provide adequate muscle relaxation. Lack of relaxation, especially in patients with a well-represented muscular plane, can create difficulties for the surgeon.

3.) Abdominal surgical maneuvers can involve visceral tractions in varying degrees, causing reflex pain, nausea and other uncomfortable sensations for the patient.

These disadvantages can be circumvented or offset by: altering acupuncture techniques, adjuvant therapy, changes of the surgical technique, and improvement of the physician-patient relationship.

a) Completion of the Analgesia

- Insertion of two acupuncture needles of 4 cun length, parallel to the planned incision or application of two flat electrodes at the angles of incision, followed by manual or electric stimulation with high frequency currents can be used to increase the analgesic effect.

- Blockage of the ear base or of the Sympathetic nervous system point with local anesthetics or narcotics increases the analgesic effect and also has a tranquilizing effect.
- Subcutaneous injection of saline solution along the course of the planned incision, on both sides, will reduce bleeding and increase the analgesic effect.

b) Improving the Muscular Relaxation

- Strong manual or electric stimulation of points **ST 36** (Zusanli) and **SP 6** (Sanyinjiao)
- Blockage of the points **BL 17** (Geshu), **BL 21** (Weishu), and **BL 23** (Shenshu)
- Regional and peritoneal electrostimulation
- Local anesthesia with xylocaine infiltration

c) Correcting the Reflexes Caused by Visceral Tractions

- Blockage of the points **BL 17** (Geshu), **BL 21** (Weishu), **BL 22** (Sanjiaoshu), **ST 36** (Zusanli), **BL 25** (Dachangshu) with analgesic injection
- Electrostimulation of points **LI 9** (Shanglian) and **PC 6** (Neiguan)
- Electrostimulation or application of flat electrodes paravertebral, during cesarean section at 1.5 cun from T 11

As an analgesic method during surgical procedures, acupuncture is effective in the surgery of the head, throat and thorax, eyes and ears (e.g. craniotomy, thoracic surgery, cesarean section and dental extraction etc.). The efficiency is lower for abdominal surgery, mainly in the obese patient with a thick abdominal wall, because of deficient muscular relaxation and reflexes of visceral traction that cause discomfort.

Acupuncture analgesia is not an adequate method for anxious patients who have no confidence in, or cannot cooperate with, their physician. Acupuncture is seldom used in emergency cases because of the amount of time needed both to induce the analgesic effect and to explain the method to the patient. Finally, it is important to note that acupuncture analgesia is not a substitute for other components of general anesthesia.

SELECTION OF THE PATIENTS

At present it is believed that only 15% to 20% of all surgical cases are suitable for acupuncture analgesia. In selecting the surgical cases that can benefit from this method, the following factors should be taken into account:

- Type of operation - acupuncture analgesia is less adequate when deep analgesia and muscular relaxation is needed, as in certain types of abdominal surgery. It also has little utility in surgical procedures, such as orthopedic surgery, that last more than two or three hours.
- Patient's age - Initially it was thought that, because of their reduced ability to cooperate with the physician, children and geriatric patients may not efficiently benefit from this method. In fact acupuncture analgesia can be useful in surgery with infants, having been found efficient in approximately 80% of all such cases where it was employed. Similarly, it may prove the preferred method with older patients for whom the administration of certain drugs can be contraindicated.
- Patient's general condition - In the past, acupuncture was not considered an adequate method in cases with excessive blood loss or profound coma. Subsequently the method has been used for treating different types of shock (hemorrhagic, toxic, traumatic) associated with surgical cases, and has been found effective in controlling breath and shortening the postoperative time of recovery.
- Physical condition and educational level of the patient - The reduced efficiency of acupuncture, when used to treat anxious patients who lack of confidence in the method and their physician, is well known. The physician-patient relationship is very important, as the efficacy of the method is directly influenced by the patient's confidence.

PREOPERATIVE PREPARATION

Because the patient using acupuncture analgesia remains conscious during the surgical procedure, the psychoemotional condition becomes very important, as it may affect the physiological functions, exacerbate pain and affect the ability to accept the surgical procedure.

In addition to the usual preoperative preparations, it is important for the patient to be acquainted with the method of acupuncture analgesia and its effects and also with the surgical procedure that will be used.

It is necessary to evaluate the acupuncture sensation, especially in those patients who have never been treated with acupuncture. The physician will simultaneously establish the patient's tolerance for pain, thus obtaining a better understanding of the method to be used and the stimulation that may be needed intraoperatively.

The patient undergoing abdominal surgery is also instructed to practice breathing exercises. Using this deep breathing technique helps to control reflex muscular spasm, nausea and vomiting.

PRINCIPLES OF SELECTING THE POINTS

Following are the methods most frequently used in selecting the points:

a) Selecting the Points According to the Theory of the Channels

This method is based upon the concept that "where a channel transverses there is a place adequate to treatment." It is expected that the point of a certain channel can act upon the areas where that channel passes.

b) Selecting the Points According to the Differentiation of Syndromes

In order to select points, signs and symptoms of a disease and their relationship to the Zang-Fu organs and the channels should be considered. Other points which correspond to associated symptoms, e.g., nausea, anxiety, dyspnea, palpitations etc., may be selected in the preoperative period and during the operation.

c) Selecting the Points According to Segmental Innervation

The segmentary integrity of the nervous system is necessary to produce acupuncture sensation and obtain the analgesic effect. Taking into account the relation between the segmental innervation of the needled place and the operative field, there are three possibilities for selecting the points:

1.) Adjacent points are selected, located in the area supplied by the same spinal nerve or an adjacent nerve that also supplies the operative field.

2.) Points located at a distance, in areas that are not supplied by the same spinal nerve or one adjacent to the operative field.

3.) The nervous trunk from the same segmentation may be stimulated in order to directly activate the peripheric nerve that supplies the operative field.

d) Selecting Auricular Points

Points located on the auricular projection areas, corresponding to different organs but related to Zang-Fu organs, are selected. Other points located on the ear, identified by sensitivity, decrease of the electrical resistance, structural deformations or color changes can also be selected.

The auricular points Shenmen and Sympathetic nervous system have sedative and analgesic effects and are widely used in acupuncture analgesia.

MANIPULATION TECHNIQUES

Manual and electrostimulation are the techniques most frequently used for acupuncture analgesia.

a) Manual Stimulation

The needles inserted in the selected points are strongly stimulated by twirling, raising and thrusting movements, aiming to "achieve the Qi," a necessary condition for obtaining the analgesic effect. The angle of the needle insertion and the depth of insertion depends upon the physical structure of the patient, the selected points and the type of the surgical procedure. The amplitude of the up and down movement of the needle is of 0.5-1 cun; this may be increased when stronger stimulation is needed. The rotation angle of the needle is approximately 180 to 360 degrees, with a frequency of 150 rotations/minute.

b) Electrostimulation

After the acupuncture sensation through the manual stimulation of the needles is obtained, their handles are attached to the electroacupuncture apparatus. Biphasic, spike and rectangular infrequent sinusoid impulses are used. There are two types of electric impulses frequency: 2-80 Hz and 40-200 Hz.

Usually acupuncture analgesia needs a stronger stimulation that is progressively increased until the limit of the patient's tolerance is reached. Prolonged electric stimulation can destroy acupuncture sensation in certain patients; therefore, when strong stimulation is necessary, an intermittent electric stimulation should be selected.

The preoperative manual or electric stimulation of the selected points is called induction. The duration of the induction is approximately 20 minutes or according to the patient's adaptation to acupuncture analgesic stimulation. The stimulation can be interrupted during the operation, with the needles left in place, when the operative stimuli are less productive of pain, and can be resumed when a stronger analgesic effect is required.

ADJUVANT THERAPY

In order to increase the analgesic effect, both preoperatively and during the operation, adjuvant therapy can be prescribed:

- Preoperative: sedatives, tranquilizers, analgesics etc.

- During the operation: local anesthetics

ACUPUNCTURE ANALGESIA
IN GYNECOLOGICAL AND OBSTETRICAL SURGERY

a) Tubal Ligation

Prescription:

ST 36 (Zusanli) + **LV 6** (Zhongdu)

ST 36 (Zusanli) + **SP 6** (Sanyinjiao) + **GB 26** (Daimai)

Acupoints located around the scar are associated. Bilateral stimulation is given for the selected points.

Auricular points: Shenmen, Ovary, Lung.

b) Cesarean Section

Prescription:

ST 36 (Zusanli) + **SP 6** (Sanyinjiao) + **GB 26** (Daimai) + **E.P.** Neimadian

The extraordinary vessel point Neimadian is located at half the distance between the point **SP 9** (Yinlingquan) and the internal malleolus.

Bilateral stimulation is given for the selected points.

Auricular points: Shenmen, Uterus, Abdomen, Lung.

c) Total Hysterectomy and Bilateral Salpingo-Oophorectomy

Prescription:

DM 2 (Yaoshu) + **DM 4** (Mingmen) + **GB 26** (Daimai)

ST 36 (Zusanli) + **SP 6** (Sanyinjiao) + **BL 33** (Zhongliao) or

BL 32 (Ciliao)

Bilateral stimulation is given to the selected points.

Auricular points: Uterus, Lung, Shenmen, Abdomen, Endocrine, External genitalia etc.

d) Episiotomy

Prescription:

SP 6 (Sanyinjiao)

LV 3 (Taichong)

e) Ovariectomy

Prescription:

DM 2 (Yaoshu)

DM 4 (Mingmen)

ST 36 (Zusanli)

BL 31 (Shangliao)

BL 32 (Ciliao)

BL 33 (Zhongliao)

BL 34 (Xiliao)

Auricular points: Kidney, Heart, Shenmen

CHAPTER 7

THE REGULAR AND EXTRA CHANNEL ACUPOINTS

THE LUNG CHANNEL

L 1 (Zhongfu) — on the upper part of the anterior thorax, between the 1st and 2nd rib, at 6 cun from the sternal midline

L 2 (Yunmen) — at the lower border of the external extremity of the clavicle, at 6 cun from the sternal midline

L 3 (Tianfu) — at 3 cun under the lower extremity of the anterior axillary fold, at the external extremity of the biceps brachi muscle

L 4 (Xiabai) — at the external extremity of biceps brachi muscle, at 1 cun below Tianfu

L 5 (Chize) — on the transverse cubital crease, at the external extremity of the tendon of the biceps muscle, with the elbow in flexion

L 6 (Kongzui) — at the radial extremity of the forearm, 7 cun above the distal wrist crease

L 7 (Lieque) — above the styloid process of the radius, 1.5 cun above the wrist crease

L 8 (Jingqu) — on the internal border of the styloid process of the radius, 1 cun above the wrist crease

L 9 (Taiyuan) — on the wrist crease, outside the radial artery

L 10 (Yuji) — at the base of the thumb, at the proximal end of the first metacarpal bone

L 11 (Shaoshang) — at 2 mm outside the nail corner of the thumb, on the radial side

See Fig. 1, The Lung Channel.

THE LARGE INTESTINE CHANNEL

LI 1 (Shangyang) — at 2 mm outside the external nail corner of the index finger

LI 2 (Erjian) — on the external border, distal to the metacarpophalangeal joint of the index finger

LI 3 (Sanjian) — on the radial side of the index finger, proximal to the metacarpophalangeal joint

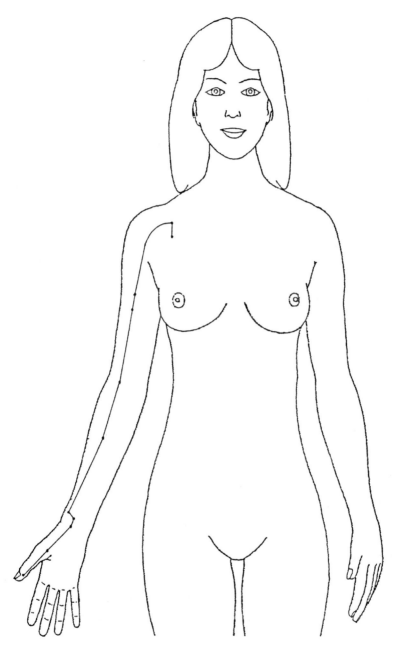

Fig. 1, The Lung Channel.

LI 4 (Hegu)	on the radial side of the index finger, midway between the 1st and 2nd metacarpal bones
LI 5 (Yangxi)	on the lower tip of the styloid process of the radius, between the two tendons
LI 6 (Pianli)	at 3 cun above Yangxi, on the posterior aspect of the forearm
LI 7 (Wenliu)	at 5 cun above Yangxi
LI 8 (Xialian)	at 4 cun below Quchi
LI 9 (Shanglian)	at 3 cun below Quchi
LI 10 (Shousanli)	at 2 cun below Quchi
LI 11 (Quchi)	at the external extremity of the elbow crease, when the forearm is in flexion
LI 12 (Zhouliao)	at 1 cun above and lateral to Quchi, below the epicondyle of the humerus
LI 13 (Wuli)	at 3 cun above the elbow crease, on the external extremity of the biceps brachi muscle
LI 14 (Binao)	at 7 cun above Quchi, at the lower border of the deltoid muscle
LI 15 (Jianyu)	on the crossing point of the acromion, clavicle and humeral bones, in the depression formed while raising the arm
LI 16 (Jugu)	in a depression above the acromion and clavicle joint
LI 17 (Tianding)	at 1 cun below Futu on the posterior border of the sternocleidomastoid muscle
LI 18 (Futu)	on the anterior border of the sternocleidomastoid muscle, at the upper border of the thyroid cartilage
LI 19 (Heliao)	at 0.5 cun lateral to Renzhong (DM 26)
LI 20 (Yingxiang)	at 0.5 cun lateral to the external border of the nostril, in the nasolabial sulcus

See Fig. 2, The Large Intestine Channel

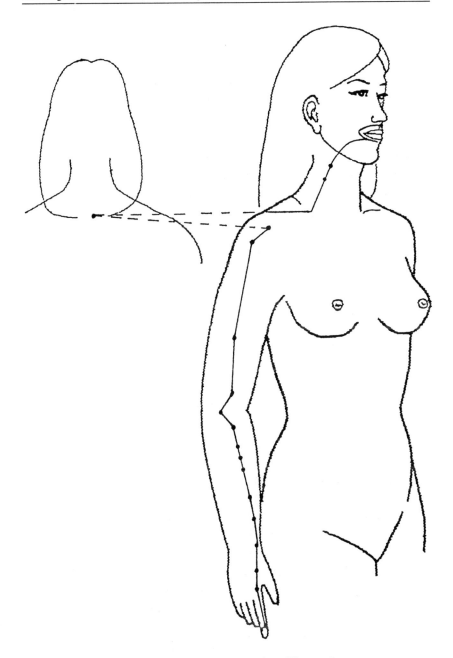

Fig. 2, The Large Intestine Channel

THE STOMACH CHANNEL

ST 1 (Chengqi)   on the vertical line of the pupil, between the eyeball and the lower border of the orbital fossa

ST 2 (Sibai)   at 0.7 cun below Chengqi

ST 3 (Juliao)   directly below Sibai, level with the lower border of the nostril, lateral to the nasolabial sulcus

ST 4 (Dicang)   at 0.4 cun lateral to the corner of the mouth

ST 5 (Daying)   proximal to the anterior angle of the mandible, on the anterior border of the masseter muscle, posterior to the facial artery

ST 6 (Jiache)   on the masseter muscle, at 0.5 cun above and anterior to the posterior angle of the mandible

ST 7 (Xiaguan)   on the lower border of the zygomatic arch, anterior to the condyle of the mandible

ST 8 (Touwei)   at 2 cun external and above the lateral extremity of the eyebrow at the border of the hairline

ST 9 (Renying)   at the upper external angle of the thyroid cartilage, on the anterior border of the sternocleidomastoid muscle

ST 10 (Shuitu)   on the lower external angle of the thyroid cartilage, between Renying and Qishe, on the anterior border of the sternocleidomastoid muscle

ST 11 (Qishe)   right below Renying on the upper border of the clavicle, between the two insertions of the sternocleidomastoid muscle

ST 12 (Quepen)   on the mammillary line in the middle of the supraclavicular fossa

ST 13 (Qihu)   at 4 cun from the median line, on the mammillary line, in the middle of the lower border of the clavicle

ST 14 (Kufang)   in the 1st intercostal space, at 4 cun lateral to the median line

ST 15 (Wuyi)	in the 2nd intercostal space, at 4 cun lateral to the median line
ST 16 (Yingchuang)	in the 3rd intercostal space, at 4 cun lateral to the median line
ST 17 (Ruzhong)	in the middle of the nipple
ST 18 (Rugen)	in the 5th intercostal space, at 4 cun lateral to the median line
ST 19 (Burong)	2 cun lateral to Juque (RM 14) and 6 cun above the umbilicus
ST 20 (Chengman)	2 cun lateral to Shangwan (RM 13) and 5 cun above the umbilicus
ST 21 (Liangmen)	2 cun lateral to Zhongwan (RM 12) and 4 cun above the umbilicus
ST 22 (Guanmen)	2 cun lateral to Jianli (RM 11) and 3 cun above the umbilicus
ST 23 (Taiyi)	2 cun lateral to Xiawan (RM 10) and 2 cun above the umbilicus
ST 24 (Huaroumen)	2 cun lateral to Shuifen (RM 9) and 1 cun above the umbilicus
ST 25 (Tianshu)	2 cun lateral to the umbilicus
ST 26 (Wailing)	2 cun lateral to Yinjiao (RM 7) and 1 cun below the umbilicus
ST 27 (Daju)	2 cun lateral to Shimen (RM 5) and 2 cun below the umbilicus
ST 28 (Shuidao)	2 cun lateral to Guanyuan (RM 4) and 3 cun below the umbilicus
ST 29 (Guilai)	2 cun lateral to Zhongji (RM 3) and 4 cun below the umbilicus
ST 30 (Qichong)	2 cun lateral to Qugu (RM 2) and 5 cun below the umbilicus
ST 31 (Biguan)	below the anterior-superior iliac spine
ST 32 (Futu)	at 6 cun above the upper border of the patella, on the line between the external extremity of the patella with the anterior-superior iliac spine

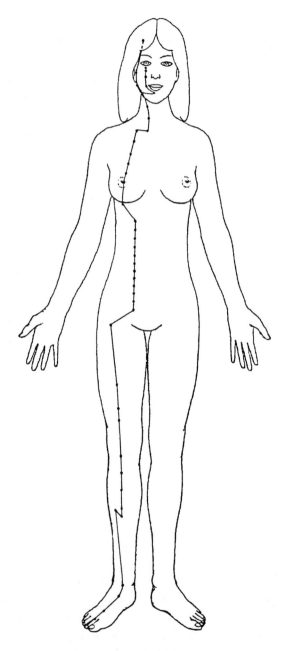

Fig. 3, The Stomach Channel.

ST 33 (Yinshi)	at 3 cun above the upper border of the patella
ST 34 (Liangqiu)	at 2 cun above the superior external border of the patella
ST 35 (Dubi)	in the depression below the patella, lateral to the knee ligament with the knee in flexion
ST 36 (Zusanli)	at 3 cun below Dubi and 1 cun outside the tibial crease in the anterior tibial muscle
ST 37 (Shangjuxu)	at 6 cun below the patella and 1 cun outside the tibial border
ST 38 (Tiaokou)	at 8 cun below the patella and 1 cun outside the tibial border
ST 39 (Xiajuxu)	at 9 cun below the patella and 1 cun outside the tibial border
ST 40 (Fenglong)	at 8 cun below the patella and 2 cun outside the tibial border
ST 41 (Jiexi)	on the anterior angle of the ankle joint, midway between the two malleoli and between the tendons of extensor muscle halluces longus and digitorum longus
ST 42 (Chongyang)	at 1.5 cun below Jiexi (ST 41) on the dorsal artery of the foot
ST 43 (Xiangu)	in the angle between the 2nd and 3rd metatarsophalangeal joint
ST 44 (Neiting)	at 0.5 cun anterior to the joint of the 2nd and 3rd toe
ST 45 (Lidui)	at 2 mm from the outer corner of the nail of the 2nd toe

See Fig. 3, The Stomach Channel.

THE SPLEEN CHANNEL

SP 1 (Yinbai)	at 2 mm from the medial corner of the 1st toe
SP 2 (Dadu)	on the internal side of the 1st toe, anterior to the metatarsophalangeal joint
SP 3 (Taibai)	on the internal aspect of the foot, posterior to the metatarsophalangeal joint

SP 4 (Gongsun)	on the internal aspect of the foot, in the depression anterior to the joint of the 1st metatarsal with the cuneiform bone
SP 5 (Shangqiu)	in the fossa located below and anterior to the medial malleolus
SP 6 (Sanyinjiao)	at 3 cun above the tip of the medial malleolus, on the posterior border of the tibia
SP 7 (Lougu)	at 6 cun above the tip of the medial malleolus, on the posterior border of the tibia
SP 8 (Diji)	at 3 cun below Yinlingquan
SP 9 (Yinlingquan)	below the internal condyle of the tibia, on the posterior border
SP 10 (Xuehai)	at 2 cun above the internal border of the patella, in the middle of the protuberance of the vastus medialis muscle
SP 11 (Jimen)	on the medial aspect of the tibia, at 6 cun above Xuehai (SP 10), at the extremity of the vastus medialis muscle
SP 12 (Chongmen)	at 3, 5 cun lateral to midline, at the level of the upper border of the pubis symphysis
SP 13 (Fushe)	at 0.7 cun above Chongmen (SP 12) and 4 cun lateral to the midline
SP 14 (Fujie)	at 1.3 cun below Daheng (SP 15)
SP 15 (Daheng)	4 cun lateral to the umbilicus
SP 16 (Fuai)	at 3 cun above the umbilicus and at 4 cun from the midline
SP 17 (Shidou)	6 cun lateral to the midline in the 5th intercostal space
SP 18 (Tianxi)	6 cun lateral to the midline in the 4th intercostal space
SP 19 (Xiongxiang)	6 cun lateral to the midline in the 3rd intercostal space
SP 20 (Zhourong)	6 cun lateral to the midline in the 2nd intercostal space

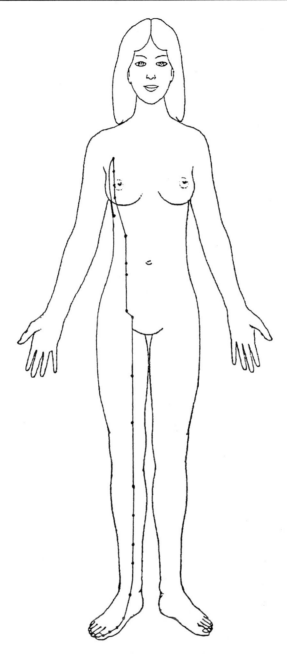

Fig. 4, The Spleen Channel.

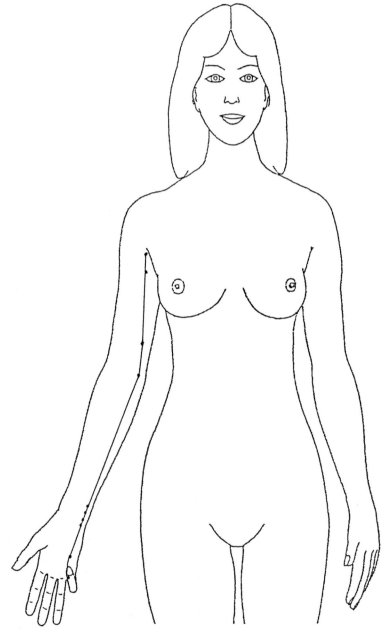

Fig. 5, The Heart Channel.

| SP 21 (Dabao) | on the medio-axillary line in the 7th intercostal space |

See Fig. 4, The Spleen Channel.

THE HEART CHANNEL

H 1 (Jiquan)	in the center of the axilla, on the medial side of the axillary artery
H 2 (Qingling)	on the internal border of the biceps brachi muscle, 3 cun above Shaohai
H 3 (Shaohai)	on the internal extremity of the elbow fold, with the arm flexed
H 4 (Lingdao)	at 1.5 cun above the wrist crease, (H 7) on the internal border of the cubital artery
H 5 (Tongli)	at 1 cun above Shenmen (H 7)
H 6 (Yinxi)	at 0.5 cun above Shenmen (H 7)
H 7 (Shenmen)	slightly below the wrist crease, on the internal border of the pisiform bone
H 8 (Shaofu)	between the 4th and 5th metacarpal bones, in the place where the 5th finger touches the palm in flexion
H 9 (Shaochong)	2 mm outside the external corner of the nail of the little finger

See Fig. 5, The Heart Channel.

THE SMALL INTESTINE CHANNEL

SI 1 (Shaoze)	2 mm posterior to the external corner of the nail of little finger
SI 2 (Qiangu)	on the cubital border of the little finger, distal to the metacarpophalangeal joint
SI 3 (Houxi)	on the cubital side of the hand, proximal to the metacarpophalangeal joint of the 5th finger, in the depression formed when the wrist is closed
SI 4 (Wangu)	on the cubital side of the hand, in the fossa between the pyramidal bone and the 5th metacarpal

SI 5 (Yanggu)	on the cubital side of the wrist joint, in the fossa between the styloid process of the ulna and the triangular bone, on the wrist crease
SI 6 (Yanglao)	above the styloid process of the ulna, on the external side
SI 7 (Zhizheng)	at 5 cun above Yanggu (SI 5), on the border of the ulna
SI 8 (Xiaohai)	in the fossa between the ulnar olecranon and the medial epicondyle of the humerus
SI 9 (Jianzhen)	at 1 cun above the extremity of the axillary fold, posterior and inferior to the scapular humeral joint
SI 10 (Naoshu)	in the fossa below the spine of the scapula
SI 11 (Tianzong)	in the fossa below the spine of the scapula, level with the apophysis of T4 vertebra
SI 12 (Bingfeng)	in the middle of the fossa above the scapular spine, 1 cun above the upper border of the scapula
SI 13 (Quyuan)	1 cun lateral to the internal extremity of the scapula, on its upper border
SI 14 (Jianwaishu)	3 cun lateral to the apophysis of T1 vertebra
SI 15 (Jianzhongshu)	2 cun lateral to the depression below the C 7 vertebra
SI 16 (Tianchuang)	on the posterior border of the sternocleido-mastoid muscle, level with the laryngeal prominence
SI 17 (Tianrong)	posterior to the mandible angle, on the anterior border of the sternocleidomastoid muscle
SI 18 (Quanliao)	on the lower border of the malar bone
SI 19 (Tinggong)	between the middle of the tragus and the temporomandibular joint, in the depression formed when the mouth is open

See Fig. 6, The Small Intestine Channel.

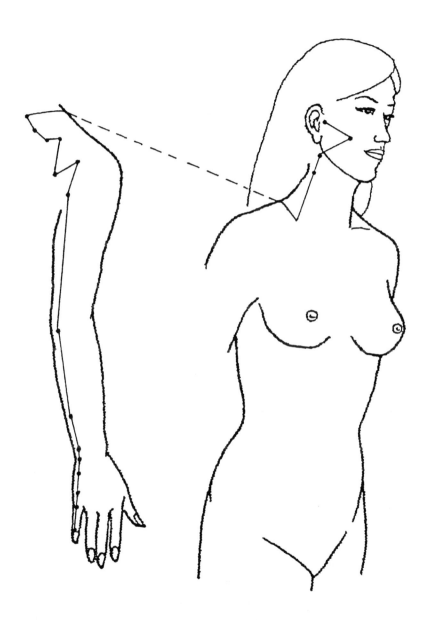

Fig. 6, The Small Intestine Channel.

THE URINARY BLADDER CHANNEL

BL 1 (Jingming)   on the internal border of the orbital fossa, at 2 mm above the inner canthus

BL 2 (Zanzhu)   on the vertical of Jingming (BL 1) at the internal extremity of the eyebrow

BL 3 (Meichong)   on the vertical of BL 1 and 2, at the hairline

BL 4 (Quchai)   at 0.5 cun above and lateral to Meichong (BL 3)

BL 5 (Wuchu)   posterior to Quchai (BL 4),1 cun from the hairline and 1.5 cun lateral to the midline

BL 6 (Changguang)   at 1.5 cun posterior to Wuchu (BL 5)

BL 7 (Tongtian)   at 1.5 cun posterior to Changguang (BL 6)

BL 8 (Luoque)   at 1.5 cun posterior to Tongtian (BL 7)

BL 9 (Yuzhen)   lateral to the upper border of the occipital protuberance, at 1.3 cun lateral to midline

BL 10 (Tianzhu)   at 1.3 cun lateral to the midline, (RM 15) at the base of the occiput, on the internal aspect of the trapezius muscle

BL 11 (Dazhu)   at 1.5 cun lateral to the apophysis of T 1 vertebra, in the 1st intercostal space

BL 12 (Fengmen)   at 1.5 cun lateral to the apophysis of T 2 vertebra

BL 13 (Feishu)   at 1.5 cun lateral to the apophysis of T 3 vertebra

BL 14 (Jueyinshu)   at 1.5 cun lateral to the apophysis of T 4 vertebra

BL 15 (Xinshu)   at 1.5 cun lateral from the apophysis of T 5 vertebra

BL 16 (Dushu)   at 1.5 cun lateral to the apophysis of T 6 vertebra

BL 17 (Geshu)   at 1.5 cun lateral to the apophysis of T 7 vertebra

BL 18 (Ganshu)   at 1.5 cun lateral to the apophysis of T 8 vertebra

BL 19 (Danshu)	at 1.5 cun lateral to the apophysis of T 10 vertebra
BL 20 (Pishu)	at 1.5 cun lateral to the apophysis of T 11 vertebra
BL 21 (Weishu)	at 1.5 cun lateral to the apophysis of T 12 vertebra
BL 22 (Sanjiaoshu)	at 1.5 cun lateral to the apophysis of L 1 vertebra
BL 23 (Shenshu)	at 1.5 cun lateral to the apophysis of L 2 vertebra
BL 24 (Qihaishu)	at 1.5 cun lateral to the apophysis of L 3 vertebra
BL 25 (Dachangshu)	at 1.5 cun lateral to the apophysis of L 4 vertebra
BL 26 (Guanyuanshu)	at 1.5 cun lateral to the apophysis of L 5 vertebra
BL 27 (Xiaochangshu)	at 1.5 cun lateral to the apophysis of S 1 vertebra, on the sacroiliac joint
BL 28 (Pangguangshu)	at 1.5 cun lateral to the apophysis of S 2 vertebra, on the sacroiliac joint
BL 29 (Zhonglushu)	at 1.5 cun lateral to the apophysis of S 3 vertebra, on the sacroiliac joint
BL 30 (Baihuanshu)	at 1.5 cun lateral to the lower opening of the sacral channel
BL 31 (Shangliao)	midway between the posterior-superior iliac spine, on the first sacral hollow
BL 32 (Ciliao)	at 1 cun lateral to the midline, on the second sacral hollow
BL 33 (Zhongliao)	at 1 cun lateral to the midline, on the 3rd sacral hollow
BL 34 (Xialiao)	at the 4th sacral hollow
BL 35 (Huiyang)	at 0.5 cun lateral to the tip of the coccyx
BL 36 (Chengfu)	in the middle of the gluteal fold
BL 37 (Yinmen)	at 6 cun below Chengfu (BL 36)

BL 38 (Fuxi)	on the external extremity of the popliteal fossa, on the internal flexion crease
BL 39 (Weiyang)	on the external extremity of the popliteal fossa, on the internal side of the tendon of the biceps femoris muscle
BL 40 (Weizhong)	in the middle of the popliteal fossa
BL 41 (Fujeng)	at 3 cun lateral to the apophysis of T 2 vertebra
BL 42 (Pohu)	at 3 cun lateral to the apophysis of T 3 vertebra
BL 43 (Gaohuang)	at 3 cun lateral to the apophysis of T 4 vertebra
BL 44 (Shentang)	at 3 cun lateral to the apophysis of T 5 vertebra
BL 45 (Yixi)	at 3 cun lateral to the apophysis of T 6 vertebra
BL 46 (Geguan)	at 3 cun lateral to the apophysis of T 7 vertebra
BL 47 (Hunmen)	at 3 cun lateral to the apophysis of T 8 vertebra
BL 48 (Yanggang)	at 3 cun lateral to the apophysis of T 10 vertebra
BL 49 (Yishe)	at 3 cun lateral to the apophysis of T 11 vertebra
BL 50 (Weicang)	at 3 cun lateral to the apophysis of T 12 vertebra
BL 51 (Huangmen)	at 3 cun lateral to the apophysis of L 1 vertebra
BL 52 (Zhishi)	at 3 cun lateral to the apophysis of L 2 vertebra
BL 53 (Baohuang)	at 3 cun lateral to the midline of the back, at level with the 2nd sacral hollow
BL 54 (Zhibian)	at 3 cun lateral to the lower opening of the sacral channel
BL 55 (Heyang)	at 2 cun below Weizhong (BL 40)
BL 56 (Chengjin)	midway between BL 55 and BL 57
BL 57 (Chengshan)	below the gastrocnemius muscle, at 8 cun below Weizhong (BL 40)
BL 58 (Feiyang)	at 7 cun above Kunlun (BL 60), on the external side of the gastrocnemius muscle
BL 59 (Fuyang)	at 3 cun above Kunlun (BL 60)

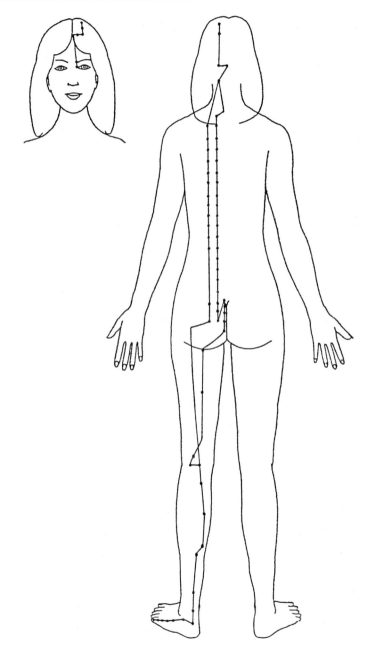

Fig. 7, The Urinary Bladder Channel.

BL 60 (Kunlun)	in the fossa between the tip of the external malleolus and the tendo calcaneus, slightly above the upper border of the calcaneus
BL 61 (Pushen)	at 1.5 cun below Kunlun (BL 60)
BL 62 (Shenmai)	in the fossa below the external malleolus
BL 63 (Jinmen)	anterior and inferior to Shenmai (BL 62) in the depression lateral to the cuboid bone
BL 64 (Jinggu)	below the tuberosity of the 5th metatarsal bone
BL 65 (Shugu)	on the external aspect of the foot, anterior to the metatarsophalangeal joint
BL 66 (Tonggu)	anterior and external to the metatarsophalangeal joint
BL 67 (Zhiyin)	at 2 mm posterior to the lateral corner of the nail of the 5th toe

See Fig. 7, The Urinary Bladder Channel.

THE KIDNEY CHANNEL

K 1 (Yongquan)	at the junction of the anterior and middle third of the sole, in the fossa formed after the flexion of the toes
K 2 (Rangu)	on the internal aspect of the foot, below the tuberosity of the navicular bone
K 3 (Taixi)	in the fossa between the internal malleolus and tendo calcaneus
K 4 (Dazhong)	at 0.5 cun posterior to Taixi (K 3), in the angle between the tendo calcaneus and calcaneus
K 5 (Shuiquan)	at 1 cun below Taixi (K 3), on the upper and internal border of the calcaneus
K 6 (Zhaohai)	at 1 cun below the tip of the medial malleolus
K 7 (Fuliu)	at 2 cun above Taixi (K 3), on the internal border of the tendo calcaneus
K 8 (Jiaoxin)	at 2 cun above Taixi (K 3), on the posterior border of the tibia
K 9 (Zhubin)	at 5 cun above Taixi (K 3), on the posterior

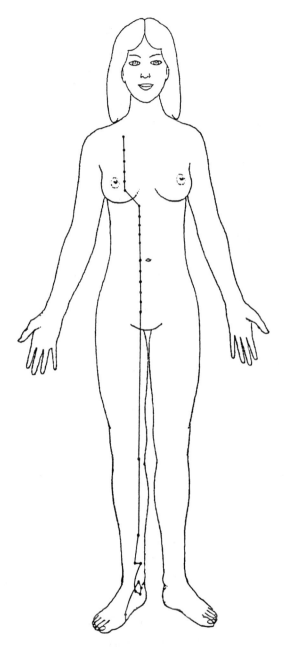

Fig. 8, The Kidney Channel.

	border of the tibia, below the gastrocnemius muscle on the line between K 3 and K 10
K 10 (Yingu)	on the popliteal flexion crease, between the tendon of the semitendinosus and semimembranosus muscles
K 11 (Henggu)	on the upper border of the pubis symphyses, at 0.5 cun from RM 2
K 12 (Dahe)	at 4 cun below the umbilicus, at 0.5 cun lateral to RM 3
K 13 (Qixue)	at 3 cun below the umbilicus, at 0.5 cun lateral to RM 4
K 14 (Siman)	at 2 cun below the umbilicus, at 0.5 cun lateral to RM 5
K 15 (Zhongzhu)	at 1 cun below the umbilicus, at 0.5 cun lateral to RM 7
K 16 (Huangshu)	at 0.5 cun lateral to the umbilicus
K 17 (Shangqu)	at 2 cun above the umbilicus, at 0.5 cun lateral to RM 10
K 18 (Shiguan)	at 3 cun above the umbilicus, at 0.5 cun lateral to RM 11
K 19 (Yindu)	at 4 cun above the umbilicus, at 0.5 cun lateral to RM 12
K 20 (Futonggu)	at 5 cun above the umbilicus, at 0.5 cun lateral to RM 13
K 21 (Youmen)	at 6 cun above the umbilicus, at 0.5 cun lateral to RM 14
K 22 (Bulang)	at 2 cun lateral to RM 16
K 23 (Shenfeng)	at 2 cun lateral to RM 17
K 24 (Lingxu)	at 2 cun lateral to RM 18
K 25 (Shencang)	at 2 cun lateral to RM 19
K 26 (Yuzhong)	at 2 cun lateral to RM 20
K 27 (Shufu)	at 2 cun lateral to RM 21

See Fig. 8, The Kidney Channel.

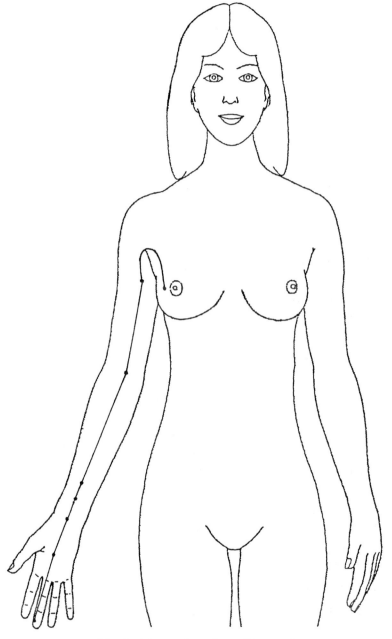

Fig. 9, The Pericardium Channel.

THE PERICARDIUM CHANNEL

PC 1 (Tianchi)   at 1 cun lateral to the nipple

PC 2 (Tianquan)   at 2 cun below the upper extremity of the anterior axillary fold

PC 3 (Quze)   on the transverse cubital crease, on the internal border of the tendon of the biceps brachi muscle

PC 4 (Ximen)   at 5 cun above Daling (PC 7)

PC 5 (Jianshi)   at 3 cun above Daling (PC 7), between the tendons of the palmaris longus and the flexor carpi radialis muscles

PC 6 (Neiguan)   at 2 cun above Daling (PC 7), between the tendons of the palmaris longus and flexor carpi radialis muscles

PC 7 (Daling)   in the middle of the wrist crease, between the tendons of the palmaris longus and flexor carpi radialis muscles

PC 8 (Laogong)   between the 2nd and 3rd metacarpal bones, where the 2nd finger touches the palm in flexion

PC 9 (Zhongchong)   2 mm posterior to the external corner of the nail of the 3rd finger

See Fig. 9, The Pericardium Channel.

THE SAN JIAO CHANNEL

SJ 1 (Guanchong)   at 2 mm posterior and external to the corner of the nail of the 4th finger

SJ 2 (Yemen)   between the 4th and 5th metacarpal bones, anterior to the metacarpophalangeal joint

SJ 3 (Zhongzhu)   in the angle between the 4th and 5th metacarpal bones, proximal to the metacarpophalangeal joint

SJ 4 (Yangchi)   on the dorsal aspect of the wrist, in the depression between the 5th metacarpal and the pyramidal bones, on the wrist crease

SJ 5 (Waiguan)	at 2 cun above the wrist crease, between the radius and ulna
SJ 6 (Zhigou)	at 3 cun above the dorsal wrist crease, between the radius and ulna
SJ 7 (Huizong)	at 3 cun above the dorsal wrist crease, on the radial border of the ulna, on the same line with Zhigou (SJ 6)
SJ 8 (Sanyangluo)	at 4 cun above the dorsal wrist crease, between the radius and the ulna
SJ 9 (Sidu)	at 5 cun below the olecranon, between the radius and ulna
SJ 10 (Tianjing)	at 1 cun above the olecranon, in the depression formed by the flexion of the elbow
SJ 11 (Qinglengyuan)	at 1 cun above Tianjing (SJ 10)
SJ 12 (Xiaoluo)	midway between SJ 11 and SJ 13
SJ 13 (Naohui)	on the vertical of SJ 14, on the posterior border of the deltoid muscle
SJ 14 (Jianliao)	posterior and inferior to the acromion, 1 cun posterior to LI 15
SJ 15 (Tianliao)	above the upper internal angle of the scapula, midway between GB 21 and SI 13
SJ 16 (Tianyou)	posterior to the mandible angle, on the posterior border of the sternocleidomastoid muscle, slightly above GB 17
SJ 17 (Yinfeng)	posterior to the ear lobe, in the fossa between the mastoid process and the mandible
SJ 18 (Qimai)	on the anterior-inferior aspect of the mastoid process
SJ 19 (Luxi)	on the anterior-superior aspect of the mastoid process
SJ 20 (Jiaosun)	on the fold in front of the auricle, right above the auricular apex
SJ 21 (Ermen)	anterior to the supratragic notch, in the depression formed when opening the mouth

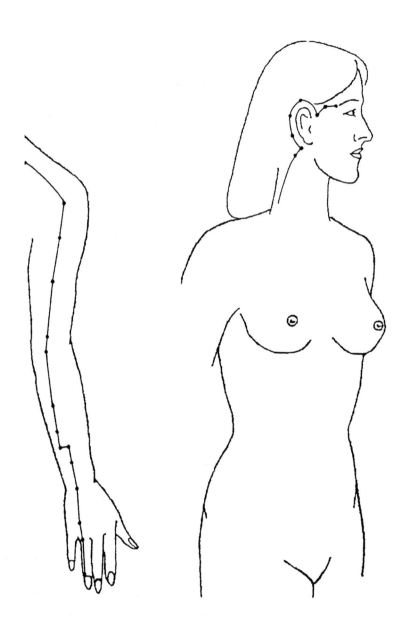

Fig. 10, The San Jiao Channel.

SJ 22 (Heliao)	anterior to the ear, on the border of the zygomatic arch, posterior to the temporal artery
SJ 23 (Sizhukong)	at the external extremity of the eyebrow

See Fig. 10, The San Jiao Channel.

THE GALL BLADDER CHANNEL

GB 1 (Tongziliao)	at 0.5 cun lateral to the external angle of the orbital fossa
GB 2 (Tinghui)	on the anterior-inferior insertion of the ear lobe
GB 3 (Shangguan)	anterior to the ear, on the upper border of the zygomatic arch, 1 cun lateral to its midpoint
GB 4 (Hanyan)	above the angle of the hairline, midway between ST 8 and GB 5
GB 5 (Xuanlu)	at 0.5 cun posterior to the hairline, midway between ST 8 and GB 7
GB 6 (Xuanli)	midway between GB 5 and GB 7
GB 7 (Qubin)	level with the auricle apex, at 1 cun anterior to SJ 20
GB 8 (Shuaigu)	above the ear, at 1 cun above the hairline
GB 9 (Tianchong)	at 0.5 cun posterior to and slightly above GB 8, on the vertical of the posterior border of the mastoid process
GB 10 (Fubai)	at 1 cun below GB 9 and above the mastoid process, posterior to the auricle insertion
GB 11 (Qiaoyin)	on the posterior border of the mastoid process, on the line between GB 10 and GB 12
GB 12 (Wangu)	on the posterior border of the tip of the mastoid process
GB 13 (Benshen)	anterior to the parietal joint, at 0.5 cun anterior to the hairline
GB 14 (Yangbai)	on the pupil vertical, 1 cun above the eyebrow
GB 15 (Linqi)	on the pupil vertical, at 0.5 cun from the hairline
GB 16 (Muchuang)	at 1.5 cun above Linqi (GB 15)

GB 17 (Zhengying)   at 1.5 cun above Muchuang (GB 16)

GB 18 (Chengling)   at 1.5 cun posterior to Zhengying (GB 17)

GB 19 (Naokong)   above Fengchi (GB 20), at the level of T 17 vertebra, on the lateral aspect of the external occipital protuberance

GB 20 (Fengchi)   below the occipital protuberance, in the fossa between the insertion of the trapezius and sternocleidomastoid muscles

GB 21 (Jianjing)   on the horizontal of the upper border of the thyroid cartilage

GB 22 (Yuanye)   at 3 cun below the axillary center, on the median axillary line, in the 4th intercostal space

GB 23 (Zhejin)   at 1 cun anterior and inferior to Yuanye (GB 22), in the 5th intercostal space

GB 24 (Riyue)   at 1.5 cun below Qimen (LV 14), on the lower border of the 7th rib

GB 25 (Jingmen)   anterior and inferior to the end of the 12th rib

GB 26 (Daimai)   on the horizontal of the umbilicus, below the tip of the 11th rib

GB 27 (Wushu)   at 3 cun anterior-inferior to Daimai (GB 26), on the horizontal of RM 4, anterior to the anterior-superior iliac spine

GB 28 (Weidao)   at 0.5 cun anterior-inferior to Wushu (GB 27)

GB 29 (Juliao)   midway between the anterior-superior iliac spine and the trochanter

GB 30 (Huantiao)   at the junction of the medium with the lateral third of the line between the great trochanter and the lower opening of the sacral channel

GB 31 (Fengshi)   on the external aspect of the thigh, touched with the 3rd finger when in standing position

GB 32 (Zhongdu)   at 2 cun below Fengshi (GB 31)

GB 33 (Xiyangguan)   at 3 cun above Yanglingquan (GB 34), above the external femoral condyle

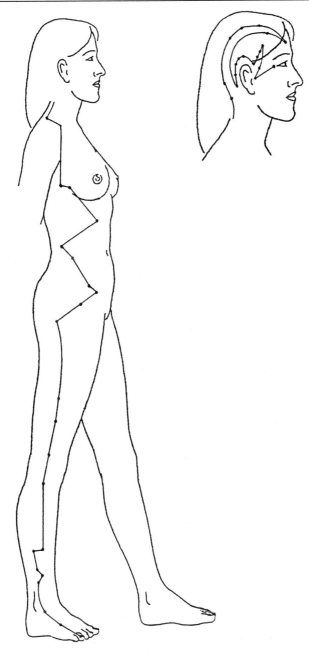

Fig. 11, The Gall Bladder Channel.

GB 34 (Yanglingquan) in the depression located anterior and inferior to the head of the fibula

GB 35 (Yangjiao)   at 7 cun above the external malleolus, on the posterior border of the fibula

GB 36 (Waiqiu)   at 7 cun above the external malleolus, on the anterior border of the fibula

GB 37 (Guangming)   at 5 cun above the external malleolus on the anterior border of the fibula

GB 38 (Yangfu)   at 4 cun above the external malleolus, on the anterior border of the fibula

GB 39 (Xuanzhong)   at 3 cun above the external malleolus, on the anterior border of the fibula

GB 40 (Qiuxu)   in the anterior-inferior fossa of the external malleolus

GB 41 (Zulinqi)   at the junction between the 4th and 5th metatarsal bones, on the lateral side of the tendon of the extensor muscle of the 5th toe

GB 42 (Diwuhui)   between the 4th and 5th metatarsal bones, at 0.5 cun anterior to GB 41 on the medial side of the tendon of the extensor muscle of the 5th toe

GB 43 (Xiaxi)   on the cleft below the 4th and 5th toes

GB 44 (Zuqiaoyin)   at 2 mm posterior and lateral to the corner of the nail of the 4th toe

See Fig. 11, The Gall Bladder Channel.

THE LIVER CHANNEL

LV 1 (Dadun)   at 2 mm posterior to the corner, at the external side of the great toe

LV 2 (Xingjian)   proximal to the cleft between the 1st and 2nd toes

LV 3 (Taichong)   posterior to the metatarsophalangeal joint between the 1st and 2nd metatarsal bones

LV 4 (Zhongfeng)   at 1 cun anterior to the internal malleolus, between the tendons of the extensor halluces

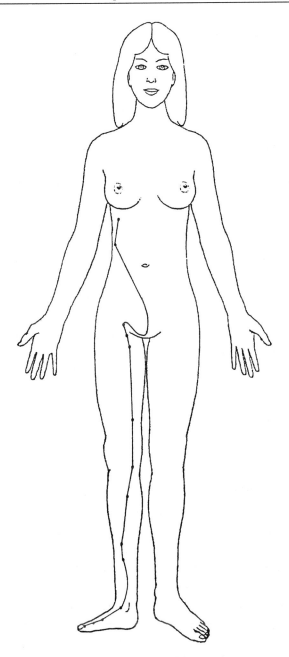

Fig. 12, The Liver Channel.

	and the anterior muscle of the shank
LV 5 (Ligou)	at 5 cun above the tip of the internal malleolus, on the medial side of the tibia
LV 6 (Zhongdu)	at 7 cun above the tip of the internal malleolus, on the medial aspect of the tibia
LV 7 (Xiguan)	at 1 cun posterior to Yinlingquan (SP 9)
LV 8 (Ququan)	at the internal extremity of the popliteal crease of flexion
LV 9 (Yinbao)	at 1 cun above the medial condyle of femur, between the vastus medialis and sartorius muscles
LV 10 (Zuwuli)	at 1 cun below Yinlian (LV 11), on the internal aspect of the thigh
LV 11 (Yinlian)	at 1 cun below Jimai (LV 12), on the external side of the femoral artery
LV 12 (Jimai)	on the femoral artery, where it meets the inguinal fold
LV 13 (Zhangmen)	below the free end of the 11th rib
LV 14 (Qimen)	on the nipple line, between the 6th and 7th ribs

See Fig. 12, The Liver Channel.

THE DU MAI VESSEL

DM 1 (Changqiang)	midway between the coccyx and anus
DM 2 (Yaoshu)	in the hiatus of the sacrum
DM 3 (Yaoyangguan)	below the apophysis of the L 4 vertebra
DM 4 (Mingmen)	below the apophysis of the L 2 vertebra
DM 5 (Xuanshu)	below the apophysis of the L 1 vertebra
DM 6 (Jizhong)	below the apophysis of the T 11 vertebra
DM 7 (Zhongshu)	below the apophysis of the T 10 vertebra
DM 8 (Jinsuo)	below the apophysis of the T 9 vertebra
DM 9 (Zhiyang)	below the apophysis of the T 7 vertebra
DM 10 (Lingtai)	below the apophysis of the T 6 vertebra
DM 11 (Shendao)	below the apophysis of the T 5 vertebra
DM 12 (Shenzhu)	below the apophysis of the T 3 vertebra

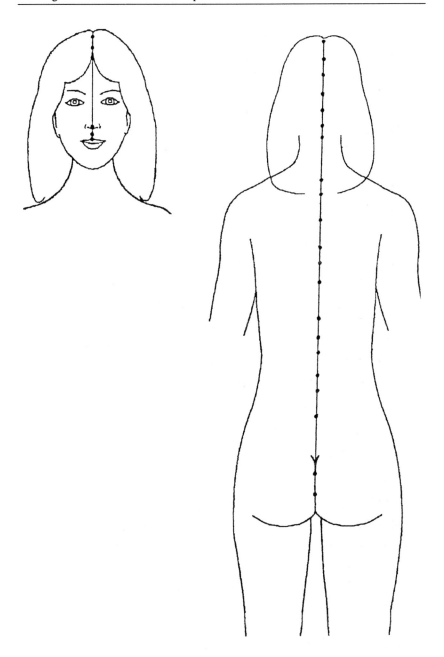

Fig. 13, The Du Mai Vessel

DM 13 (Taodao)	below the apophysis of the T 1 vertebra
DM 14 (Dazhui)	between the apophysis of the C 7 and T 1 vertebrae
DM 15 (Yamen)	on the nape, at 0.5 cun above the posterior hairline
DM 16 (Fengfu)	at 1 cun above the posterior hairline
DM 17 (Naohu)	at 1.5 cun above Fengfu (DM 16)
DM 18 (Qiangjian)	at 1.5 cun above Naohu (DM 17)
DM 19 (Houding)	at 1.5 cun above Qiangjian (DM 18)
DM 20 (Baihui)	at 7 cun above the posterior hairline and midway between the apexes of the ears
DM 21 (Qianding)	at 1.5 cun above Baihui (DM 20)
DM 22 (Xinhui)	at 3 cun above Baihui (DM 20)
DM 23 (Shangxing)	at 1 cun above the anterior hairline
DM 24 (Shenting)	at 0.5 cun above the anterior hairline
DM 25 (Suliao)	on the tip of the nose
DM 26 (Renzhong)	at the upper third of the philtrum
DM 27 (Duiduan)	at the tip of the philtrum
DM 28 (Yinjiao)	on the frenulum of the upper lip

See Fig. 13, The Du Mai Vessel.

THE REN MAI VESSEL

RM 1 (Huiyin)	in the center of the perineum
RM 2 (Qugu)	at the upper border of the symphyses pubis, on the anterior midline
RM 3 (Zhongji)	at 4 cun below the umbilicus
RM 4 (Guanyuan)	at 3 cun below the umbilicus
RM 5 (Shimen)	at 2 cun below the umbilicus
RM 6 (Qihai)	at 1.5 cun below the umbilicus
RM 7 (Yinjiao)	at 1 cun below the umbilicus
RM 8 (Shenque)	in the center of the umbilicus
RM 9 (Shuifen)	at 1 cun above the umbilicus
RM 10 (Xiawan)	at 2 cun above the umbilicus
RM 11 (Jianli)	at 3 cun above the umbilicus

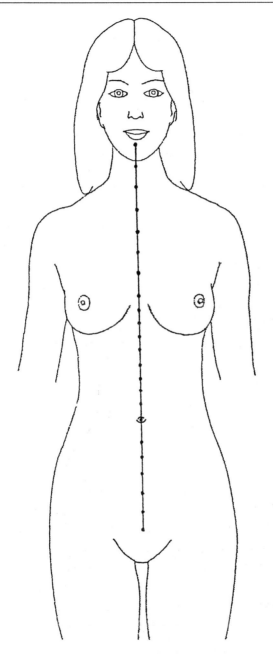

Fig. 14, The Ren Mai Vessel.

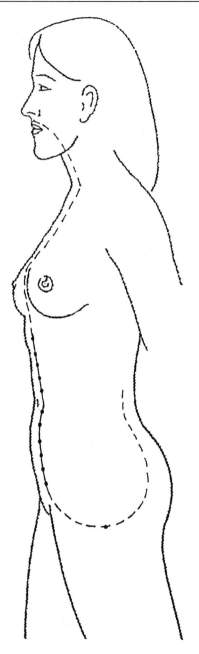

Fig. 15, The Chong Mai Vessel.

RM 12 (Zhongwan) at 4 cun above the umbilicus

RM 13 (Shangwan) at 5 cun above the umbilicus

RM 14 (Juque) at 6 cun above the umbilicus

RM 15 (Jiuwei) at 7 cun above the umbilicus

RM 16 (Zhongting) at the level of the lower border of the sternum body

RM 17 (Shanzhong) level with the 4th intercostal space, between the nipples

RM 18 (Yutang) in the 3rd intercostal space, on the median line

RM 19 (Zigong) in the 2nd intercostal space

RM 20 (Huagai) one rib above Zigong (RM 19)

RM 21 (Xuanji) one rib above Huagai (RM 20)

RM 22 (Tiantu) in the center of the suprasternal fossa

RM 23 (Lianquan) between the Adam's apple and the mandible

RM 24 (Chengjing) in the depression below the upper lip

See Fig. 14, The Ren Mai Vessel.

THE CHONG MAI VESSEL

The coalescent points are:

K 11 (Henggu)

K 12 (Dahe)

K 13 (Qixue)

K 14 (Siman)

K 15 (Zhongzhu)

K 16 (Huangshu)

K 17 (Shangqu)

K 18 (Shiguan)

K 19 (Yindu)

K 20 (Tonggu)

K 21 (Youmen)

See Fig. 15, The Chong Mai Vessel.

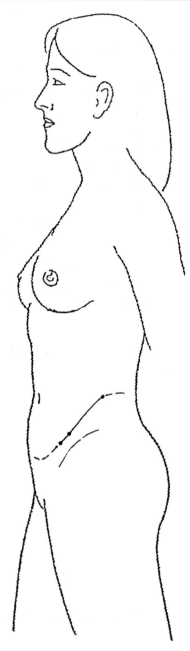

Fig. 16, The Dai Mai Vessel.

THE DAI MAI VESSEL

The coalescent points are:

GB 26 (Daimai)

GB 27 (Wushu)

GB 28 (Weidao)

See Fig. 16, The Dai Mai Vessel.

THE YIN QIAO MAI VESSEL

The coalescent points are:

K 6 (Zhaohai)

K 8 (Jiaoxin)

BL 1 (Jingming)

See Fig. 17, The Yin Qiao Mai Vessel.

THE YIN WEI MAI VESSEL

The coalescent points:

K 9 (Zhubin)

SP 13 (Fushe)

SP 15 (Daheng)

SP 16 (Fuai)

LV 14 (Qimen)

RM 22 (Tiantu)

RM 23 (Lianquan)

See Fig. 18, The Yin Wei Mai Vessel.

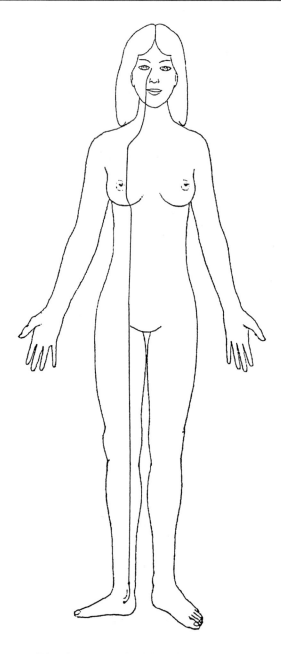

Fig. 17, The Yin Qiao Mai Vessel.

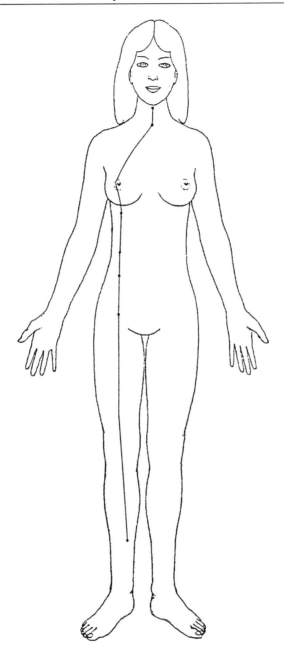

Fig. 18, The Yin Wei Mai Vessel.

REFERENCES

1. ALTHERR J.E. - Les atteintes des méridiens curieux dans les infertilités feminines. L'acupuncture, revue trimestrielle de l'organisation pour l'étude et le développment de l'acupuncture, No. 92, 1987, ppg. 9-23
2. AUSTIN M. - Acupuncture therapy, ASI Publishers Inc., New York, 1972
3. AUTEROCHE B., DUBOIS J.C., NAVAILH P.-L'examen de la langue en médecine chinoise, Méridiens, No. 57-58, 1982, ppg. 27-58
4. AUTEROCHE B., NAVAILH P., MARRONNAUD P., MULLENS E. - Acupuncture en gynécologie et obstétrique, Maloine, Paris, 1986
5. BARON B. et al. - Les hypogalacties, Mensuel du Médecin Acupuncteur, No. 78, 1981, ppg. 297
6. BATRA Y.K. - Acupuncture in the treatment of migraine, American Journal of Acupuncture, vol. 14, No. 3, 1986, ppg. 135-137
7. BENSON R.C., PERNOLL M.L. - Handbook of Obstetrics & Gynecology, 9th Ed., McGraw Hill Inc., 1994
8. BORSARELLO J.F. - Pulsologie chinoise traditionnelle, Masson, Paris, 1981
9. BOSSY J. - Bases modernes et traditionnelles de la douleur et de son traitement. Douleur-Analgésie, Séminaire d'Acupuncture A.F.E.R.A., Nimes, 1989, ppg. 5-12
10. BOSSY J. - Atlas anatomique des points d'acupuncture, Masson, Paris, 1990
11. BOSSY J., GUEVIN F., YASUI H. - Nosologie traditionnelle chinoise et acupuncture, Masson, Paris, 1990
12. CHANG S.T. - The complete book of acupuncture, Celestial Arts, Berkely, 1976
13. CHEN J.Y.P. - Acupuncture anesthesia in the People's Republic of China, DHEW Publication, 1973
14. CHEN Z., HU Q. - Recent development in research on tongue inspection, Chinese Medical Journal, No. 99, 1986, ppg. 444-456
15. CONSTANTIN D. - Chap. Acupunctura in "Medicina Naturista" under the editorial of Pavel Chirila, Ed. Medicala, Bucuresti, 1987
16. CUNNINGHAM G., MAC DONALD P., GANT N. - Williams Obstetrics, 18th Ed., Appleton & Lange, East Norwalk, 1989
17. DAO A. - Acupuncture found of major importance in depressive

syndromes, American Journal of Acupuncture, No. 8, 1990, ppg. 335-339

18. DEROC D. - Les troubles sexuel chez la femme et médecine traditionnelle chinoise. Séminaire: Actualites 1991 - Acupuncture et gynécologie-obstétrique, C.H.R.U. de Nimes, 1991

19. EYSSALET J.M. - A propos des pouls dans la practique quotidienne, Revue Française d'Acupuncture, No. 24, 1980, ppg. 31-42

20. FARA A. et al. - Acupuncture in the treatment of hypogalactia, American Journal of Acupuncture, No. 10, 1992, ppg. 333-340

21. FLAWS B. - Leukorrhea and vaginitis: their differential diagnosis and treatment, American Journal of Acupuncture, vol. 14, No. 4, 1986, ppg. 305-315

22. FORMAN A. - Acupuncture for the treatment of dysmenorrhea, American Journal of Acupuncture, No. 6, 1978, ppg. 139-141

23. FOUQUES-DUPARC V. et al. - L'acupuncture en obstétrique-déclanchement du travail par électrostimulation acupuncturale, Méridiens, No. 47-48, 1979, ppg. 125-132

24. FRESNET M. -Les troubles des régles et l'acupuncture, Revue Française d'Acupuncture, No. 30, 1973, ppg. 173

25. GAO D. et al. - Efficacy of acupuncturing the Jianjing point in 393 cases of acute mastitis, Journal of Traditional Chinese Medicine, vol. 6, No. 1, 1986, ppg. 19-20

26. GHEORGHIU N.N., DRAGOMIRESCU C., RAUT C., IONESCU-TIRGOVISTE C., CIUCA S. - Manual de acupuncutura, Ed. Medicala, Bucharest, 1974

27. GHEORGHIU N.N. et al. - Tratamentul hipogalactiilor prin acupunctura, Rev. Obstetrica si Ginecologia, No.3, 1971

28. GIRALT I., VINAS F. - Pain and other symptoms associated to scar, at the 6th International Congress of Acupuncture, Bucharest, 1991

29. GOURION A. - Régles irréguliéres, Mensuel du Médecin Acupuncteur, No. 74, 1980, ppg. 157

30. HADIDA P. - Les anuries, Mensuel du Médecin Acupunctuer, No. 4, 1982, ppg. 791

31. HAMMER L.I. - The Extraordinary acupuncture meridians. Homeostatic Vessels, American Journal of Acukpuncture, No. 8, 1989, ppg. 123-146

32. HART B.F. - Treatment of migraine headache with acupuncture,

American Journal of Acupuncture, No. 6, 1978, ppg. 73-74

33. HUANG W. et al. - 56 cases of chronic pruritus vulvae treated with acupuncture, Journal of Traditional Medicine, vol. 7, No. 1, 1987, ppg. 1-3

34. IONESCU-TIRGOVISTE C. - Bazele teoretice ale acupuncturii, vol. 1 and 2, Ed. Athaeneum, Bucharest, 1992

35. HI X.P. - Teaching round: insomnia, Journal of Traditional Chinese Medicine, vol. 7, No. 1, 1987, ppg. 73-76

36. JONES III H.W., WENTZ A.C., BURNETT L.S. - Novak's textbook of Gynecology, 11th Ed., Williams & Wilkins, Baltimore, 1988

37. KESPI J. - Examen de la langue, Revue Française d'Acupuncture, No. 5, 1976, ppg. 7-12

38. KIENER E. - Examen de la langue, Revue Française d'Acupuncture, No. 2, 1980, ppg. 27-31

39. LAVAL J. - L'acupuncture dans la depression nerveuse, Méridiens, No. 37-38, 1977, ppg. 119-137

40. LI C. et al. - Relative specificity of points in acupuncture analgesia, Journal of Traditional Chinese Medicine, vol. 7, No. 1, 1987, ppg. 29-34

41. LIANG Z. - 32 cases of acute mastitis treated with acupuncture, moxibustion and cupping, Journal of Traditional Chinese Medicine, vol. 8, No. 1, 1988, ppg. 15-18

42. LILE P.C. - Les méridiens curieux, Contrepoint, No. 20, 1986, ppg. 7-26

43. LITARCZEK G. - Anestezia chirurgicala prin acupunctura, at the 5th Acupuncture Natural Symposium, Bucharest, 1986, ppg. 190-193

44. LIU W. et al. - Acupuncture treatment of functional uterine bleeding - a clinical observation of 30 cases, Journal of Traditional Chinese Medicine, vol. 8, No. 1, 1988, ppg. 31-33

45. LOW H.L. - Acupuncture in Gynaecology and Obstetrics, Thorsons Publishers Ltd., Wellinborough, 1990

46. LUCA V. - Diagnostic si conduita in sarcina cu risc crescut, Ed., Medicala, Bucharest, 1989

47. MANAKA Y., URQUHART I.A. - The Layman's guide to acupuncture, Weatherhill Inc., New York, 1972

48. MINELLI E. - Chong Mai: Grossesse, avortement, hypogalactie, stérilité, Revue Française de Médecine Traditionnelle Chinoise, No.

119, 1986. ppg. 307-309

49. NGUYEN-RECOURS C. - L'acupuncture en obstétrique: quel avenir?, Revue Française de Médecine Traditionnelle Chinoise, No. 123, 1987, ppg. 201-204

50. NGUYEN-RECOURS C. - Nevrose gravidique, Revue Française de Médecine Traditionnelle Chinoise, No. 150, 1992, ppg. 41

51. NGUYEN VAN NGHI - Acupuncture, son passe et une de ses particularites: le systeme des "huit méridiens curieux", Mensuel du Médecin Acupuncteur, No. 44, 1977, ppg. 125-164

52. NGUYEN VAN NGHI, LANZA U., MAI VAN DONG - Théorie et practique de l'analgésie par acupuncture, Imprimerie Socedim, Marseille, 1973

53. NGUYEN VAN NGHI, BAI VAN THO - Découvertes pulsologique sous le doight, Revue Française de Médecine Traditionnele Chinoise, No. 150, 1992, ppg. 21-32

54. NGUYEN VAN NGHI, BAI VAN THO - Pouls normaux et pathologiques des organes et entrailles, Revue Française de Médecine Traditionnelle Chinoise, No. 153, 1992, ppg. 149-163

55. NOGIER P.M. - L'auriculotherapie, Maisonneuve, Paris, 1980

56. PEI D.E. - Use of acupuncture analgesia during childbirth, Journal of Traditional Chinese Medicine, No. 5 1985, ppg. 253-255

57. PION P. - Le postpartum blues. Séminaire: Actualites 1991-Acupuncture et gynécologie-obstétrique, C.H.R.U. de Nimes, 1991

58. PRAT-PRADAL D. Insomnie de la grossesse. Séminaire: Actualites 1991 - Acupuncture et gynécologie-obstétrique, C.H.R.U. de Nimes, 1991

59. PRAT-PRADAL D. - Hypertension arterielle et grossesse. Séminaire: Actualites 1991: Acupuncture et gynécologie-obstétrique, C.H.R.U. de Nimes, 1991

60. PREMARATNE A.V. - Fundamentals of Chinese pulse diagnosis, American Journal of Acupuncture, No. 9, 1981, ppg. 265

61. RADULESCU E. - Chap. Disfunctii genitale dureroase, in "Tratat de patologie chirurgicala" under the editorial of Proca E., vol. 7: Ginecologie, Ed. Medicala, Bucharest, 1983

62. RAUT C. - The treatment of hemorrhoids by acupuncture, American Journal of Acupuncture, No. 2, 1974. ppg. 109-112

63. ROMANO L. - Les dystocies. Séminaire: Actualites 1991 -

Acupuncture et gynécologie-obstétrique, C.H.R.U. de Nimes 1991

64. ROMANO L. et al. - Les hemorrhoids du postpartum. Séminaire Actualites 1991 - Acupuncture et gynécologie-obstétrique, C.H.R.U. de Nimes, 1991

65. ROSS J. - Traditional Chinese Medicine and gynecology, part one, The Journal of Chinese Medicine, No. 11, 1983, ppg. 12-21

66. ROSS J. - Traditional Chinese Medicine and gynecology, part two, The Journal of Chinese Medicine, No. 12, 1983, ppg. 8-19

67. ROUSTAN C. - Traite d'Acupuncture, Masson, Paris, 1979

68. RUBIN M. - L'acupuncture et les maladies de la femme, Libraire Le François, Paris, 1976

69. SBRIGLIO V.S. et al. - Traitement par électroacupuncture des dystocies par anomalies de la contraction uterine, Mensuel du Médecin Acupuncteur, No. 19, 1973, ppg. 335

70. SHENG C. - The treatment of urogenital diseases by acupuncture, The Journal of Chinese Medicine, No. 22, 1986, ppg. 3-12

71. SIRI A. - Le Inn Wei Mai, Les dossiers de l'obstétrique, Revue d'information médicales et professionnelles de la sage femme, No. 147, 1988, ppg. 20-21

72. STAEBLER F.E. - Clinical acupuncture in childbirth, British Journal of Acupuncture, vol. 4, No. 2, 1985, ppg. 3-12

73. STEINBERGER A. - The treatment of dysmenorrhea by acupuncture, American Journal of Chinese Medicine, No. 1, 1981, ppg. 57

74. SU X. - The treatment of hemorrhoids by acupuncture, Journal of Chinese Medicine, No. 25, 1987, ppg. 23-24

75. TRAN V.D. - The curious meridians, American Journal of Acupuncture, No. 17, 1989, ppg. 45-46

76. TUREANU L., TUREANU V.- A clinical evaluation of the effectiveness of acupuncture for insufficient lactation, American Journal of Acupuncture, vol. 22, No. 1, 1994, ppg. 23-27

77. TUREANU V., TUREANU L. - An evaluation of the effectiveness of acupuncture for the treatment of post-oral contraceptive menstrual irregularities & amenorrhea, vol. 22, No. 2, 1994, ppg. 117-121

78. TUREANU L., TUREANU V. - Microsisteme, timpi optimi si puncte extrameridian in acupunctura, Ed. All, Bucharest, 1994

79. TUREANU V., TUREANU L. - Acupuncture in gynecological diseases, Alternative Health Practitioner, vol. 2, No. 2 summer 1996,

ppg. 123-130

80. VERRET J. - Prise de poids excessive pendant la grossesse, Revue
    Française de Médecine Traditionnelle Chinoise, No. 155, 1992, ppg.
    246-257

81. VIBES J. - Cystites - Cystopathies "amicrobiennes", Acupuncture,
    No. 66, 1980, ppg. 33

82. VOISIN H. - L'acupuncture du practicien, Maloine, Paris, 1972

83. WANG X. - Observations of the therapeutic effects of acupuncture
    and moxibustion in 100 cases of dysmenorrhea, Journal of Traditional
    Chinese Medicine, No. 7, 1987, ppg. 15-17

84. WANG X. - On the therapeutic efficiency of electric acupuncture and
    moxibustion in 95 cases of chronic pelvic infectious disease, Journal
    of Traditional Chinese Medicine, No. 9, 1989, ppg. 21-24

85. YANG D. - Acupuncture treatment in 182 cases of abdominal colic
    due to calculi in the urinary system, Journal of Traditional Chinese
    Medicine, No. 9, 1989, ppg. 247-248

86. YOON S. et al. - Clinical study of the objective pulse diagnosis,
    American Journal of Chinese Medicine, No. 14, 1986, ppg. 179-183

87. YUAN S. et al. - 110 cases of mastosis treated with acupuncture,
    Journal of Traditional Chinese Medicine, No. 4, 1984 ppg. 5-6

88. ZHAN C. - Treatment of 32 cases of dysmenorrhea by puncturing
    Hegu and Sanyinjiao acupoints, Journal of Traditional Chinese
    Medicine, No. 10, 1990, ppg. 33-35

89. ZHANG Y. - A report of 49 cases of dysmenorrhea treated by
    acupuncture, Journal of Traditional Chinese Medicine, No. 4, 1984,
    ppg. 101-102

90. ZHAO C. - Lectures on formulating acupuncture prescriptions-
    selection and matching of acupoints. Hypertension. Journal of
    Traditional Chinese Medicine, No. 7, 1987. ppg. 77-78

91. ZHAO C. - Lectures on formulating acupuncture prescriptions-
    selection and matching of acupoints. Acupuncture treatment of
    insomnia, Journal of Traditional Chinese Medicine, No. 7, 1987,
    ppg. 151-152

92. ZHAO C. - Postmenopausal urinary incontinence, Journal of
    Traditional Chinese Medicine, No. 7, 1988, ppg. 305-306

93. ZHAO C. - Acupuncture treatment of menstrual pain, Journal of
    Traditional Chinese Medicine, No. 8, 1988, ppg. 73-74

94. ZHAO R. - 39 cases of morning sickness treated with acupuncture, Journal of Traditional Chinese Medicine, vol. 7, No. 1, 1987, ppg. 25-26

95. ZHARKIN N.A. - Acupuncture in obstetrics, part two, The Journal of Chinese Medicine, No. 34, 1990 ppg. 14-19

96. ZHEN J.X. - Coliques nephretiques, Mensuel du Médecin Acupuncteur, No. 74, 1980, ppg. 141

97. ZHEN J.X. - Leucorrhées, Mensuel du Médecin Acupuncteur, No. 76, 1980, ppg. 229

98. ZHEN J.X. - Vomissement de la grossesse, Mensuel du Médecin Acupuncteur, No. 76, 1980, ppg. 230

99. ZHU R. - Induction du travail par électroacupuncture. Analyse de 771 observations, Mensuel du Médecin Acupuncteur, No. 75, 1980, ppg. 179

100.   *** Anatomic atlas of Chinese acupuncture, Shandong Science and Technology Press, 1982

101.   *** Applied Chinese Acupuncture for clinical practitioner, Shandong Science and Technology Press, 1985

102.   *** Chinese Acupuncture and Moxibustion, Foreign Language Press, Beijing, 1987

103.   *** Essentials of Chinese Acupuncture, Foreign Language Press, Beijing, 1980

104.   *** Illustrated dictionary of Chinese Acupuncture, Sheep's Publications Ltd., Beijing, 1985

105.   *** Manual de acupunctura chineza, Ed. Medicala, Bucharest, 1982 (translation of "Precis d'Acupuncture Chinoise, Edition en langues etrangeres, Pekin, 1977)

INDEX

A

abdominal distension, painful: 16, 18, 19, 42, 45, 64, 88, 91, 135, 162, 163, 164, 168, 172, 180, 233, 236, 254, 307

abdominal pain, in pregnancy: 38, 43, 44, 68-72, 78, 79, 101, 132, 135, 229

abdominal tumoral masses: 163, 235

abnormal presentation of the fetus: 36, 39, 102-104, 111, 129

abnormal uterine bleeding: 47, 49, 192-196, 207

abortion: 171, 178, 217
    induced: 82-83
    threatened: 30, 36, 41, 46, 78-82, 158

acne: 170

accumulation of Damp-Heat in Lower Jiao: 217, 301

accumulation of Heat in San Jiao: 25

accumulation of Phlegm in Lower Jiao: 260

acupuncture analgesia: 314
    action mechanism: 314-316
    advantages and disadvantages: 316-318
    induction of: 314, 322
    in Obstetrics & Gynecology surgery: 322-323
    principles of selecting the points: 320-321

acupuncture treatment and pregnancy: 158-159

afterpains: 6, 134-137

amenorrhea: 6, 11, 12, 13, 39, 45, 199-207, 240, 251, 285
    postpill: 262-263

amniotomy:106, 108, 115

analgesia during childbirth: 127-131

anorgasmia: 281-282

antedated menstruation: 173, 177, 180, 185-187, 254

antipathogenic Qi: 5, 24, 33, 35, 62

anxiety: 55, 59, 63, 109, 111, 131, 151, 170, 197, 207, 214, 223, 226, 265, 277, 287, 302

ascendance of Liver Fire: 11, 90, 269

Ashi points: 130, 136, 272, 300

asthenia: 36, 73, 79, 87, 100, 116, 125, 138, 149, 151, 180, 201, 218, 223, 226, 247, 254, 264, 279, 307

excess: 63

M

manipulation techniques: 321-322
mastitis, acute: 37, 264-267
memory disorders: 13, 173, 208, 210, 215
menopause: 7, 10, 11, 13, 17, 41, 42, 48, 207, 215, 223, 246, 279, 285
  mental disorders: 48
  ovarian cyst in: 236
menorrhagia: 176, 192
menstrual cycle: 7-8, 24
  disorders: 10, 11, 12, 17, 20, 35, 36, 37, 40, 43, 176-185, 208,
    226, 230, 237, 244, 251, 252, 253, 254, 269, 272
menstruation: 6, 7, 8, 18, 22, 78, 162, 170, 200, 236
  antedated: 173, 177, 185-187, 254
  ceasing of: 7, 10, 16, 207
  irregular: 7, 37, 44, 48, 177, 180, 218, 240, 254
  postdated: 13, 18, 39, 172, 177, 180, 187-190, 254
metrorrhagia: 6, 11, 18, 19, 28, 40, 42, 193, 196
Middle Jiao: 5, 12, 21, 36, 151, 154
  Qi of: 185, 216
migraine: 168-169
milk formation: 9, 14, 143
miscarriage: 7, 12, 16, 17, 19, 20, 28, 31, 78, 109, 251
morning sickness: 19, 38, 43, 44, 46, 52-54, 55, 158
moxibustion: 57, 76, 89, 112, 114, 132, 139, 141, 142, 143, 146, 151,
    156, 158, 176, 182, 192, 195, 214, 220, 234, 260, 283, 286, 294,
    300, 312
musculoskeletal pathology in pregnancy: 83-86

N

nausea: 37, 52, 88, 111, 116, 132, 138, 153, 164, 169, 202, 237, 265
nervousness: 73, 93, 94, 173, 205, 210, 247, 254
newborn resusciation: 122
nipple: 264, 265
nymphomania: 288